A practical approach
to clinical arrhythmology

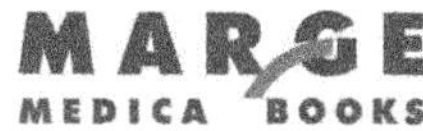

A practical approach to clinical arrhythmology

Editors
Dr. Lluís Mont
Dr. Josep Brugada

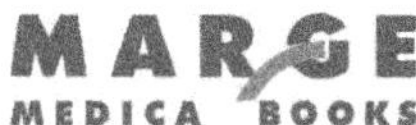

Collection: ARRHYTHMIA AND CARDIAC STIMULATION

A PRACTICAL APPROACH TO CLINICAL ARRHYTHMOLOGY
Editors: Dr. Lluís Mont, Dr. Josep Brugada
1st. edition 2010
2nd. edition 2012

© of this edition, ICG Marge, SL

Publisher: Marge Médica Books - València, 558, ático 2.ª - 08026 Barcelona (Spain)
www.marge.es - Tel. +34-932 449 130 - Fax +34-932 310 865

Publishing director: Hèctor Soler
Managing editors: Ana Soto, Anna Palacios
Editing: Kike Juanico, Rosa Serra, David Soler
Technical back-up: Alice Corson, Leanne Fairley
Make-up editor: Rosa Grafisme
Printed by: Service Point (El Prat de Llobregat)

ISBN: 978-84-15340-47-8

Index

Authors

Cristina Basso
Department of Cardiac, Thoracic
and Vascular Science
University of Padua Medical School
Padua, Italy

David Andreu
Thorax Institute
Hospital Clinic, University of Barcelona
Barcelona, Spain

Begoña Benito
Montreal Heart Institute
Montreal, Canada

Antonio Berruezo
Thorax Institute
Hospital Clinic, University of Barcelona
Barcelona, Spain

Michele Brignole
Department of Cardiology
Ospedali del Tigullio
Lavagna, Italy

Georgia Sarquella-Brugada
Arrhythmia Unit, Cardiology Section
Sant Joan de Déu Hospital
Barcelona, Spain

Josep Brugada
Thorax Institute
Hospital Clinic, University of Barcelona
Barcelona, Spain

Pedro Brugada
Cardiovascular Division
UZ Brussel-VUB
Brussels, Belgium

Ramón Brugada
Cardiovascular Genetics Center
University of Girona
Girona, Spain

Margherita Calcagnino
Institute of Cardiovascular Science
and The Heart Hospital
University College London Partners
London, United Kingdom

Oscar Campuzano
Cardiovascular Genetics Center
University of Girona
Girona, Spain

Marina Cerrone
Division of Cardiology
New York University School of Medicine
New York, USA

K.R. Julian Chun
Department Head
II. Medizinische Abteilung
Asklepios Klinik St. Georg
Hamburg, Germany

Domenico Corrado
Department of Cardiac, Thoracic
and Vascular Science
University of Padua Medical School
Padua, Italy

Franciso G. Cosio
Cardiology Service and Arrhythmia Unit
Hospital Universitario de Getafe
Madrid, Spain

Michel Haïssaguerre
Service de Rythmologie
Hôpital Cardiologique du Haut-Lévêque
Université Victor Segalen Bordeaux II
Bordeaux, France

Mélèze Hocini
Service de Rythmologie
Hôpital Cardiologique du Haut-Lévêque
Université Victor Segalen Bordeaux II
Bordeaux, France

Anna Iglesias
Cardiovascular Genetics Center
University of Girona
Girona, Spain

Pierre Jaïs
Service de Rythmologie
Hôpital Cardiologique du Haut-Lévêque
Université Victor Segalen Bordeaux II
Bordeaux, France

Jonathan M. Kalman
Department Of Cardiology, Department
of Medicine
Royal Melbourne Hospital and University
of Melbourne
Melbourne, Australia

Peter M. Kistler
Department Of Cardiology, Department
of Medicine
Royal Melbourne Hospital and University
of Melbourne
Melbourne, Australia

Karl-Heinz Kuck
Department Head
II. Medizinische Abteilung
Asklepios Klinik St. Georg
Hamburg, Germany

William J. McKenna
Institute of Cardiovascular Science and The
Heart Hospital
University College London Partners
London, United Kingdom

Caroline Medi
Department Of Cardiology, Department
of Medicine
Royal Melbourne Hospital and University
of Melbourne
Melbourne, Australia

Lluís Mont
Thorax Institute
Hospital Clínic, University of Barcelona
Barcelona, Spain

Stephan Andreas Müller- Burri
Heart Rhythm Management Centre
UZ Brussel-VUB
Brussels, Belgium

Mercè Nadal
Thorax Institute
Hospital Clínic, University of Barcelona
Barcelona, Spain

Stanley Nattel
Department of Medicine and Research
Center
Montreal Heart Institute and Université
de Montréal
Quebec, Canada

Ambrosio Núñez
Cardiology Service and Arrhythmia Unit
Hospital Universitario de Getafe
Madrid, Spain

Feifan Ouyang
Cardiac Electrophysiology Laboratory
II. Medizinische Abteilung
Asklepios Klinik St. Georg
Hamburg, Germany

Carlo Pappone
Department of Arrhythmology
Villa Maria Cecilia Hospital
Ravenna, Italy

Agustín Pastor
Cardiology Service and Arrhythmia Unit
Hospital Universitario de Getafe
Madrid, Spain

Martina Perazzolo Marra
Department of Cardiac, Thoracic
and Vascular Science
University of Padua Medical School
Padua, Italy

Silvia G. Priori
Molecular Cardiology Laboratories
Fondazione S. Maugeri IRCC
Pavia, Italy
Cardiovascular Genetics Program
Leon H. Charney Division of Cardiology
Universita' degli Studi di Pavia
Pavia, Italy
Division of Cardiology
New York University School of Medicine
New York, USA

Ilaria Rigato
Department of Cardiac, Thoracic
and Vascular Science
University of Padua Medical School
Padua, Italy

Vincenzo Santinelli
Department of Arrhythmology
Villa Maria Cecilia Hospital
Ravenna, Italy

Boris Schmidt
Department Head
II. Medizinische Abteilung
Asklepios Klinik St. Georg
Hamburg, Germany

William G. Stevenson
Cardiovascular Divison
Brigham and Women's Hospital
Boston, USA

Usha B. Tedrow
Cardiovascular Divison
Brigham and Women's Hospital
Boston, USA

Gaetano Thiene
Department of Cardiac, Thoracic
and Vascular Science
University of Padua Medical School
Padua, Italy

Kurt Roberts-Thomson
Department Of Cardiology, Department
of Medicine
Royal Melbourne Hospital and University
of Melbourne
Melbourne, Australia

Andrew W. Teh
Department Of Cardiology, Department
of Medicine
Royal Melbourne Hospital and University
of Melbourne
Melbourne, Australia

Erik Wissner
Staff Physician
II. Medizinische Abteilung
Asklepios Klinik St. Georg
Hamburg, Germany

Matthew Wright
Service de Rythmologie
Hôpital Cardiologique du Haut-Lévêque
Université Victor Segalen Bordeaux II
Bordeaux-Pessac
St Thomas' Hospital
London, United Kingdom

Sanam Yaghoubian
Division of Cardiology
New York University School of Medicine
New York, USA

Introduction

This book is a celebration. Let us explain. We started medical school in 1975, the same year Franco died, and along with many other young people at that time, we wanted to change our country and to change the world. We lived those exciting, turbulent years in an environment of important change, and certainly we were deeply influenced by the enormous expectations of those times.

Many years later, in 1989, we met again in Maastricht, where we began a lasting friendship along with our careers in electrophysiology. We have been working together ever since, with brief interruptions, and have been fortunate to learn from many people whose contributions have expanded the field of electrophysiology. We consider all who have participated not only as colleagues and friends but also as members of a growing family that has accompanied us along our career paths to date. As in any family, there have been conflicts and misunderstandings, but looking back over the past 20 years, the contributions to medicine and to individual health have been huge . Our "family photo" tells the story of a great success.

It occurred to us that a great way to celebrate our 20th anniversary of friendship and collaboration would be to invite some of our best friends and colleagues to contribute to a sort of family history. We would like to explain the principles of clinical arrhythmology, in a very practical and understandable way, in a book intended for young cardiologists who sometimes get lost in the complexities of the field and fail to organize their knowledge in an efficient way.

With this goal in mind, we have selected a number of topics and then selected authors based on two criteria: first of all for friendship as well as for their contributions and experience in the field. Although more people certainly could have been included under these criteria, we have imposed some limitations so that the result can be a book that is concise, manageable, and easy to read.

In this era of the Internet and computers, some would argue that books are really out of fashion, and they may be right! However, being 'too old for rock'n roll, too young to die' (in the lyrics of an old Jethro Tull song) means we still like old-fashioned things. We have secured some funding and a publisher to support this initiative. We sincerely hope the readers will enjoy this very personal celebration of friendship and electrophysiology.

Dr. Lluís Mont, Dr. Josep Brugada

Chapter 1. What should a clinician know about basic mechanisms of arrhythmia?

S. Nattel

Dept. of Medicine and Research Center
Montreal Heart Institute and Université de Montréal
Montreal, Canada

Address for correspondence:
Montreal Heart Institute and
Université de Montréal
Dr. Stanley Nattel
stanley.nattel@icm-mhi.org

Introduction

Clinical electrophysiology is probably the clinical medicine area with the closest link between basic science and clinical practice. In this chapter, I will try to provide everything I consider a physician needs to know to understand the basic mechanisms underlying the main points of the contents of the rest of this book.

1 The action potential

The key to understanding cardiac cellular activity, and the base of cardiac electrophysiology, is the action potential (see figure 1).[1] The "engine" driving cardiac electrical function is the electrical field across the cardiac cell membrane. Normally, cardiac cells are negative intracellularly (relative to the extracellular space), or "polarized" at rest. When they fire, they "depolarize", going from a negative to a positive intracellular voltage. Then they subsequently go through a series of highly regulated steps in which the intracellular voltage becomes more and more negative ("repolarization") until they finally reach their initial negative state at which they are fully "repolarized". Although the voltages across the cardiac cell membrane (also called the "sarcolemma"), seem pretty small (about ~80 mV, or $80/1000^{th}$ of a volt at rest; +40 mV, $40/1000^{th}$ of a volt at peak) they are exerted over a tiny distance (the sarcolemmal thickness), resulting in enormously powerful electrical fields. It is these fields and their changes that drive ions into and out of the cell during the action potential. Strong ionic fluxes provide important electrical forces, generating the energy for cardiac conduction and driving a variety of other cellular processes.

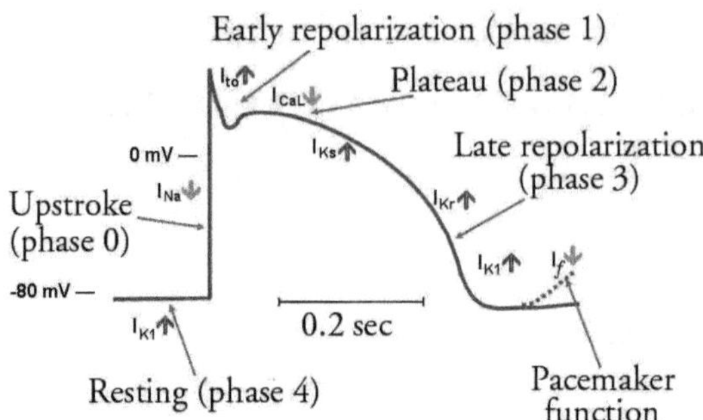

Figure 1. The cardiac action potential. Phases of the action potential and most important associated currents are shown. Inward currents are indicated by upward blue arrows and outward currents by downward red arrows.

The cardiac action potential is a recording of cardiac cellular electrical potential, as seen from the inside of heart cells, over time. Ions move across the cell membrane in the direction of their chemical gradient, ruled by the law that indicates that when a membrane is permeable to a molecule, it moves in a way so as to equalize its concentration on both sides of the membrane. The movement of ions is controlled by their relative intracellular versus extracellular concentrations and the "permeability" of the membrane to each ion (ability to allow the ion to pass across), which is very selective and highly regulated. Since intracellular potassium (K^+) concentration is about 25-30 times extracellular, K^+ tends to move from inside the cell to the extracellular space, leaving a negative intracellular charge. At rest the cell is quite permeable to K^+ (and not permeable to much else), so the resting cardiac cell has quite a negative intracellular charge (the "resting potential") because of the K^+ ions that are left inside of the cell. When a cell is fired, the rapid depolarization opens sodium (Na^+) "gates", which greatly increase the cell's Na^+ permeability. Since there is about 15 times more Na^+ outside the cell than inside, a large and rapid influx of Na^+ is caused. The great number of Na^+ ions that enters the cell creates a powerful electrical current, providing energy for rapid electrical conduction and creating a relatively positive intracellular potential. Current movement direction is defined by convention as the direction of positive-ion movement, so K^+, which leaves the cell, carries "outward current" whereas Na^+ and Ca^{2+} carry "inward current". The phases of the cardiac action potential involve discrete processes, and are numbered sequentially from 0 to 4. Phase 0 is the phase of rapid Na^+ entry. Na^+ channel gates close quickly at positive potentials, terminating phase 0. The rest of the action potential is then dominated by the opening of K^+ channels, which allow K^+ to leave the cell and eventually restore the cell's original intracellular negativity. There is an early rapid repolarizing phase called phase 1, carried by a rapidly opening but then rapidly inactivating K^+ current called "transient outward" current, I_{to} ("I" is the standard electrical symbol for current). This phase is ended by inactivation of I_{to} and is followed by the "plateau phase" or phase 2. The membrane voltage changes very slowly during phase 2 (forming a "plateau"), because there is a fairly large inward calcium (Ca^{2+}) current during phase 2. Like Na^+, Ca^{2+} is more concentrated outside the cell than inside, and tends to enter the cell to make it more positive intracellularly. The phase 2 Ca^{2+} current balances remaining outward K^+ currents, keeping the voltage fairly constant. Finally, time-dependent K^+ currents begin to overwhelm the Ca^{2+} current to produce rapid phase 3 repolarization, bringing the cell back to its resting state (phase 4). The delayed activation of the phase 3 K^+ current is a critical determinant of cell repolarization, and due to this characteristic property this current is called the "delayed rectifier" current. The resting state is normally dominated by a very large background K^+ permeability, carrying a current called "I_{K1}" or "inward-rectifying" background current due to its particular electrical characteristics.

For most cardiac cells, the resting phase (4) is flat, making them quiescent. Certain electrically specialized parts of the heart (the sinoatrial or "SA" and atrioventricular or "AV" nodes, as well as the His-Purkinje system) show spontaneous phase 4 inward depolarization, which can bring them to their threshold potential for firing, resulting in the property of "automaticity" (ability to act as a pacemaker tissue). A key mechanism underlying automaticity is an unusual current that has mixed permeability to Na^+ and K^+. This current, called the "funny current" or "If" because of its unusual properties, is activated by repolarization and its gradual increase makes the cell become more and more positive intracellularly. In spontaneously depolarizing (automatic) tissue, there is no true "resting potential" because the cell never rests at a stable phase 4 voltage: in this case, the equivalent of the resting potential is the maximum diastolic potential, the most negative voltage achieved by the cell immediately after repolarization.

2　Coupling of cardiomyocytes to create a syncytium

In order for the heart to work as an electrically continuous syncytium, heart cells have to be coupled to one another (see figure 2A). This is achieved via specialized intercellular connections called "gap junctions" located at the interfaces between cell-ends.[2] Electrical communication between cells is provided by specialized ion-channel proteins called "connexins", which form half-channels ("hemichannels") in cell-ends. When attached to corresponding hemichannels in the adjacent cell, connexins constitute fully functional large-pore ion channels that allow

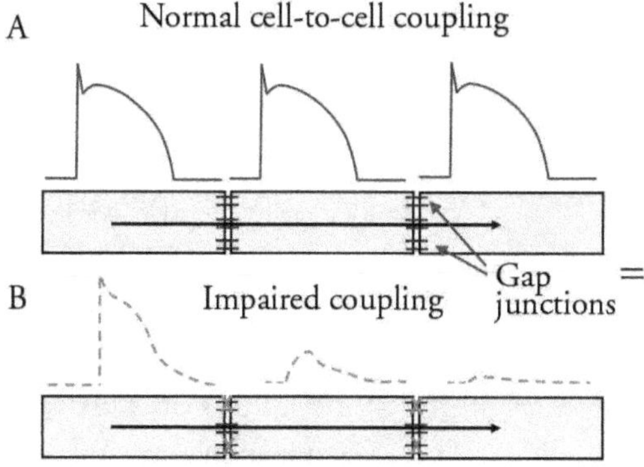

Figure 2. The role of cell to cell coupling. Cardiomyocytes are shown as pink boxes, with corresponding action potentials shown above.
A = importance of normal cell-to-cell coupling by gap junctions to permit electrical continuum and smooth action potential propagation; B = results of loss of connexin-expression that causes impaired gap junction function.

ions and some larger molecules to pass between adjacent cells. Connexins play similar cell-communication roles throughout the body and organ-specific communication is produced by having different types of connexin proteins. The main connexins in the heart are connexin43 (Cx43), connexin40 (Cx40) and connexin45 (Cx45). Abnormalities in connexin function play key roles in a variety of arrhythmia syndromes. When connexin-coupling is poor, electrical activity has difficulty activating adjacent cells and conduction can become decremental to the point of failing (see figure 2B). The intracellular acidosis produced by acute myocardial causes connexin channels to close, uncoupling cells from each other and causing conduction barriers that promote arrhythmogenesis.

3 Tissue-specific electrical activity

An important aspect of cardiac bioelectricity is regional-specific electrical specialization.[3] Figure 3 illustrates some of the more important differences in action potential properties in different parts of the heart. Differences in action potentials are created by different amounts, sometimes even by types of ion currents in different parts of the heart, and subserve specific local functional and electrical needs. There are subtle but significant differences between atrial, ventricular subendo-, mid-, and subepicardium, and Purkinje cells from the specialized conducting system. In contrast, the action potential types in the SA and AV nodes are very different from those in all the other parts of the heart.

Cardiac tissue is divided broadly into two large categories (see figure 4). Action potentials that depend on Na^+ channels for firing, as discussed in the "Action Potential" section, are called "fast-channel" because of the rapid rate of Na^+ channel opening and closure. They are found in working atrial and ventricular muscle, as well as the His-Purkinje system. SA and AV nodes contain a second type of tissue, which depends on current through Ca^{2+} channels for phase 0 activation, called "slow-channel" tissue. Slow-channel action potentials have very little or no I_{K1} background current, so their resting potentials are much less negative (around ~50 to ~60

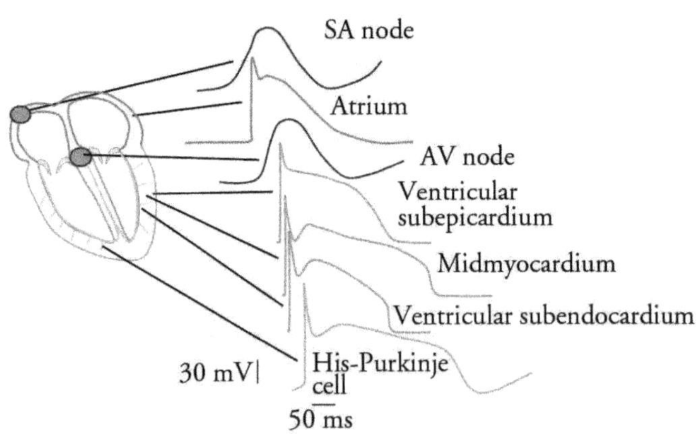

Figure 3. Electrical heterogeneity in the heart. Different electrically specialized regions are shown along with their corresponding action potential properties. Each action potential is a plot of intracellular voltage (vertical axis) versus time (horizontal axis); voltage and time scales are shown.

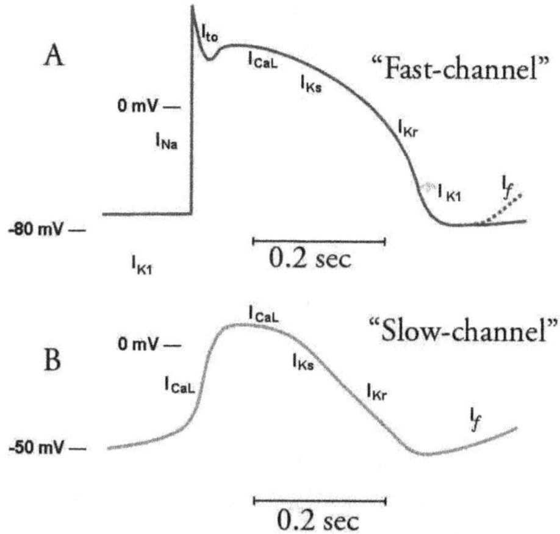

Figure 4. General types of cardiac action potentials.
A = fast-channel action potential typical of working atrial and ventricular myocardium and His-Purkinje system; B = typical slow-channel action potential of SA and AV node.

mV) than in fast-channel cells. They also have very little or no Na^+ current, due to their positive resting potential (which inactivates Na^+ current, I_{Na}) and because they express very few Na^+ channels. Ca^{2+} current activates, inactivates and recovers from inactivation much more slowly, and is much smaller than Na^+ current. These properties explain why SA and AV node cells conduct very slowly and require additional time after full repolarization to reactivate ("post-repolarization refractoriness"). SA and AV node cells also typically have large I_f, which is very important for their pacemaking function. Ca^{2+} current is very sensitive to autonomic neurotransmitters, accounting for the much greater autonomic sensitivity of nodal cells compared to atrial and ventricular muscle or the His-Purkinje conducting system.

Within the ventricle, there is also significant transmural heterogeneity. The subepicardial layer differs from deeper layers in having a much smaller I_{to}. In conditions like Brugada syndrome with reductions in I_{Na}, I_{to} can produce early repolarization in deeper layers, causing arrhythmogenic repolarization gradients. The midmyocardium and Purkinje network have longer action potentials, promoting repolarization dispersion and early afterdepolarizations (EADs, see below) that play a major role in long QT syndrome.

Connexin subtype distribution is also tissue-selective. Cx43 is by far the most important type in ventricular tissue. Atrial tissue has an important contribution from Cx43 but Cx40 also plays a prominent role, and SA node/compact AV node tissue have little Cx43 and more Cx40/Cx45. The Purkinje-fiber network has strong Cx43 expression, but also expresses significant Cx40 and a smaller quantity of connexin43.

4   Arrhythmia mechanisms

The principle mechanisms underlying clinical arrhythmias include enhanced automaticity, delayed afterdepolarizations (DADs), early afterdepolarizations (EADs) and reentry,[1] as illustrated in figure 5. Focal arrhythmia mechanisms (see figures 5A-C) manifest as enhanced local firing. Cardiac reentry (see figure 5D) depends on variability in refractory properties and interactions among tissues in order to generate arrhythmia. Recordings of intracellular electrical activity within the arrhythmia-generating zone would directly show the cellular arrhythmia mechanisms illustrated in figures 5A-C, whereas multiple recordings to provide the sequence of electrical activity would be required to identify the mechanism shown in figure 5D.

Enhanced automaticity (see figure 5a) occurs when normal automaticity is enhanced or when spontaneous phase 4 depolarization begins to manifest in normally non-automatic tissues. Automaticity is enhanced when phase 4 depolarization is accelerated, or when the cell's maximum diastolic potential (MDP) becomes closer to the threshold potential for firing. Acute myocardial infarction is an example of a clinical context for enhanced automaticity. Extracellular K^+ increases in the infarct zone, resulting in a reduced chemical driving force for K^+, reducing background K^+ current and causing less negative MDP (in example, MDP approaches threshold potential). In addition, norepinephrine is released from sympathetic nerve endings in the infarct zone, accelerating phase 4 depolarization in local Purkinje cells. Consequently, automaticity is enhanced, causing ventricular ectopic beats and tachycardias.

Delayed afterdepolarizations (DADs, see figure 5B) are caused by spontaneous diastolic intracellular Ca^{2+} concentration ($[Ca^{2+}]_i$) increases.[4] $[Ca^{2+}]_i$ rises substantially during systole to cause cell contraction. The systolic $[Ca^{2+}]_i$-rise is mainly due to Ca^{2+} release from the sarcoplasmic reticulum (the SR) through specialized Ca^{2+}-release channels, also called ryanodine receptors (RyRs: so-called because they were first identified by their affinity for the toxin ryanodine). RyRs are sensitive to $[Ca^{2+}]_i$ and are initially opened by the entry of Ca^{2+} through the cell-membrane Ca^{2+}-channel during phase 2 of the action potential. Once RyRs open and release SR Ca^{2+}, they close and remain refractory to prevent abnormal diastolic Ca^{2+} releases, which would otherwise cause DADs. Abnormal RyR diastolic Ca^{2+} releases occur when the SR gets Ca^{2+}-overloaded, which disturbs RyR function and causes RyRs to leak Ca^{2+} in diastole. Cellular Ca^{2+} overload occurs in pathological conditions like acute myocardial infarction and excessive

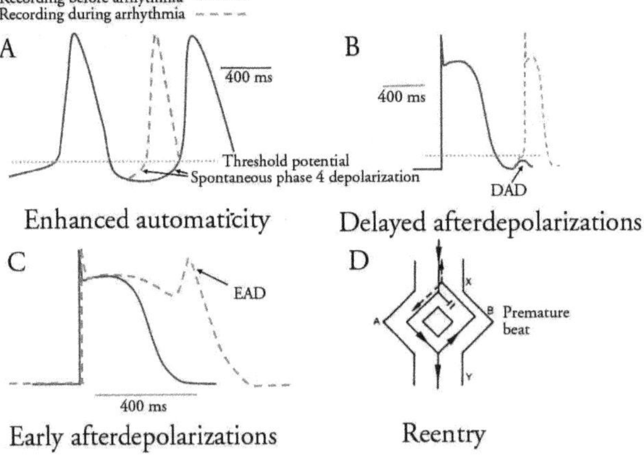

Figure 5. Principal cardiac arrhythmia mechanisms.
A = enhanced automaticity; B = delayed afterdepolarizations; C = early afterdepolarizations; D = reentry.

hypertrophy, most notably hypertrophic cardiomyopathies. Diastolic Ca^{2+} release can also result from abnormal RyR function, as caused by RyR channel mutations that render RyRs leaky in diastole, or by excessive phosphorylation of RyR channels, which can occur in heart failure.

Early afterdepolarizations (EADs, see figure 5C) are seen when the action potential becomes excessively prolonged, most typically by a mutation that impairs the functioning of a repolarizing K^+-channel or causes Na^+- or Ca^{2+}-channel inactivation deficiency to cause persistent inward current during the plateau.[5] Because the electrocardiographic T-wave corresponds to ventricular repolarization, ventricular EADs (which are associated with excess action potential prolongation) almost always accompany QT prolongation. Ventricular cells of different types show differing susceptibility to action potential prolongation. Midmyocardial cell (often called M-cells) and Purkinje cell action potentials prolong much more than those of subendocardial or subepicardial cells, causing important variations in action potential duration (and consequently refractory period) in different transmural regions. This transmural dispersion of refractoriness creates a substrate for reentry. In addition, the differential susceptibility to action-potential prolongation causes EADs in midmyocardial and Purkinje fiber cells when adjacent subendocardial and subepicardial cells repolarize normally (albeit with some repolarization slowing).

EADs in Purkinje or midmyocardial cells can depolarize adjacent tissue to threshold, causing propagated extrasystoles and inducing transmural reentry.[5,6] This sequence of events is illustrated in figure 6. Panel "A" shows a subendocardial cell recording (blue) and Purkinje cell

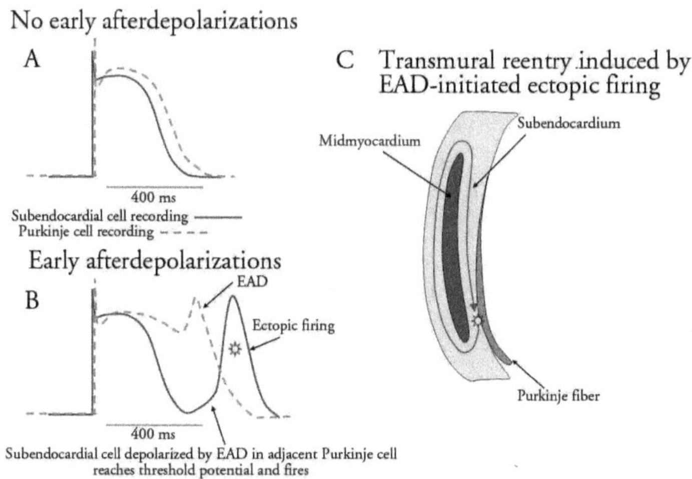

Figure 6. Mechanism of arrhythmia associated with EADs.
A = subendocardial ventricular muscle (blue) and connected Purkinje cell (red) action potentials
in the absence of EADs; B = corresponding recordings under condition provoking EADs.
The Purkinje fiber shows an EAD, whereas the subendocardial muscle does not. However, the EAD
depolarizes the subendocardial tissue to which it is coupled, causing it to depolarize and reach threshold,
generating an ectopic beat; C = the subendocardial ectopic beat propagates around still-refractory
midmyocardial tissue (dark blue) to produce transmural reentry.

recording (red) under conditions that do not lead to EADs. Panel "B" shows recordings when EADs occur and lead to arrhythmias. Purkinje cell action potential prolongation leads to the indicated EAD. The adjacent subendocardial muscle cells have repolarized by the time the Purkinje EAD arises, so the EAD depolarizes the adjacent tissue. When the EAD-induced depolarization is large enough to reach threshold, the subendocardial tissue fires, producing ectopic activity. Panel "C" shows how subendocardial ectopic activation can propagate around the refractory barrier of still-depolarized midmyocardium (which, like Purkinje tissue has prolonged action potentials) and reenter, producing additional ectopic beats or tachycardias.

Figure 5D illustrates the general determinants of reentry. Reentry occurs when an impulse reaches two zones of tissue, one of which can conduct (designated "A" here) and the other ("B") is still refractory. If conditions are right, the impulse can reenter tissue "B" at its distal end, propagating backwards in the retrograde direction. If pathway "A" has recovered excitability by the time the reentering impulse reaches its proximal end, it will be reexcited, and this process can then continue indefinitely. The occurrence of reentry requires particular refractoriness and conduction conditions to be sustained. The time for the reentering impulse to travel throughout the circuit (the circuit time, CT) has to be greater than the longest refractory period (RP) in the circuit for reentry to be maintained. The circuit time is given by the length of the circuit (L) divided by conduction velocity (CV), and RP>L/CV is necessary for sustained reentry. Thus, shorter refractory periods and slower conduction favor reentry maintenance. This notion explains why reentry in the AV node (with its slow conduction properties) is one of the more common forms of reentry in otherwise normal hearts.

Premature beats are much more likely than regular sinus beats to encounter variably refractory tissue and induce reentry. The presence of alternate pathways with differing refractory and conduction properties greatly facilitates the induction and maintenance of reentry. Many forms of clinical reentrant arrhythmias depend on discrete pathways for reentry, like AV node reentry via dissociable AV nodal pathways and AV reentrant tachycardias involving bypass tracts. These arrhythmia syndromes can be cured by destroying one of the pathways required for arrhythmia generation. Other forms of arrhythmia require a critical zone of slowly conducting tissue to maintain reentry, like the cavotriscupid isthmus in atrial flutter. Here, too, destroying the critical anatomical component for reentry can prevent arrhythmia recurrence. Atrial fibrillation (AF) is a complex arrhythmia of varying mechanism.[7] Paroxysmal AF is often due to rapid firing from pulmonary vein ectopic foci and can be treated effectively by isolating the pulmonary veins from the rest of the atria. Persistent AF is likely maintained by multiple functional reentry circuits, and the creation of multiple ablation lines in critical anatomical regions may be needed to eliminate the underlying mechanism.

5 Conclusions

Much is known about the relationship between basic electrophysiological mechanisms and arrhythmia occurrence and prevention. A good understanding of these mechanisms is very helpful for an appreciation of the determinants of clinical arrhythmias and the principles of arrhythmia therapy.

References

1. Nattel S, Maguy A, Le Bouter S, Yeh YH. Arrhythmogenic ion-channel remodeling in the heart: heart failure, myocardial infarction, and atrial fibrillation. Physiol Rev 2007 Apr; 87(2): 425-56.

2. van Rijen HV, van Veen TA, Gros D, Wilders R, de Bakker JM. Connexins and cardiac arrhythmias. Adv Cardiol 2006; 42: 150-60.

3. Schram G, Pourrier M, Melnyk P, Nattel S. Differential distribution of cardiac ion channel expression as a basis for regional specialization in electrical function. Circ Res 2002 May 17; 90(9): 939-50.

4. Eisner DA, Kashimura T, Venetucci LA, Trafford AW. From the ryanodine receptor to cardiac arrhythmias. Circ J 2009 Sep; 73(9): 1561-7.

5. Antzelevitch C, Shimizu W. Cellular mechanisms underlying the long QT syndrome. Curr Opin Cardiol 2002 Jan; 17(1): 43-51.

6. Nattel S, Carlsson L. Innovative approaches to anti-arrhythmic drug therapy. Nat Rev Drug Discov 2006 Dec; 5(12): 1034-49.

7. Nattel S. New ideas about atrial fibrillation 50 years on. Nature 2002 Jan 10; 415(6868): 219-26.

Chapter 2. Electrophysiological study in the diagnosis of syncope

M. Brignole

Arrhythmologic Centre and Syncope Unit
Department of Cardiology
Ospedali del Tigullio, Italy

Address for correspondence:
Arrhythmologic Centre and
Syncope Unit
Dr. M. Brignole
mbrignole@asl4.liguria.it

Key points: identifying the mechanism of uncertain syncope by means of electrophysiological study
Electrophysiological study is indicated when cardiac arrhythmic syncope is suspected at initial evaluation in patients with the following: • Ischemic heart disease, unless there is already an established indication for an ICD • Bundle branch block • Suspected sinus node dysfunction (rare) • Syncope is preceded by sudden and brief palpitations if prolonged ECG monitoring is inconclusive (rare)
Electrophysiological findings are able to establish the cause of syncope (and therefore to guide specific therapy) in the case of: • Sinus bradycardia and very prolonged SNRT (SNRT >2 sec or corrected SNRT >800 msec) • Bundle brunch block and either a baseline HV interval of 100 ms, or 2nd or 3rd degree His-Purkinje block demonstrated during incremental atrial pacing, or with pharmacological challenge • Induction of sustained monomorphic VT in patients with previous myocardial infarction • Induction of rapid SVT which reproduces hypotensive or spontaneous symptoms
Other abnormal findings are of uncertain interpretation and further tests (e.g., implantable loop recorder) are usually required for diagnosis. This is, for example, the case of: • Bundle brunch block and HV interval between 70 and 100 ms • Induction of polymorphic VT or ventricular fibrillation in patients with Brugada syndrome, arrhythmogenic right ventricular cardiomyopathy and hypertrophic cardiomyopathy

Electrophysiological study (EPS) is indicated in patients with structural heart disease when cardiac arrhythmic syncope is suspected at initial evaluation. The minimal protocol suggested for the evaluation of uncertain syncope is shown in table 1.[1] In essence, the aim of EPS is to reproduce in the laboratory the arrhythmia which is thought to have been responsible for the spontaneous syncope. The diagnostic efficacy of the invasive EPS is, like all test procedures, highly dependent on the degree of suspicion of abnormality (pretest probability), and the criteria used for diagnosing the presence of clinically significant abnormalities.

There are four areas of special relevance to electrophysiological testing in syncope patients: suspected sinus node disease (suspected intermittent bradycardia), bundle branch block (impending high degree AV block), suspected tachycardia in normal heart and suspected ventricular tachycardia in structural heart disease.

Measurement of sinus node recovery time and corrected sinus node recovery time by repeated sequences of atrial pacing for 30-60 sec with at least one low (10-20 bpm higher than sinus rate) and two higher pacing rates.*

Assessment of the His-Purkinje system includes measurement of the HV interval at baseline and His-Purkinje conduction with stress by incremental atrial pacing. If the baseline study is inconclusive, pharmacological provocation with slow infusion of ajmaline (1 mg/kg i.v.), procainamide (10 mg/kg i.v.), or disopyramide (2 mg/kg i.v.) is added unless contraindicated.

Assessment of ventricular arrhythmia inducibility performed by ventricular programmed stimulation at two right ventricular sites (apex and outflow tract), at two basic drive cycle lengths (100 or 120 bpm and 140 or 150 bpm), with up to two extrastimuli.**

Assessment of supraventricular arrhythmia inducibility by any atrial stimulation protocol.

Table 1. Minimal suggested electrophysiological protocol for diagnosis of syncope.
*When sinus node dysfunction is suspected autonomic blockade may be applied,
and measurements repeated.
**A third extrastimulus may be added. This may increase sensitivity, but reduces specificity.
Ventricular extrastimulus coupling intervals below 200 ms also reduce specificity.

1 Suspected sinus node disease (suspected intermittent bradycardia)

Sick sinus syndrome is a descriptive term which refers to a constellation of signs and symptoms defining sinus node dysfunction found in a clinical setting. The most frequent electrocardiographic sign is persistent sinus bradycardia. Although persistent clinical manifestations of bradycardia (due to the consequent reduction in cerebral and peripheral perfusion), such as subtle symptoms of fatigue, irritability, lassitude, inability to concentrate, lack of interest, forgetfulness and dizziness can be expected, it is more difficult to explain intermit-

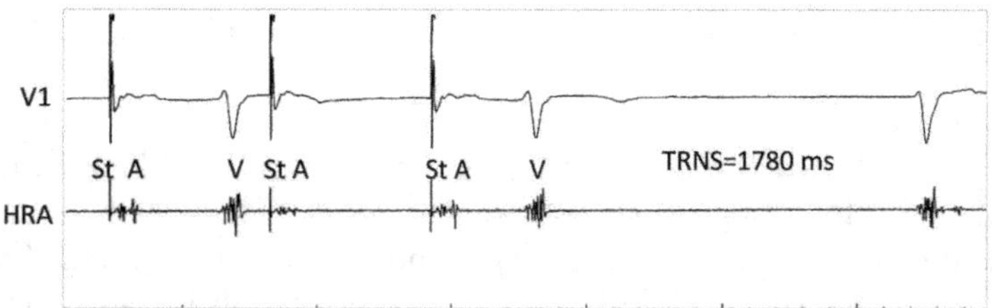

Figure 1. Abnormal sinus node recovery time (SNRT). At the cessation of rapid right atrial pacing (St) at a rate of 100 bpm, a pause of 1780 ms occurs which is followed by an escape junctional beat which obscures the recovery of a normal sinus beat. Therefore, the SNRT is longer than that interval. Note that there is also decreased conductive properties of the AV node as evidenced by the induction of a second degree Weckebach AV block during atrial pacing, which indicates a clinical diagnosis of binodal atrial disease.
St = stimulus; HRA = high right atriogram; A = atrial wave; V = ventricular wave.

tent symptoms (syncope and presyncope). The diagnosis of intermittent symptoms requires the concurrent documentation of intermittent severe sinus bradycardia or sinus-atrial block (cause-effect relationship). In bradycardia patients in whom syncope is the only symptom, this type of correlation can be made in a minority of patients who show ECG documentation of prolonged pause or pauses following the termination of a tachycardia. A prolonged sinus node recovery time (SNRT) induced by incremental atrial pacing (see figure 1) is associated with a higher likelihood of syncope due to sinus arrest. The pause induced by atrial pacing has the same meaning as the spontaneous pause observed at the cessation of a paroxysmal atrial tachyarrhythmia

The pretest probability of a transient symptomatic bradycardia is relatively high when there is asymptomatic sinus bradycardia (<50 bpm [beats per minute]), or sinoatrial block and syncope has occurred suddenly, without premonitory symptoms, and is independent of posture and physical activity, short-lasting, and followed by rapid recovery.

A prolonged sinus node recovery time reflects abnormal sinus node automaticity, sinoatrial conduction, or both. The sensitivity of SNRT >1500-1720 ms and/or CSNRT (SNRT corrected for heart rate) >525 ms is approximately 50 to 80%, whereas specificity is >95%.[2,3] Pharmacological challenge has a place in increasing the sensitivity of the EPS, when the baseline study is inconclusive.[4-7] Complete autonomic blockade of the sinus node activity can be achieved by the administration of intravenous propranolol (0.2 mg/kg body weight) and intravenous atropine sulphate (0.04 mg · kg⁻¹ body weight) according to the seminal work by Jose and Collison,[4] defining the so-called intrinsic heart rate. Normal values for intrinsic heart rate can be determined by using a linear regression equation, which associates predicted intrinsic heart rate (IHRp) with age; IHRp = 118.1 − (0.57 · age).

The prognostic value of prolonged sinus node recovery time is largely unknown. One observational study, however, found a relationship between the presence of prolonged recovery time at EPS and the effect of pacing on symptoms.[8] More recently, Menozzi *et al.*[9] addressed a related issue in a small prospective study, showing that the patients with a CSNRT of ≥800 ms had an 8-fold higher risk of syncope than patients with a CSNRT below this value. According to ESC guidelines[1,10] in the presence of an SNRT >2 sec or CSNRT ≥800 msec, sinus node dysfunction may be the cause of syncope.

2   Syncope in patients with bundle branch block (impending high degree AV block)

The most alarming ECG sign in a patient with syncope is probably alternating complete left and right bundle branch block, or alternating right bundle branch block with left anterior or posterior fascicular block, suggesting trifascicular conduction system disease and intermittent or impending high degree AV block. This finding is rarely observed. The most common finding is bifascicular block (right bundle branch block plus left anterior or left posterior fascicular block, or left bundle branch block). Since not all the patients with bifascicular bundle branch block will develop high-degree AV block, and also that syncope may have a different mechanism even in presence of bifascicular block, EPS is useful in order to identify the patients at higher risk. The prognostic value of the HV interval was prospectively studied by Scheinman *et al.,*[11] indicating that the progression rate to AV block at 4 years was 4%, 2%, 12%, and 24% respectively, for patients with an HV interval of <55 ms (normal), 55-69 ms, 70-100 ms and >100 ms. In order to increase the diagnostic yield of the electrophysiological evaluation, incremental atrial pacing and pharmacological provocation were added (see figure 2). The development of intra- or infra-His block at incremental atrial pacing,[12] is highly predictive of impending AV block, but is rarely observed and has low sensitivity. For example, in the study by Gronda *et al.*[13] in 131 patients, an HV prolongation of >10 ms was observed in 6% of cases and 2nd-degree AV block in 5% of cases. Complete AV block developed in 40% of these patients during a mean follow-up of 42 months. In the study by Dini *et al.,*[14] in 85 patients, pacing induced AV block in 7% with progression to complete AV block in 30% within two years. Acute intravenous pharmacological stress testing of the

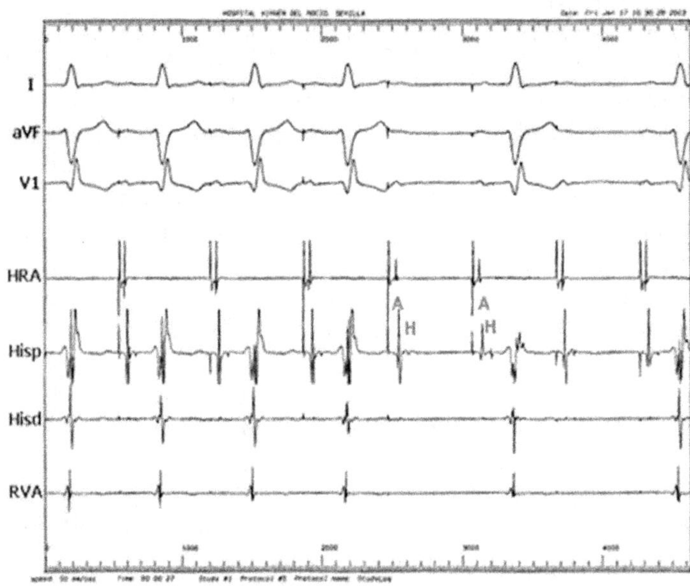

Figure 2. Infra-His second degree AV block during incremental atrial pacing. The fourth paced beat show an H deflection not followed by V wave, indicating that the site of block is distal to His deflection inside the His-Purkinje conduction system.

His-Purkinje system has been performed with several class IA antiarrhythmic drugs: ajmaline, at a dosage of 1 mg/kg,[13-15] procainamide at a dosage of 10 mg/kg,[16] and disopyramide at a dosage of 2 mg/kg.[17] In five studies[13-17] evaluating the diagnostic value of pharmacological stress testing for a total of 333 patients, high degree AV block was induced in 50 (15%) of the patients. During the follow-up, wich ranged between 24 and 63 months, 68% (range 43-100) of these patients developed spontaneous AV block. Thus, the induction of AV block during the test is highly predictive of the subsequent development of AV block. The prognostic value of a pharmacologically prolonged HV interval to a value of >120 ms or >50% of the baseline value without induction of AV block is uncertain. In three studies[13,14,18] AV block progression was observed in 18%, 29% and 75% of positive patients, respectively. By combining the above mentioned parts of the electrophysiological protocol, it was possible to identify most of the patients who developed high-degree AV block. For example, the positive predictive value was 87% in the study by Gronda *et al.*[13] and 80% in that by Bergfeldt *et al.*[18] On the other hand, in patients with negative electrophysiological studies, Link *et al.* [19] observed the development of permanent AV block in 18 % (after 30 months), and Gaggioli *et al.*[20] observed this in 19% (at 62 months); and intermittent or stable atrioventricular block was documented by an implantable loop recorder in 33% of patients (within 15 months).[21]

In conclusion, in patients with syncope and bifascicular block, a positive electrophysiological result is highly predictive of the cause of syncope. However, a negative EPS cannot rule out paroxysmal AV block as the cause of syncope and further investigation using, for example, an implantable loop recorder, is recommended.

3   Suspected tachycardia in structural normal heart

Sudden-onset palpitations immediately followed by syncope in patients without structural heart disease suggests a paroxysmal undocumented supraventricular or ventricular tachycardia. In this circumstance, ECG documentation of the episode is usually feasible with prolonged ECG monitoring (external or implantable loop recorder) and is diagnostic. In selected cases, EPS may be used to evaluate the hemodynamic effects of an induced tachycardia, especially when combined with the administration of isoprenaline or atropine. In general, EPS is indicated only if catheter ablation of the induced arrhythmia is planned during the same procedure. Electrophysiological study is used to stratify risk in patients affected by Brugada syndrome independently of the presence of syncope, although its usefulness is controversial.[22] The inducibility rate of ventricular tachyarrhythmias is similar in patients with and without syncope.[23,24] There are no data in the literature on the use of EPS for the diagnosis of unexplained syncope in Brugada syncope and in long QT syndrome.[25]

4   Suspected ventricular tachycardia in structural heart disease

Ventricular tachycardia may present as syncope with or without palpitations or other accompanying symptoms. The major concern with programmed electrical stimulation (see figure 3) as part of an EPS for inducing clinically significant ventricular arrhythmia is its varying sensitivity (and specificity) in different clinical settings.

Programmed electrical stimulation is a sensitive tool in patients with chronic ischemic heart disease (previous myocardial infarction). In this setting, the induction of a monomorphic ven-

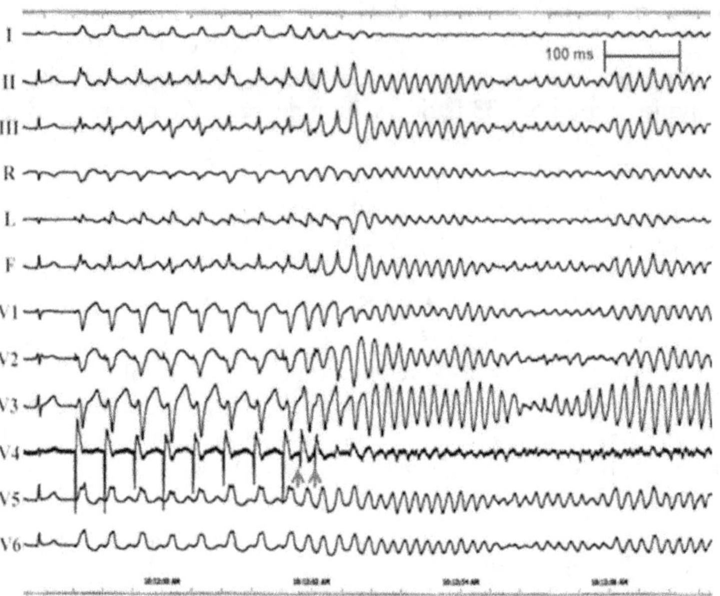

Figure 3. Programmed ventricular stimulation results in induction of ventricular fibrillation. Eight ventricular paced beats are followed by two premature ventricular beats (arrow) that induce ventricular fibrillation.

tricular tachycardia is thought to be a specific event that should guide therapy. For example, in the ESVEM trial,[26] syncope, associated with induced ventricular tachyarrhythmias at electro-physiological testing, indicated a high risk of death, similar to that of patients with document-ed spontaneous ventricular tachyarrhythmias. The predictive value of EPS has been confirmed by studies of patients with an ICD, and showed a good correlation between recurrent syncope and spontaneous ventricular tachyarrhythmias[27] and an appropriate ICD discharge rate simi-lar to that of the patients with documented spontaneous ventricular tachycardia.[27,28] Conversely, in patients with coronary artery disease and preserved cardiac function, noninducibility at EPS predicted a low risk of sudden death and ventricular arrhythmias.[19] The specificity of the in-duction of polymorphic ventricular tachycardia and ventricular fibrillation in patients with coronary artery disease is open to question because the follow-up of patients with and without inducible polymorphic ventricular tachycardia or fibrillation demonstrated no difference in survival.[29] However, patients with heart failure and an established indication for ICD accord-ing to current guidelines should receive this therapy before and independently of the evalua-tion of the mechanism of syncope. This is the case, for example, of patients with ischemic or dilated cardiomyopathy and low ejection fraction (<30% or 35% and NYHA class II).

Programmed ventricular stimulation has low predictive value in patients with non-ischemic dilated cardiomyopathy and its use is discouraged.[30,31] In a study[30] on patients affect-ed by idiopathic dilated cardiomyopathy who received an ICD, there was a high incidence of appropriate shocks both in the inducible sustained monomorphic ventricular tachycardia group and in the non-inducible sustained monomorphic ventricular tachycardia group. In another study,[31] the patients with unexplained syncope and negative EPS who recived an ICD had a high incidence of tachyarrhythmic episodes during the follow-up. The specificity of induction of ventricular tachycardia has been questioned in patients with syncope and bifascicular block.[32] Kuck *et al.*[33] performed EPS in 54 consecutive patients with HCM. The type and incidence of induced ventricular arrhythmias did not differ between the "symptomatic" (syncope) and "asymptomatic" (no syncope) groups. Therefore EPS is not indicated in patients with hypertrophic cardiomyopathy.[34] Neither is programmed ventricular stimulation of value in identifying patients at risk of tachyarrhythmias in patients with arrhythmogenic right ventricular dysplasia and syncope (positive predictive value 49%, negative predictive value 54%).[35]

In conclusion, programmed ventricular stimulation is indicated only in patients with undocumented syncope, coronary artery disease and depressed systolic function. In these patients, the inducibility of sustained monomorphic ventricular tachycardia is diagnostic of the cause of the syncope; conversely non-inducibility predicts a more favorable outcome.

5　Clinical perspectives

Electrophysiological study has been used in the diagnosis of unexplained syncope since the 1980s. After the initial enthusiasm, not only its usefulness but also its limitations became evident. Consequently, in recent years, its indications have been restricted to the few well-defined areas described above. More extensive use and a more liberal interpretation of the results than that described above yields unacceptably low diagnostic accuracy and runs the risk of misdiagnosis.

Similar to all the other provocation tests aimed at inducing syncope or related abnormalities in an artificial setting (e.g., laboratory), EPS has a suboptimal diagnostic accuracy. In an overview of eight studies including 625 patients with syncope undergoing EPS, Linzer *et al.*[36] assessed the association between organic heart disease and an abnormal test result. Ventricular tachycardia was induced in 21%, and abnormal indices of bradycardia were found in 34% of patients with organic heart disease or an abnormal standard ECG. The corresponding figures were 1% and 10%, respectively, in patients with an apparently normal heart ($p<0.001$ for both comparisons). Thus, positive results at EPS occur almost exclusively in patients with overt heart disease or conduction defects, with the exception of patients with supraventricular tachycardias, and its use in patients without structural heart disease is inappropriate. However, it must be emphasized that, even in patients with structural heart disease, normal electrophysiological findings cannot completely exclude an arrhythmic cause of syncope. When an arrhythmia is likely, further evaluations (e.g., loop recording) are recommended.

Since false-positive responses are not uncommon, the interpretation of a positive response requires knowledge of the clinical context in which the spontaneous syncope occurred; in more scientific terms, the pretest probability largely influences the interpretation of a positive response. Depending on the clinical context, even apparently abnormal electrophysiological findings (e.g., relatively long HV interval, inducible atrial arrhythmias and ventricular fibrillation with aggressive stimulation) may not be diagnostic of the cause of syncope. For example, Fujimura *et al.*[37] compared the findings of a positive EPS with the arrhythmia documented during a spontaneous syncopal episode by ECG monitoring and found that EPS suggested the correct diagnosis in only 15% of patients, who had syncope due to transient bradycardia. Admittedly, their study had some limitations because pharmacological provocation was not used and bradycardic syncope due to an abnormal vagal reflex was not excluded. In the same study, unrelated ventricular tachyarrhthmias and atrial tachyarrhythmias, that may have been mistakenly designated as the cause of syncope, were induced in 24% of patients. Brignole *et al.*[38] found a similar 20% rate of false-positive responses. Finally, Lacroix *et al.*[39] showed that, whereas an EPS reproduced the spontaneous arrhythmia in 13 of 17 cases, a nonspecific atrial or ventricular arrhythmia was also induced in 31 of 44 cases.

For the above reasons, the appropriate selection of patients is crucial. In particular, the best diagnostic accuracy is observed in patients with ischemic heart disease, bundle branch block or syncope preceded by sudden and brief palpitations. Inappropriate indications increase the risk of false-positive results. If appropriate indications are applied, only a small number of patients (probably <10% of those with uncertain syncope) need an EPS. In a large multicenter study,[40] performed in patients referred for syncope to eleven emergency departments in Italy, EPS was appropriately performed according to the indications of the ESC guidelines in 9% of the patients in whom the cause of syncope had remained uncertain after the initial evaluation. In another multicenter study,[41] performed in patients referred to nine specialized syncope facilities, EPS was appropriately performed according to the indications of the ESC guidelines in 6% of the patients in whom the cause of syncope had remained uncertain after the initial evaluation. When the selection criteria are appropriate, the diagnostic value is very good, and resulted in a diagnosis in 30% and 35% of patients in the two studies above, respectively.

In conclusion, 30 years after its introduction into clinical practice, the electrophysiological techniques, indications and interpretation of results have been refined. Electrophysiological study has an established and important role for the diagnosis of unexplained syncope, albeit limited to a selected minority of patients provided that it is used appropriately.

References

1. Brignole, M, Alboni, P, Benditt, D, Bergfeldt L, et al. Guidelines on management (diagnosis and treatment) of syncope: Update 2004. Europace 2004; 6: 467-537.

2. Narula O, Samet P, Javier RP. Significance of the sinus node recovery time. Circulation 1972; 45: 55-61.

3. Benditt DG, Gornick C, Dunbar D, et al. Indications for electrophysiological testing in diagnosis and assessment of sinus node dysfunction. Circulation 1987; 75 (Suppl III): 93-99.

4. Jose AD, Collison D. The normal range and determinants of the intrinsic heart rate in man. Cardiovasc Res 1970; 4: 160-6.

5. Vallin H, Edhag O, Sowton E. Diagnostic capacity of sinus node recovery time after inhibition of autonomous neural tone. Eur J Cardiol 1980; 12: 81-93.

6. Alboni P, Malacarne C, Pedroni P, et al. Electrophysiology of normal sinus node with and without autonomic blockade. Circulation 1982; 65: 1236-42.

7. Bergfeldt L, Vallin H, Rosenqvist M, et al. Sinus node recovery time assessment revisited: role of pharmacological blockade of the autonomic nervous system. J Cardiovasc Electrophysiol 1996; 7: 95-101.

8. Gann D, Tolentino A, Samet P. Electrophysiologic evaluation of elderly patients with sinus bradycardia. A long-term follow-up study. Ann Intern Med 1979;90: 24-29.

9. Menozzi C, Brignole M, Alboni P, et al. The natural course of untreated sick sinus syndrome and identification of the variables predictive of unfavourable outcome. Am J Cardiol 1998; 82: 1205-1209.

10. Moya A, Sutton R, Ammirati F, et al. Guidelines for the Diagnosis and Management of Syncope (Version 2009). Eur Heart J 2009; 30: 2631–2671.

11. Scheinman MM, Peters RW, Sauvé MJ, et al. Value of the H-Q interval in patients with bundle branch block and the role of prophylactic permanent pacing. Am J Cardiol 1982; 50: 1316-1322.

12. Dhingra RC, Wyndham C, Bauernfeind R, et al. Significance of block distal to the His bundle induced by atrial pacing in patients with chronic bifascicular block. Circulation 1979; 60: 1455-1464.

13. Gronda M, Magnani A, Occhetta E, et al. Electrophysiologic study of atrio-ventricular block and ventricular conduction defects. G Ital Cardiol 1984; 14: 768-773.

14. Dini P, Iaolongo D, Adinolfi E, et al. rognostic value of His-ventricular conduction after ajmaline administration. In: Masoni A, Alboni P (eds). Cardiac electrophysiology today. Academic press, London 1982: 515-522.

15. Kaul U, Dev V, Narula J, et al. Evaluation of patients with bundle branch block and "unexplained" syncope: a study based on comprehensive electrophysiologic testing and ajmaline stress. PACE 1988; 11: 289-297.

16. Twidale N, Heddle W, Tonkin A. Procainamide administration during electrophysiologic study – Utility as a provocative test for intermittent atrioventricular block. PACE 1988; 11: 1388-1397.

17. Englund A, Bergfeldt L, Rosenqvist M. Pharmacological stress testing of the His-Purkinje system in patients with bifascicular block. PACE 1998; 21: 1979-1987.

18. Bergfeldt L, Edvardsson N, Rosenqvist M, *et al.* Atrioventricular block progression in patients with bifascicular block assessed by repeated electrocardiography and a bradycardia-detecting pacemaker. Am J Cardiol 1994; 74: 1129-1132.

19. Link M, Kim KM, Homoud M, *et al.* Long-term outcome of patients with syncope associated with coronary artery disease and a no diagnostic electrophysiological evaluation. Am J Cardiol 1999; 83: 1334-1337.

20. Gaggioli G, Bottoni N, Brignole M, *et al.* Progression to second or third-degree atrioventricular block in patients electrostimulated for bundle branch block: a long-term study. G Ital Cardiol 1994: 24: 409-416.

21. Brignole M, Menozzi C, Moya A, *et al.* The mechanism of syncope in patients with bundle branch block and negative electrophysiologic test. Circulation 2001; 104: 2045-50.

22. Antzelevitch C, Brugada P, Borggrefe M, *et al.* Brugada Syndrome: Report of the Second Consensus Conference: Endorsed by the Heart Rhythm Society and the European Heart Rhythm Association Circulation 2005; 111: 659-670.

23. Paul M, Gerss J, Schulze-Bahr E, *et al.* Role of programmed ventricular stimulation in patients with Brugada syndrome: a meta-analysis of worldwide published data. Eur Heart J 2007; 28: 2126-2133.

24. Sacher F, Probst V, Iesaka Y, *et al.* Outcome after implantation of a cardioverter-defibrillator in patients with Brugada syndrome: a multicenter study. Circulation 2006; 114: 2317-24.

25. Roden DM. Clinical practice. Long-QT syndrome. N Engl J Med 2008; 358: 169-76.

26. Olshansky B, Hahn EA, Hartz VL, *et al.* Clinical significance of syncope in the electrophysiologic study versus electrocardiographic monitoring (ESVEM) trial. Am Heart J 1999; 137: 878-886.

27. Pires L, May L, Ravi S, *et al.* Comparison of event rates and survival in patients with unexplained syncope without documented ventricular tachyarrhythmias versus patients with documented sustained ventricular tachyarrhythmias both treated with implantable cardioverter-defibrillator. Am J Cardiol 2000; 85: 725-728.

28. Andrews N, Fogel R, Pelargonio G, *et al.* Implantable defibrillator event rates in patients with unexplained syncope and inducible sustained ventricular tachyarrhythmias. J Am Coll Cardiol 1999; 34: 2023-2030.

29. Mittal S, Hao S, Iwai S, *et al.* Significance of inducible ventricular fibrillation in patients with coronary artery disease and unexplained syncope. J Am Coll Cardiol 2001; 38: 371-376.

30. Brilakis E, Shen W, Hammill S, *et al.* Role of programmed ventricular stimulation and implantable cardioverter defibrillators in patients with idiopathic dilated cardiomyopathy and syncope. PACE 2001; 24: 1623-1630.

31. Knight B, Goyal R, Pelosi F, *et al.* Outcome of patients with nonischemic dilated cardiomyopathy and unexplained syncope treated with an implantable defibrillator. J Am Coll Cardiol 1999; 33: 1964-1970.

32. Englund A, Bergfeldt L, Rehnqvist N, *et al.* Diagnostic value of programmed ventricular stimulation in patients with bifascicular block: a prospective study of patients with and without syncope. J Am Coll Cardiol 1995; 26(6): 1508-1515.

33. Kuck KH, Kunze KP, Schluter M *et al.* Programmed electrical stimulation in hypertrophic cardiomyopathy. Results in patients with and without cardiac arrest or syncope. Eur Heart J 1988;9:177–85.

34. Williams L, Frenneaux M. Syncope in hypertrophic cardiomyopathy: mechanisms and consequences for treatment. Europace 2007; 9: 817-22.

35. Corrado D, Leoni L, Link MS, *et al.* Implantable cardioverter-defibrillator therapy for prevention of sudden death in patients with arrhythmogenic right ventricular cardiomyopathy/dysplasia. Circulation 2003; 108: 3084-3091.

36. Linzer M, Yang E, Estes M, *et al.* Diagnosing syncope. Part II: Unexplained syncope. Ann Intern Med 1997; 127: 76-86.

37. Fujimura O, Yee R, Klein G, *et al.* The diagnostic sensitivity of electrophysiologic testing in patients with syncope caused by transient bradycardia. N Engl J Med 1989; 321: 1703-1707.

38. Brignole M, Menozzi C, Bottoni N, *et al.* Mechanisms of syncope caused by transient bradycardia and the diagnostic value of electrophysiologic testing and cardiovascular reflexivity maneuvers. Am J Cardiol 1995; 76: 273-278.

39. Lacroix D, Dubuc M, Kus T, *et al.* Evaluation of arrhythmic causes of syncope: correlation between Holter monitoring, electrophysiologic testing, and body surface potential mapping. Am Heart J 1991; 122: 1346-1354.

40. Brignole M, Menozzi C, Bartoletti A, *et al.* A new management of syncope: prospective systematic guideline-based evaluation of patients referred urgently to general hospitals. Eur Heart J 2006; 27: 76-82.

41. Brignole M, Ungar A, Casagranda I, *et al.* Prospective multicentre systematic guideline-based management of patients referred to the Syncope Units of general hospitals. Europace 2010; 12(1): 109-18.

Chapter 3. Pacing maneuvers and ablation of sustained ventricular tachycardia

U.B. Tedrow,[1] W.G. Stevenson[2]

[1]Clinical Cardiac Electrophysiology Program
Brigham and Women's Hospital
Harvard Medical School
Boston, USA

[2]Clinical Cardiac Electrophysiology Program
Brigham and Women's Hospital
Harvard Medical School
Boston, USA

Address for correspondence:
Cardiovascular Divison
Brigham and Women's Hospital
Dr. Usha B. Tedrow
utedrow@partners.org

Introduction

Sustained ventricular tachycardia (VT) can occur with or without structural heart disease. Idiopathic VT typically occurs in the absence of heart disease, and in this situation, sudden death is rare, but ablation is used to prevent symptomatic VT (see chapter 5).[1] When structural heart disease is present, sustained VT is associated with a risk of sudden death, and implantable cardioverter-defibrillators (ICDs) are warranted in most of these patients. ICDs do not prevent VT and some patients have symptoms or syncope prior to VT termination by the device. ICD shocks are painful, reduce quality of life, and are markers for increased risk of heart failure and mortality.[2] Catheter ablation for VT is an important adjunct to the management of these patients, reducing shocks and reducing the need for potentially toxic anti-arrhythmic drugs.[1]

The type of VT and underlying heart disease direct the approach to mapping and ablation. Most VTs that are considered for ablation are monomorphic, indicating that ventricular activation is the same from beat to beat and that a structural substrate or focus is present that can be targeted for ablation. When VT has a focal origin, the site of earliest activation during VT identifies the focus and pacing at the site ("pace-mapping") reproduces the ventricular activation sequence during VT, and therefore the QRS morphology of the VT (see chapter 5). Sustained monomorphic VT with structural heart disease is most often due to reentry through regions of ventricular scar. Scars are most commonly due to prior myocardial infarction, but also occur in idiopathic and familial cardiomyopathies, right ventricular dysplasia, sarcoidosis, and surgical incisions, such as after repair of tetralogy of Fallot.[3] Scar-related reentry requires a different approach to mapping and ablation than that for focal VTs.

1   Scar-related reentry

Ventricular scars causing monomorphic VT are comprised of variable regions of dense fibrosis with interposed surviving myocyte bundles and interstitial fibrosis. Diminished cellular coupling produces circuitous paths and zones of slow conduction that along with more discrete areas of conduction block, promote reentry.[4] These circuits can be modelled as having an isthmus or channel comprised of a small mass of tissue that does not contribute to the surface ECG (see figure 1). The QRS complex begins when the excitation wave front emerges from an exit along the border of the scar and spreads across the ventricles. The narrow width of the channel makes it a desirable target for catheter ablation. After the reentry wavefront emerges from the exit, it may return to the channel by propagating along the border of the scar, referred to as an outer loop and back to the entrance to the channel. Outer loops are often broad and difficult to interrupt with ablation. Alternatively inner loops through the scar may be present (see figure 1). Both inner and outer loops may even be present. These reentry circuits are often large, extending over several square centimeters. Sites that are not part of the reentry circuit are des-

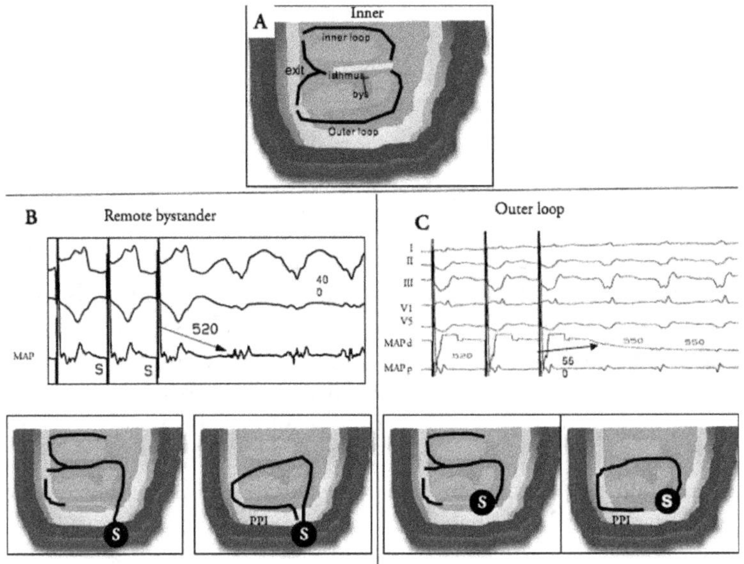

Figure 1. A model of scar-related reentry and findings during entrainment.
Panel A shows a schematic of a region of ventricle. Orange represents the region with the lowest amplitude electrogram; signals increase in amplitude at yellow and green regions. Purple represents normal myocardium. Grey regions are dense fibrosis that is electrically unexcitable. The reentry circuit has an exit region, from which wavefronts propagate across the ventricles to produce the QRS complex, then return to an isthmus in the scar by propagating through an outer loop on the border of the scar, or an inner loop through the scar. A bystander (bys) region is attached to the isthmus.
Panel B shows entrainment from a remote bystander site with a schematic illustrating the findings below the tracing. Pacing changes the QRS morphology consistent with fusion. The post-pacing interval (PPI) of 520 ms exceeds the VT cycle length by 120 ms.
Panel C shows entrainment from an outer loop site. Pacing subtly changes the QRS morphology (most noticeable as the narrower R wave in lead I). The post pacing interval is 550 ms indicating that the site is in this VT circuit.

ignated bystanders. Bystander sites in scars can be difficult to distinguish from reentry circuit sites. Multiple potential reentry circuits are usually present, giving rise to multiple inducible VTs, with different cycle lengths and QRS morphologies, in a single patient. Multiple VTs can originate from the same region of the scar, such that ablation at one region abolishes more than one VT.[5-10] Multiple reentry circuits from widely separated areas also occur. Scars causing VT often border a valve annulus (e.g., the mitral annulus for inferior wall left ventricular scars) that forms a border for part of the circuit.[8,11] Although reentry circuits are commonly subendocardial, portions of the circuit, and even entire circuits, can be intramural or subepicardial in location.

Extensive mapping in VT is often limited by hemodynamic intolerance. One approach to targeting scar-related VTs is shown in figure 2. Substrate mapping is used during stable sinus rhythm, or stable VT, to identify the region of scar that is likely to contain the reentry circuit. The mapping catheter is placed at a site of interest in that region and VT is then induced. If VT is stable for mapping, a combination of activation sequence mapping and entrainment mapping is used to identify ablation sites in the scar region. If VT is unstable, entrainment may be performed quickly followed by ablation if the site is a channel in the circuit. Alternatively the VT is terminated by pacing or cardioversion, and ablation is performed guided by substrate

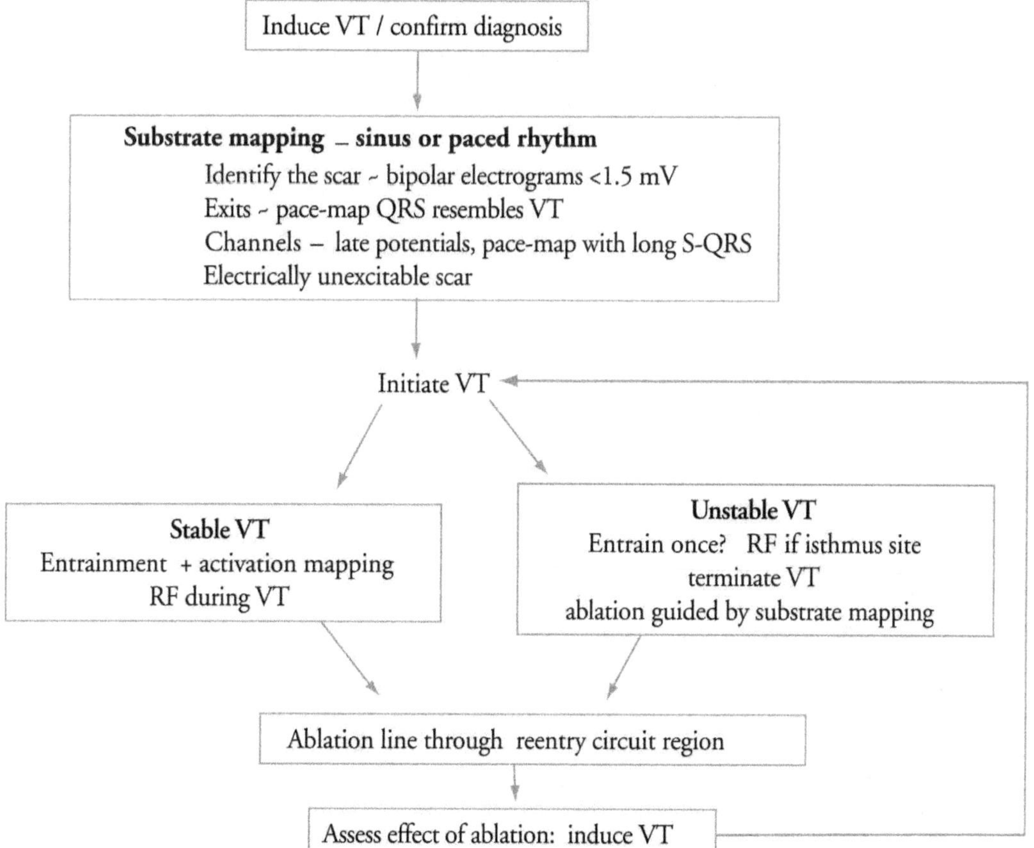

Figure 2. One approach to mapping and ablation of scar-related VTs (see text for discussion).

mapping. Failure of ablation is often related to anatomic obstacles that would potentially benefit from further technological advances.

2   Substrate mapping for scar-related VT

The delineation of the likely arrhythmogenic substrate and reentry circuit sites during a stable sinus or paced rhythm is called *substrate mapping*.[8,10,12] Areas of ventricular scar are characterized by low amplitude bipolar electrograms (<1.55 mV). Plots of peak to peak electrogram amplitude displayed in electroanatomic mapping reconstructions are referred to as "voltage maps" (see figure 3).[10,12] The low voltage region is likely to contain the reentry circuit, but is often extensive, exceeding 20 cm in circumference in many patients.[8] Ablation of the entire region is typically not possible. Additional analyses of electrograms, voltage, or pace-mapping are used to identify exits or channels within the scar or along the border of the scar, where electrogram amplitude is typically between 1.5 and 0.5 mV.

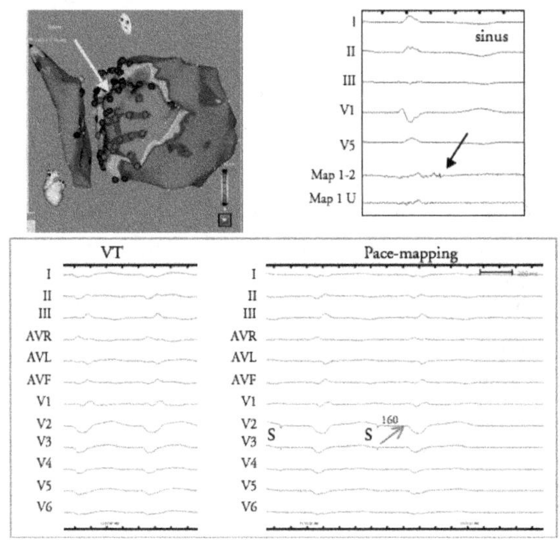

Figure 3. Findings during mapping in a patient with prior anterior wall myocardial infarction.
At top left an electroanatomic endocardial voltage map is shown as viewed from an LAO projection. A limited right ventricular map is on the left; the left ventricle is seen on the right. The His bundle is indicated by the orange dot in the right ventricle. Purple indicates a bipolar electrogram amplitude of 1.5 mV or greater; electrogram amplitude diminishes from blue, to green, to yellow, to red. Grey indicates electrically unexcitable scar (EUS). A low amplitude region of scar is present extending along the anterior and septal walls. The arrow indicates a potential scar channel where the findings in the other panels were observed. Dark red spots indicate ablation lesion sites. At the right are recordings during sinus rhythm. The bipolar recording from the mapping catheter shows low amplitude multicomponent signals that extend beyond the end of the QRS complex, consistent with abnormal conduction in the infarct scar. The bottom panel shows 12-lead ECGs. The induced VT has a right bundle configuration in lead V1, and negative deflections in I, aVL. Pace-mapping at the site designated in electroanatomic map produces a QRS similar to that of VT. The S-QRS interval is 160 ms consistent with pacing in an isthmus for the VT. Ablation through this region resulted in non-inducibility of VT.

2.1 QRS morphology and pace-mapping

Assessment of QRS morphology during VT and pace-mapping (see below) suggests the location of the reentry circuit exit.[13] A left bundle branch blocklike configuration in lead V1 (dominant S-wave) indicates an exit in the right ventricle or interventricular septum; dominant R-waves in V1 indicate a left ventricular exit. The frontal plane axis points away from the exit. A superiorly directed axis indicates an inferior wall exit. An inferiorly directed axis indicates an anterior wall exit. The closer an exit is to a precordial lead, the more negative the S-wave in that lead, providing an indication of exit location between the base and apex. Apical exits generate dominant S-waves in leads V3 and V4. Basal exits generate dominant R-waves in these leads.

The QRS morphology only suggests a starting point for localization of the VT circuit. Areas of scars, conduction block and abnormal ventricular anatomy can render the QRS morphology misleading. Pace-mapping (see below) can suggest the relation between anatomic location and anticipated QRS morphology is as expected in an individual patient.

Pacing from the mapping catheter while in stable sinus or paced rhythm is called "pace mapping". In the VT exit region along the border of the scar, pace mapping usually replicates the QRS morphology of VT.[14,15] During pacing in the scar border and in normal myocardium, the interval between the stimulus and QRS onset is typically short ($\leq$40 ms) indicating rapid conduction away from the pacing site. Long S-QRS intervals are consistent with slow conduction, which is an important substrate for reentry (see figure 3). Pace-mapping in an isthmus proximal to the exit, the paced QRS morphology may also resemble VT, but with a longer S-QRS interval consistent with the increased conduction time from the pacing site to the exit.[14,16] If the wavefront leaves the scar by another path, however, such as the entrance to a channel, the paced QRS morphology may differ from VT, or resemble a different VT. Thus a paced-QRS that resembles VT is helpful; a QRS that does not match VT does not exclude a region from consideration for ablation.

Pace-mapping also allows the identification of electrically unexcitable areas of scar (EUS) that are regions of fixed conduction block that can be border-forming for the reentry path. EUS has been defined as a pacing threshold >10 mA at 2 ms pulse width with unipolar pacing. Narrow bands of fibrosis likely escape detection with this method. Inadequate electrode myocardial contact is also a potential source of error. EUS can not be reliably detected based on electrogram amplitude alone. Pacing captures at many sites with very low electrogram amplitude of 0.25 mV. In contrast, some EUS sites have electrogram amplitude >0.5 mV, due to the presence of large far field potentials. Thus, electrogram characteristics and pacing techniques provide complimentary information during substrate mapping.

2.2 Electrograms

Fractionated multicomponent electrograms are markers of slow conduction. Delayed local activation of a channel during sinus or paced rhythm can create isolated potentials inscribed after the end of the QRS (see figure 5).[16-19] Some potential channels have greater amplitude than surrounding tissue, allowing them to be exposed by assessing the relative electrogram amplitudes in a low voltage region.[20,21]

2.3 Ablation

Substrate-guided ablation usually involves placing a series of RF lesions through regions that have one or more of the features of reentry circuit channels or isthmuses, confining the ablation to the low voltage scar area to avoid damage to functioning myocardium, followed by retesting for inducible VT.[8,10,15] These areas are often large. Even for unstable VT, limited activation mapping and entrainment mapping VT can be helpful to confirm that an identified region is in a reentry circuit and to facilitate successful ablation with fewer ablation lesions.[8] These approaches have not been directly compared.

3 Mapping during VT

3.1 Activation mapping and electrograms

During VT, the QRS onset is typically used as a reference point for mapping. The QRS onset occurs after the wavefront has emerged from the exit. Electrograms at the exit precede the QRS onset and are described as "presystolic" (see figure 4). Activation is progressively earlier at sites in the isthmus proximal to exit, occurring in electrical diastole (between QRS complexes) (see figure 5, panel A), and at very proximal and loop sites activation occurs during the QRS complex (systolic). Sites that are proximal in the circuit can be activated at the end of the QRS complex, without diastolic electrical activity, but can be identified by entrainment (see below).[22] Electrograms often have multiple rapid components due to asynchronous activation of my-

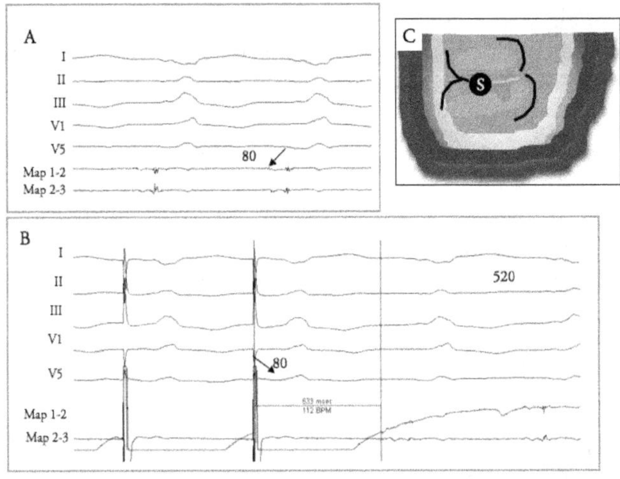

Figure 4. Mapping in scar-related VT in a patient with prior infarction.
Panel A shows sustained VT. Fractionated presystolic electrograms are recorded
from the mapping catheter.
Panel B shows the entrainment with concealed fusion with a stimulus to QRS of 80 ms and post-
pacing interval of 533 ms and tachycardia cycle length of 520 ms, consistent with pacing in the exit
region of an isthmus. Ablation at this site terminated the tachycardia.

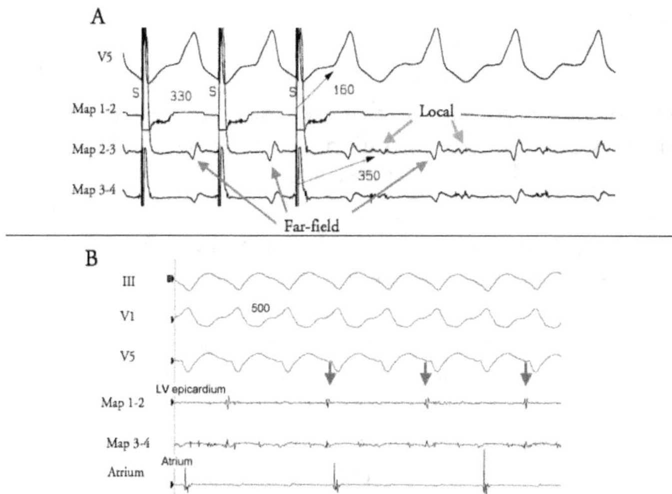

Figure 5. Examples of potential misleading findings during mapping of scar-related VTs.
In panel A entrainment is performed during sustained monomorphic VT. No signal is visible on the distal mapping catheter recordings due to saturation of the recording amplifier by the pacing stimuli, therefore the mid (map 2-3) and proximal (map 3-4) recordings are analyzed. During VT (last three complexes) a double potential with additional fractionated components is present. During pacing, the larger component is visible preceding the stimulus artifact, and is therefore a far-field potential. The low amplitude signal reflects local activation, and the PPI is measured to the local signal, indicating that the site is in the reentry circuit.
In panel B recordings are from an epicardial region of scar. The proximal electrodes of the mapping catheter (map 3-4) record fractionated diastolic and systolic electrograms. In the distal recordings (map 1-2) an isolated potential with 2:1 conduction into this region of the scar is present, indicating that site is not participating in the reentry circuit.

ocyte bundles separated by fibrosis consistent with abnormal conduction and scar. Isolated diastolic potentials are often recorded at isthmus sites.

Multielectrode and non-contact mapping systems that assess activation over broad areas can be helpful for evaluating brief episodes of VT. The low amplitude signals in the VT isthmus are usually not detected, but exit regions can usually be identified, particularly if combined with voltage map data to delineate the scar border.[7] However, electrogram timing alone, particularly at individual sites, does not reliably indicate reentry circuit location. Presystolic and diastolic electrograms can also occur at bystander sites that are not in the circuit. Pacing maneuvers and entrainment are useful for further characterizing potential reentry circuit sites.

3.2 Entrainment mapping

Confirmation that a site is in the reentry circuit can be obtained by entrainment mapping.[8,23-25] During entrainment, pacing at a rate faster than the VT continuously resets the reentry circuit (see figure 1, panels B and C). Each stimulated wavefront propagates to the reentry circuit and splits into two components. An antidromic wavefront travels in the direction opposite to that of the tachycardia wavefronts and collides with a returning orthodromic wavefront. The stimulated orthodromic wavefront propagates through the circuit to reset the circuit. Entrainment is confirmed by the criteria developed by Waldo and co-workers, that includes evidence of constant fusion between paced orthodromic and antidromic wavefronts, and progressive fusion due to proportionately greater activation of the ventricles by paced antidromic wavefronts as the pacing rate is increased.[26] The demonstration of entrainment indicates that reentry with an excitable gap in the circuit is the tachycardia mechanism.

Pacing with capture indicates electrode contact with excitable tissue. Entrainment may be performed with bipolar or unipolar pacing. Unipolar pacing from the distal electrode of the mapping catheter has the advantage of restricting direct capture to tissue beneath the electrode that will be used for ablation, but produces a large stimulus artifact. With bipolar pacing capture may occur at the distal or proximal ring electrode, however, with narrow interelectrode spacing of 1-2 mm, this effect does not seem to be clinically important. It is necessary to ensure that stable capture was achieved and that the VT continues with stable QRS and cycle length after termination of pacing. Pacing is typically performed at cycle lengths 10-30 ms faster than the VT to reduce altering conduction in the circuit or terminating VT, as is more likely with faster pacing rates.

3.2.1   *Post-pacing interval*

The post-pacing interval is an indication of the conduction time between the pacing site and the reentry circuit. After the last capturing stimulus the stimulated orthodromic wavefront propagates through the reentry circuit and back to the pacing site (see figure 1, panel B). Thus the time from the last stimulus to the next activation at the pacing site reflects the sum of the conduction times from the pacing site to the circuit, revolution through the circuit (tachycardia cycle length), and from the circuit back to the pacing site. At sites in the reentry circuit the PPI equals the tachycardia cycle length (see figure 1, panel B and figure 4). Ablation is more likely to terminate VT at sites with a PPI – TCL difference <30 ms as opposed to those with longer differences.[27] The PPI can be misleading if pacing changes the reentry circuit. Conduction slowing during pacing prolongs the PPI. The PPI alone does not indicate whether the pacing site is in a narrow isthmus in the reentry circuit; it does not distinguish between an outer loop and an isthmus site.

The PPI must be measured to the local potential. Far-field potentials due to depolarization of tissue that is remote from the pacing site and not directly captured by pacing are often present in electrograms recorded from scar regions (see figure 5, panel A).[28] Most far-field potentials can be recognized during pacing, because they are visible during pacing and not obscured by the stimulus artifact (see figure 5). In contrast, the local potential is obscured by the stimulus artifact and reappears after pacing.

It is desirable to measure the PPI to the electrogram recorded in the same electrodes that are used for pacing. With many recording systems, however, the stimulus artifact saturates the recording amplifier, obscuring these electrograms (see figure 5, panel A). The PPI can be measured to an electrogram recorded from the adjacent bipoles or filtered unipolar electrode, provided that this electrogram is also present on the distal bipolar recording. The PPI – TCL difference can also be determined by measuring the time from the last stimulus to a consistent QRS or ventricular electrogram on the beat falling two cycles after the last stimulus (the n+1 beat) and relating this interval to the electrogram of interest visible after the recording amplifier has recovered from the stimulus artifact.[29]

3.2.2 Entrainment with concealed fusion

Reentry circuit isthmuses are detected from assessment of fusion. QRS fusion occurs if the stimulated wavefronts alter ventricular activation over a sufficiently large region to alter the ECG. Pacing in a reentry circuit isthmus, the stimulated antidromic wavefronts are contained in or near the circuit by collision with the returning orthodromic wavefronts and by areas of conduction block that define the reentry path (see figure 4). The stimulated orthodromic wavefront emerges from the reentry circuit exit, producing the same ventricular activation as during VT. Collision of antidromic and orthodromic wavefronts (fusion) is concealed, although it may be evident in electrograms recorded from near the pacing site. During entrainment with concealed fusion, the S-QRS interval indicates the conduction time between the pacing site and the reentry circuit exit, and matches the electrogram to QRS interval during VT.

At broad portions of the reentry circuit, such as outer loops along the border of the scar, entrainment occurs with QRS fusion due to propagation of stimulated wavefronts away from the pacing site, but the PPI still indicates that the pacing site is in the circuit (see figure 1, panel C).[27] At sites remote from the circuit, QRS fusion occurs with a PPI that exceeds the tachycardia cycle length. It is important to assess QRS fusion in the 12-lead ECG, subtle degrees of fusion can easily be missed.

Entrainment with concealed fusion is occasionally seen at bystander sites that are in the scar, but not actually in the circuit (adjacent bystander sites). These may be bystander loops or "dead end" pathways that connect to the circuit. At these sites the S-QRS interval during entrainment exceeds the electrogram to QRS during VT and the PPI exceeds the VT cycle length.

3.2.3 Termination without global capture and mechanical termination

A stimulus that terminates VT without producing a QRS often indicates that the catheter is in a reentry circuit isthmus. The mechanism is likely local capture with block of the simulated wavefront between the pacing site and the reentry circuit exit, and collision of the antidromic wavefront with the returning orthodromic wavefront. Termination of VT during mapping can also occur by catheter-induced mechanical pressure at an isthmus site.[24,30] Assessing reproducibility of the finding is warranted as it can be mimicked by spontaneous VT termination.

4 Special substrate considerations

4.1 The Purkinje system and VT

Approximately 8% of patients with sustained monomorphic VT associated with structural heart disease have bundle branch reentry as the cause of one of their VTs, although scar-related reentry is often also present.[3] Most, but not all have a prolonged HV interval in sinus rhythm and interventricular conduction delay or bundle branch block, in which case, VT can resemble the sinus rhythm QRS morphology in sinus rhythm. Most commonly the reentry circuit involves anterograde conduction over the right bundle branch and retrograde conduction over the left bundle branch, giving rise to VT with a left bundle branch block configuration. The PPI at the apical septum indicates that this region is in or near the circuit.[31] A right bundle potential and/or His bundle electrogram preceding and linked to the QRS helps establish the diagnosis. Ablation of the right bundle branch typically eliminates this VT. Occasionally interfascicular reentry requires ablation of left bundle fascicles.

Portions of the Purkinje system can also be involved in scar-related reentry circuits, particularly after myocardial infarction.[32,33] These VTs can have a relatively narrow QRS duration of $\leq$145 ms with Purkinje potentials present in the exit region.

Rarely, focal automaticity in the Purkinje system is the cause of VT in patients with structural heart disease.[3]

An idiopathic left ventricular VT, referred to as intrafascicular reentry, appears to be due to reentry involving the distal ramifications of the left ventricular Purkinje system, can often be effectively treated by ablation.[1]

4.2   *Ablation for polymorphic VT and ventricular fibrillation*

Recurrent polymorphic VT causing "electrical storm" that is not due to ongoing acute ischemia is rare, but occurs in idiopathic ventricular fibrillation, the long QT syndrome, Brugada syndrome, and early and late after myocardial infarction. VT is often initiated by premature beats from one or a few foci that can be targeted for ablation if they occur with sufficient frequency. Sharp potentials consistent with Purkinje activation are often recorded from foci in the left or right ventricles. Less frequently an RVOT focus is a trigger. Storms can be intermittent. Immediate patient transport to the laboratory when the arrhythmia is active is warranted if ablation is to be attempted. In selected patients, approximately 90% of patients are free from recurrences during follow-up.[34]

4.3   *Preprocedure preparation to minimize complications*

Catheter ablation of VT can be challenging. Careful attention to risks and potential complications is warranted. Procedure-related mortality in patients with structural heart disease is approximately 2-3%, with most deaths related to uncontrollable VT that likely reflects failure of the procedure.

Preprocedure planning is essential to minimize risks. Underlying heart disease should be carefully defined. The potential for myocardial ischemia should be assessed. Although ischemia is not usually the cause of monomorphic VT, it may contribute to hemodynamic instability and increase procedure risk. Consideration of fluid balance, electrolyte abnormalities, anemia, and metabolic abnormalities, such as hyperthyroidism, that might contribute to hemodynamic deterioration or development of uncontrollable arrhythmias during the procedure is important. Hemodynamic support with intraaortic balloon counterpulsation and other devices may be considered for patients with severe disease. Some patients warrant consideration of longer term ventricular assist devices and transplantation if VT is not controlled.

Cerebral or systemic embolism is reported in 0-2.7% of patients.[1] If endocardial left ventricular mapping is planned echocardiography should be performed. A mobile LV thrombus is a contraindication to endocardial LV mapping. During endocardial LV mapping and ablation systemic anticoagulation is achieved with heparin. After ablation continued anticoagulation with aspirin or warfarin is recommended depending on the extent of ablation performed.

LV access is usually achieved with a retrograde aortic approach. Damage to the valve or coronary artery ostia are possible, but rare.[35] Significant vascular access complications occur in 2.1%

of patients.[35] A transseptal approach to the left atrium allows access to the LV through the mitral valve for patients with peripheral vascular disease, or a mechanical aortic valve.

5 Outcomes

Studies of scar related VTs are in patient populations characterized by recurrent episodes of VT despite antiarrhythmic drug therapy, the majority of whom also have ICDs. Following ablation at least one VT is no longer inducible in 73-100% of patients and no monomorphic VT of any type can be induced in 38-95% of patients.[1] Remaining inducible VTs are often faster and initiated by more aggressive stimulation than the initial VTs. Acute failure often appears to be due to anatomic obstacles, such as epicardial or intramural reentry circuits.

When the targeted VT remains inducible after ablation the recurrence risk exceeds 60%.[1,36] Absence of any inducible VT has been associated with a lower, but still significant incidence of recurrence ranging from less than 3-27%.[1] Healing of initial ablation lesions and reduction of antiarrhythmic medications likely contribute to recurrences. Some patients benefit from a repeat procedure.

Multicenter trials including patients with VT due to prior myocardial infarction approximately 50% of patients are free from any recurrent VT during follow-ups of 6-12 months.%[1]. Frequent episodes of VT or incessant VT are markedly reduced in over 70% of patients (scientific statement, Calkins, Thermocool).

Data for ablation in nonischemic cardiomyopathies is largely from small case series.[1,37] These VTs are more difficult to ablate and more often require epicardial techniques (see chapter 4), but benefit is achieved in a substantial majority of patients. Although high recurrence rates during follow-up have been observed in patients with arrhythmogenic RV cardiomyopathy, suggesting disease progression, recent use of epicardial mapping and ablation in this disease may achieve better outcomes for palliation.[38]

Small case series of VT in valvular heart disease and repaired congenital heart disease show that these VTs can often be ablated using the approaches to scar-related VTs defined above.[1,39]

Conclusion

Catheter ablation of VT has an important role in reducing VT episodes in patients with ICDs. It can be life saving in patient with incessant VT and electrical storms. Present techniques enable ablation for multiple and hemodynamically unstable VTs. Failure is often related to anatomic obstacles that would potentially benefit from further technological advances.

References

1. Aliot EM, Stevenson WG, Almendral-Garrote JM, *et al.* EHRA/HRS Expert Consensus on Catheter Ablation of Ventricular Arrhythmias: developed in a partnership with the European Heart Rhythm Association (EHRA), a Registered Branch of the European Society of Cardiology (ESC), and the Heart Rhythm Society (HRS); in collaboration with the American College of Cardiology (ACC) and the American Heart Association (AHA). Heart Rhythm Jun 2009; 6(6): 886-933.

2. Poole JE, Johnson GW, Hellkamp AS, *et al.* Prognostic importance of defibrillator shocks in patients with heart failure. N Engl J Med 2008; 359(10): 1009-17.

3. Lopera G, Stevenson WG, Soejima K, *et al.* Identification and ablation of three types of ventricular tachycardia involv-

ing the His-purkinje system in patients with heart disease. J Cardiovasc Electrophysiol 2004; 15(1): 52-8.

4. de Bakker JM, van Capelle FJ, Janse MJ, *et al.* Slow conduction in the infarcted human heart. 'Zigzag' course of activation. Circulation 1993; 88(3): 915-26.

5. Della Bella P, Riva S, Fassini G, *et al.* Incidence and significance of pleomorphism in patients with postmyocardial infarction ventricular tachycardia. Acute and long-term outcome of radiofrequency catheter ablation. Eur Heart J 2004; 25(13): 1127-38.

6. Bogun F, Li YG, Groenefeld G, *et al.* Prevalence of a shared isthmus in postinfarction patients with pleiomorphic, hemodynamically tolerated ventricular tachycardias. J Cardiovasc Electrophysiol 2002; 13(3): 237-41.

7. Klemm HU, Ventura R, Steven D, *et al.* Catheter ablation of multiple ventricular tachycardias after myocardial infarction guided by combined contact and noncontact mapping. Circulation 2007; 115(21): 2697-704.

8. Soejima K, Suzuki M, Maisel WH, *et al.* Catheter ablation in patients with multiple and unstable ventricular tachycardias after myocardial infarction: short ablation lines guided by reentry circuit isthmuses and sinus rhythm mapping. Circulation 2001; 104(6): 664-9.

9. de Chillou C, Lacroix D, Klug D, *et al.* Isthmus characteristics of reentrant ventricular tachycardia after myocardial infarction. Circulation 2002; 105(6): 726-31.

10. Marchlinski FE, Callans DJ, Gottlieb CD, *et al.* Linear ablation lesions for control of unmappable ventricular tachycardia in patients with ischemic and nonischemic cardiomyopathy. Circulation 2000; 101(11): 1288-96.

11. Marchlinski FE, Zado E, Dixit S, *et al.* Electroanatomic substrate and outcome of catheter ablative therapy for ventricular tachycardia in setting of right ventricular cardiomyopathy. Circulation 2004; 110(16): 2293-8.

12. Reddy VY, Neuzil P, Taborsky M, *et al.* Short-term results of substrate mapping and radiofrequency ablation of ischemic ventricular tachycardia using a saline-irrigated catheter. J Am Coll Cardiol 2003; 41(12): 2228-36.

13. Josephson ME, Callans DJ. Using the twelve-lead electrocardiogram to localize the site of origin of ventricular tachycardia. Heart Rhythm 2005; 2(4): 443-6.

14. Brunckhorst CB, Delacretaz E, Soejima K, *et al.* Identification of the ventricular tachycardia isthmus after infarction by pace mapping. Circulation 2004; 110(6): 652-9.

15. Kottkamp H, Wetzel U, Schirdewahn P, *et al.* Catheter ablation of ventricular tachycardia in remote myocardial infarction: substrate description guiding placement of individual linear lesions targeting noninducibility. J Cardiovasc Electrophysiol 2003; 14(7): 675-81.

16. Bogun F, Good E, Reich S, *et al.* Isolated potentials during sinus rhythm and pace-mapping within scars as guides for ablation of post-infarction ventricular tachycardia. J Am Coll Cardiol 2006; 47(10): 2013-9.

17. Arenal A, Glez-Torrecilla E, Ortiz M, *et al.* Ablation of electrograms with an isolated, delayed component as treatment of unmappable monomorphic ventricular tachycardias in patients with structural heart disease. J Am Coll Cardiol 2003; 41(1): 81-92.

18. Harada T, Stevenson WG, Kocovic DZ, *et al.* Catheter ablation of ventricular tachycardia after myocardial infarction: relation of endocardial sinus rhythm late potentials to the reentry circuit. J Am Coll Cardiol 1997; 30(4): 1015-23.

19. Brunckhorst CB, Stevenson WG, Jackman WM, *et al.* Ventricular mapping during atrial and ventricular pacing. Relationship of multipotential electrograms to ventricular tachycardia reentry circuits after myocardial infarction. Eur Heart J 2002; 23(14): 1131-8.

20. Arenal A, del Castillo S, Gonzalez-Torrecilla E, *et al.* Tachycardia-related channel in the scar tissue in patients with sustained monomorphic ventricular tachycardias: influence of the voltage scar definition. Circulation 2004; 110(17): 2568-74.

21. Hsia HH, Lin D, Sauer WH, *et al.* Anatomic characterization of endocardial substrate for hemodynamically stable reentrant ventricular tachycardia: identification of endocardial conducting channels. Heart Rhythm 2006; 3(5): 503-12.

22. Bogun F, Knight B, Goyal R, *et al.* Discrete systolic potentials during ventricular tachycardia in patients with prior myocardial infarction. J Cardiovasc Electrophysiol 1999; 10(3): 364-9.

23. Delacretaz E, Stevenson WG. Catheter ablation of ventricular tachycardia in patients with coronary heart disease: part I: Mapping. Pacing Clin Electrophysiol 2001; 24(8 Pt 1): 1261-77.

24. Bogun F, Kim HM, Han J, *et al.* Comparison of mapping criteria for hemodynamically tolerated, postinfarction ventricular tachycardia. Heart Rhythm 2006; 3(1): 20-6.

25. El-Shalakany A, Hadjis T, Papageorgiou P, *et al.* Entrainment/mapping criteria for the prediction of termination of ventricular tachycardia by single radiofrequency lesion in patients with coronary artery disease. Circulation 1999; 99(17): 2283-9.

26. Henthorn RW, Okumura K, Olshansky B, *et al.* A fourth criterion for transient entrainment: the electrogram equivalent of progressive fusion. Circulation 1988; 77(5): 1003-12.

27. Stevenson WG, Friedman PL, Sager PT, *et al.* Exploring postinfarction reentrant ventricular tachycardia with entrainment mapping. J Am Coll Cardiol 1997; 29(6): 1180-9.

28. Tung S, Soejima K, Maisel WH, et al. Recognition of far-field electrograms during entrainment mapping of ventricular tachycardia. J Am Coll Cardiol 2003; 42(1): 110-5.

29. Soejima K, Stevenson WG, Maisel WH, et al. The N + 1 difference: a new measure for entrainment mapping. J Am Coll Cardiol 2001; 37(5): 1386-94.

30. Bogun F, Good E, Han J, *et al.* Mechanical interruption of postinfarction ventricular tachycardia as a guide for catheter ablation. Heart Rhythm 2005; 2(7): 687-91.

31. Merino JL, Peinado R, Fernandez-Lozano I, *et al.* Bundle-branch reentry and the postpacing interval after entrainment by right ventricular apex stimulation: a new approach to elucidate the mechanism of wide-QRS-complex tachycardia with atrioventricular dissociation. Circulation 2001; 103(8): 1102-1108.

32. Hayashi M, Kobayashi Y, Iwasaki YK, *et al.* Novel mechanism of postinfarction ventricular tachycardia originating

in surviving left posterior Purkinje fibers. Heart Rhythm 2006; 3(8): 908-18.

33. Bogun F, Good E, Reich S, *et al.* Role of Purkinje fibers in post-infarction ventricular tachycardia. J Am Coll Cardiol 2006; 48(12): 2500-7.

34. Wright M, Sacher F, Haissaguerre M. Catheter ablation for patients with ventricular fibrillation. Curr Opin Cardiol 2009; 24(1): 56-60.

35. Calkins H, Epstein A, Packer D, *et al.* Catheter ablation of ventricular tachycardia in patients with structural heart disease using cooled radiofrequency energy: results of a prospective multicenter study. Cooled RF Multi Center Investigators Group. J Am Coll Cardiol 2000; 35(7): 1905-14.

36. van der Burg AE, de Groot NM, van Erven L, *et al.* Long-term follow-up after radiofrequency catheter ablation of ventricular tachycardia: a successful approach- J Cardiovasc Electrophysiol 2002; 13(5): 417-23.

37. Soejima K, Stevenson WG, Sapp JL, *et al.* Endocardial and epicardial radiofrequency ablation of ventricular tachycardia associated with dilated cardiomyopathy: the importance of low-voltage scars. J Am Coll Cardiol 2004; 43(10): 1834-42.

38. Garcia FC, Bazan V, Zado ES, *et al.* Epicardial substrate and outcome with epicardial ablation of ventricular tachycardia in arrhythmogenic right ventricular cardiomyopathy/dysplasia. Circulation 2009; 120(5): 366-75.

39. Zeppenfeld K, Schalij MJ, Bartelings MM, *et al.* Catheter ablation of ventricular tachycardia after repair of congenital heart disease: electroanatomic identification of the critical right ventricular isthmus. Circulation 2007; 116(20): 2241-52.

Chapter 4. Epicardial ventricular tachycardias. Diagnosis and treatment

A. Berruezo, D. Andreu

Thorax Institute
Cardiology Department, Arrhythmia Section
Hospital Clinic, University of Barcelona
Barcelona, Spain

Address for correspondence:
Thorax Institute. Hospital Clínic
University of Barcelona
Dr. Antonio Berruezo
berruezo@clinic.ub.es

Introduction

The first description of the epicardial mapping and ablation technique was published in 1996, by Sosa *et al.*[1] The technique was developed for mapping and ablation in patients with Chagas disease, which typically produces an arrhythmogenic epicardial substrate. Later, epicardial catheter ablation was demonstrated to be useful in patients with recurrent VT after myocardial infarction (MI)[2] and to be of great value in patients with incessant ventricular tachycardia.[3] Since that time, a significant number of research papers have provided information about the usefulness of the epicardial approach in various clinical settings, as in some idiopathic LV outflow tract VTs, idiopathic LV aneurysms, right ventricular dysplasia, idiopathic dilated cardiomyopathy and other substrates. Electrocardiographic methods for identifying epicardial VTs were also developed[4-6] to help in case selection and procedure indication. However, important questions, including the true incidence of epicardial VTs in the different substrates, concerns about risks and complications, and the high level of operator skill required, limit the widespread implementation of the technique. The procedure is currently performed in reference centers with well-established VT ablation programs, although it continues to evolve and further refinement of the technique is needed. Finally, although the exact role of epicardial catheter ablation is not well defined, a large body of available information suggests that the technique will become part of the routine procedures performed in electrophysiology laboratories.

1 Incidence of epicardial ventricular tachycardias

Although several studies have shown that the probability of having an epicardial VT may vary depending on the substrate, its true incidence is unknown. Idiopathic LV outflow tract VTs more frequently require an epicardial approach than do RV outflow tract VTs. Some kind of cardiomyopathies are more prone to produce epicardial reentry circuits. Epicardial mapping and ablation is needed more often in patients with non-ichemic dilated cardiomyopathy; in ischemic patients, inferolateral infarcts are the ones most frequently associated with epicardial VTs. Chagas disease is known to have a tendency to cause epicardial reentry circuits.[7] Epicardial VT circuits are also frequent in arrhythmogenic right ventricular dysplasia, in our experience.

The higher the incidence of epicardial VTs in a given substrate, the higher the probability of needing an epicardial approach for a given patient with such a substrate. Therefore, it is crucial to know as much as possible about the epidemiological profile of epicardial VTs. This information may help in making decisions about when to perform an epicardial access procedure, although other tools providing more precise information should also be taken into account.

1.1 Chagas disease

Two years after first describing the technique, Sosa *et al.* published the results of epicardial ablation in the first series of patients. In this study, 10 consecutive patients with Chagas disease were submitted to simultaneous endocardial and epicardial RF ablation.[7] Epicardial ablation was required in 6 (60%) of 10 patients and an epicardial circuit was found in 14 of 18 mappable inducible VTs, revealing a high incidence of epicardial circuits in Chagas disease.

1.2 Ischemic cardiomyopathy

The prevalence of epicardial VTs in ischemic cardiomyopathy seems to be lower than in Chagas disease. Data from simultaneous endocardial and epicardial mapping during the surgical treatment of VTs revealed that around 20% of VTs could have earliest epicardial activation rather than endocardial activation (e.g., an epicardial origin of ventricular activation).[8] However, the fact that the epicardial exit site of a circuit is located at the epicardium does not imply that the circuit is completely located at the subepicardial layer. Theoretically, it is possible that epicardial re-entry VTs with part of the circuit at the subendocardium could be treated by endocardial ablation. The existence of complete reentry circuits at either the subendocardial or the subepicardial layer, and the presence of circuits with only a part of the isthmus at the subendocardial layer, was also demonstrated in patients with chronic myocardial infarction. Complete subendocardial reentry circuits were observed in 25% of patients (15% of VTs) and complete subepicardial reentry circuits in 14% of patients (9% of VTs). Incompletely mapped circuits (multilayer) with an endocardial LV breakthrough were observed in 75% of patients (53% of VTs) and incompletely mapped circuits with an epicardial LV breakthrough in 11% of patients (6% of VTs). Right ventricular epicardial breakthrough was observed in 25% of patients (17% of VTs), representing circuits in the deep septal layers. Therefore, LV endocardial reentry substrates accounted for 68% of VTs, with an additional 6% of VTs having part of the circuit in an endocardial location with an epicardial exit. Thus, from a practical point of view, around 15% of ischemic patients will have complete subepicardial VT circuits inaccessible to endocardial VT ablation.[9]

Intraoperative mapping studies have also shown that patients with inferior free-wall myocardial infarctions seem to have a higher prevalence of epicardial VTs than those with other infarct locations.[10,11] In one of these studies, one-third of patients required epicardial ablation.

In addition, an aneurysm was present in 70% of patients with successful endocardial ablation, but only present in 10% of patients requiring epicardial ablation, 90% of whom had a right or left circumflex coronary artery-related infarction.[11]

Detailed 3D electroanatomical high-density endocardial and epicardial mapping has shown that myocardial scars in patients with ischemic cardiomyopathy have a scar area 3 times greater in the endocardium than in the epicardium. Epicardial mapping revealed that small islands of viable myocardium can be identified in regions corresponding to endocardial scar tissue.[12] These observations are in agreement with data showing that the wavefront of myocardial damage after coronary occlusion starts at the endocardium and extends toward the epicardium, with a variable amount of transmurality.[13]

Data from catheter ablation studies also suggest a higher prevalence of epicardial circuits in patients with post-infarction VTs related to an inferior MI. In the study by Sosa *et al.*, 39% of all mappable VTs in patients with inferior MI were interrupted by epicardial RF applications.[14] Consistent with previous studies, only 1 of 14 patients had an inferior aneurysm, suggesting that most of the patients had non-transmural MI. In the study by Brugada *et al.*, 75% of epicardial VTs in ischemic patients with incessant VTs were related to an inferior or inferolateral MI.[15]

In conclusion, despite overall low prevalence, epicardial VTs in ischemic cardiomyopathy may be present in up to one-third of patients, particularly in those with non-transmural inferior or inferolateral infarcts without aneurysms.

1.3 Non-ischemic cardiomyopathy

The success rate of endocardial ablation in patients with non-ischemic cardiomyopathy (NICM) is generally lower than in ischemic patients. Reentry circuits deep in the endocardium and epicardium appear to be a likely explanation. When epicardial ablation is attempted after a failed endocardial approach, the success rate is higher.

In the study by Soejima *et al.*,[16] in a series of 28 consecutive patients with NICM and VTs, only 6 (27%) were successfully ablated from the endocardium; ablation was not attempted in 2 patients (9%) and in 14 patients (64%) endocardial ablation failed, although epicardial ablation was then performed in 7 of them and succeeded in 6 patients (85%). Small low-voltage areas were identified and related to the VT origin. The underlying mechanism in most patients was re-entry. The majority of scar areas (63%) extended to a valve annulus both at the endocardium and at the epicardium, being larger at the epicardial surface. This propensity for a basal location of abnormal endocardial electrograms was also observed by Hsia *et al.*[17] and remains unexplained. Recently, in a consecutive series of 22 patients with NICM, Cano *et al.* found that 18 of them (82%) required epicardial ablation. Confluent low-voltage areas were present in 18 epicardial maps (82%) and 12 endocardial maps (54%) and were typically over the basal lateral LV. Epicardial low-voltage areas were greater than the endocardial ones.

Therefore, basal and lateral scars adjacent to a valve annulus that can be transmural and greater in extent at the epicardium are the common substrate for reentrant VTs in NICM. The predominant location of the scar in the subepicardium explains the low success rate of classic endocardial catheter ablation in NICM. Although the precise incidence is not known, it seems that more than half of the patients could have epicardial VTs. Thus, a combined endocardial and epicardial mapping procedure is likely to improve the success rate of ablation in NICM.

1.4   Arrhythmogenic right ventricular cardiomyopathy

Arrhythmogenic right ventricular cardiomyopathy/dysplasia (ARVC/D) is a genetically determined myocardial disease characterized by right ventricular (RV) myocardial atrophy and fibrofatty replacement. The disease predisposes to ventricular arrhythmias and sudden death. Arrhythmogenic right ventricular cardiomyopathy/dysplasia is a familial disease in at least 50% of cases and is mostly transmitted as an autosomal dominant trait with variable penetrance, affecting the intercellular mechanical junction (desmosomal proteins) of the cardiomyocytes.[18] Its molecular diagnosis is problematic and clinical diagnosis may also be difficult because of the lack of sensitivity (for early disease) and specificity of ECG abnormalities and RV arrhythmias, as well as the limitations of current imaging techniques.[19]

Three-dimensional electroanatomical mapping (3D-EAM) can identify low-voltage areas and delayed activation in zones corresponding to the fibrofatty tissue replacing the myocardium. 3D-EAM has been shown to assist in the differential diagnosis of diseases that mimic ARVC/D, such as inflammatory cardiomyopathy and idiopathic RVOT tachycardia.[20,21]

In ARVC/D patients, fibrofatty replacement of the myocardium starts at the epicardium or midmyocardium and extends until becoming transmural. Left ventricular involvement may be present in up to 75% of patients, and is usually confined to the posterolateral subepicardium.[22,23] This fibrofatty replacement creates the substrate for ventricular arrhythmias. Therefore, from a pathophysiological point of view, the epicardium is the most probable location of the VT circuits in ARVC/D.

On the other hand, catheter ablation of VT in ARVC/D has a variable acute success rate, ranging from 60-90%, and relapses are frequent, with a VT recurrence rate of up to 90% during 3-year follow-up.[24] Therefore, a convincing explanation for the lack of effectiveness is that the presence of epicardial VT circuits may preclude endocardial VT ablation success. In addition, the progressive nature of the disease can play a role in increasing the probability of long-term recurrences.

In this line, ARVC/D patients who have undergone a previous failed endocardial ablation procedure have been shown to have a more extensive epicardial scar area.[25] Available histological information suggests this also may be true in the general population of ARVC/D patients. However, the percentage of ARVC/D patients needing an epicardial ablation procedure is not known because there are no studies evaluating the results of simultaneous endocardial and epicardial mapping and ablation as a first-line therapy for VT ablation in this subset of patients. An example of an ARVD case in which an epicardial VT ablation procedure was performed is shown in figure 1.

1.5   Idiopathic left ventricular outflow tract ventricular tachycardias

Three locations have been described as a possible origin for left ventricular outflow tract ventricular tachycardias (LVOT VTs): the endocardium of the LV, aortic sinus of Valsalva (AOSV) and epicardium of the LVOT. The prevalence of idiopathic LVOT VTs has been reported to form up to one-third of all outflow tract VTs and up to one-third of them may be epicardial in origin. Idiopathic outflow tract VTs originating from the LV are more likely to arise from the epicardium than are RV outflow tract VTs. A predominantly perivascular origin for epicardial LVOT VTs has been described, although the reason for this remains unknown.[5] Ablation

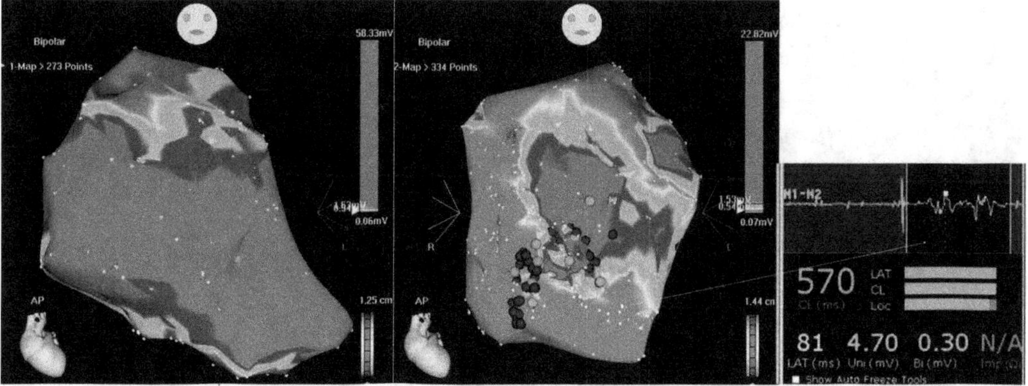

Figure 1. Endocardial (left) and epicardial (right) voltage maps of a patient with a right ventricular cardiomyopathy, submitted for VT ablation due to recurrent sustained monomorphic VTs. The VT circuit and exit was epicardial, at the middle third of the right ventricular free wall. At this location the endocardial bipolar voltage map was normal. The scar areas were larger at the epicardium. Scar areas show low voltage, fractionated electrograms.

can be performed in most cases from inside the coronary venous system, and the most frequent location for successful ablation is the zone surrounding the junction of the distal great cardiac vein and the anterior interventricular vein (see figure 2).

The LVOT origin of a VT can be inferred from ECG analysis. A transition (R>S) in V1 or V2 is considered highly specific for a successful ablation outside the RV outflow tract. Conversely, a transition in V4 or later is considered highly specific for successful RV ablation. However, when an R>S transition is observed in V3 (a feature present in more than 50% of patients with outflow tract VTs) the value of surface ECG criteria is limited.[26] Therefore, the precise location of a VT origin and the access route necessary to perform ablation must be determined by intracardiac mapping. However, although no ECG pattern is specific for an epicardial LV outflow tract, slowed initial precordial QRS activation, as quantified by the "maximum deflection index" (MDI), might be of use. The MDI is the result of dividing the earliest time to maximum deflection in any of the precordial leads by the total QRS duration. A delayed MDI ≥0.55 identified epicardial VT remote from the AOSV with an excellent level of discrimination.[5]

The LVOT VTs from the AOSV appear to arise from the epicardium underlying the valve leaflets, most frequently the left coronary cusp. This anatomic landmark is closely associated with the distal great cardiac vein and proximal anterior interventricular vein, although the distance is usually >1 cm. The ECG appearance at these two locations is similar to that of the AOSV but resembles that of the septal RVOT when the origin is more distal in the anterior interventricular vein. Local activation time during coronary venous mapping usually precedes endocardial activation time by ≥10 ms.[5]

In our laboratory, the following stepwise mapping strategy is used for outflow tract VTs with a transition in V3 or in case of ablation failure in the RVOT. Mapping starts at the RV and pulmonary artery (given that half of these VTs are right-sided). In case of inadequate activation or pace mapping, the coronary sinus is mapped up to the distal great cardiac vein and the first part of the anterior interventricular vein. If unsuitable for ablation, the LVOT (endocardial LVOT and AOSV) should be mapped via retrograde aortic access. A comparison between the earliest activation times in the different structures is of crucial importance at this

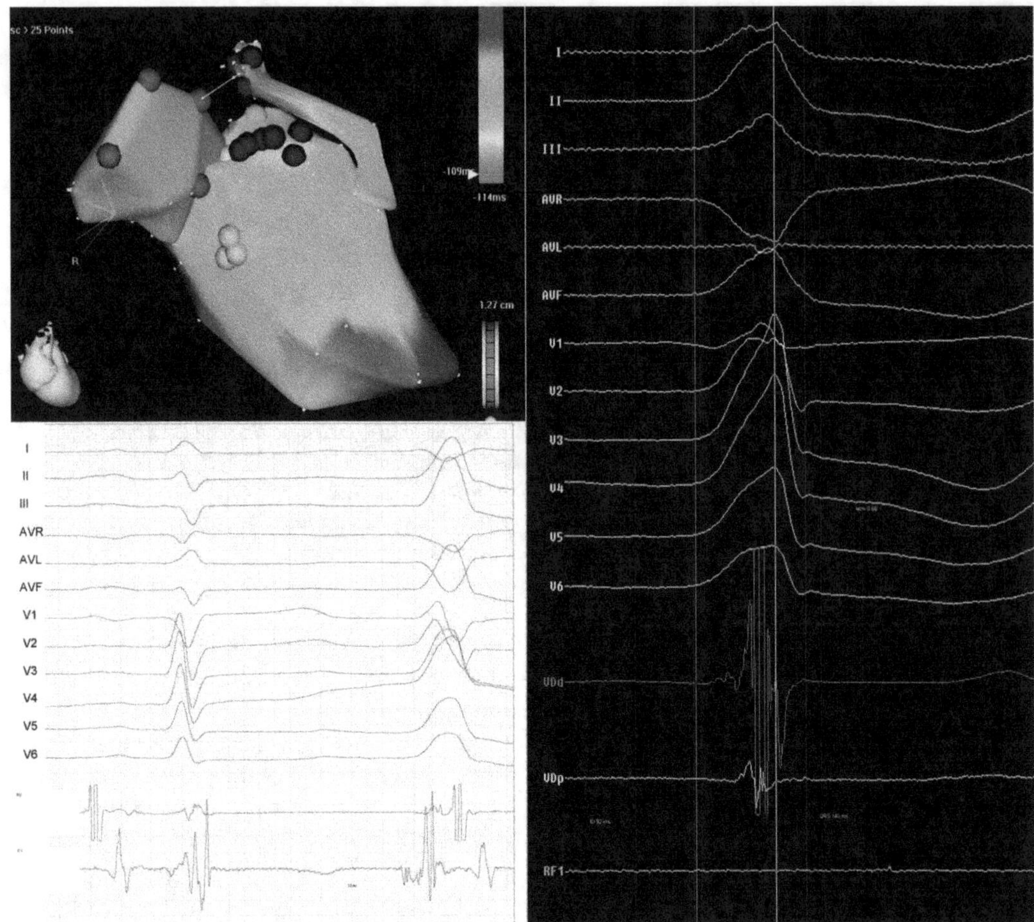

Figure 2. Epicardial left ventricular outflow tract VT. The 12-lead ECG (right) shows a premature ventricular complex with a dominant R wave in V1, suggesting a left ventricular outflow tract VT. A 3D electroanatomical activation map (upper, left) of the aortic root and endocardial left ventricular outflow tract showed greater precocity in the left ventricle, just below the aortic valve. Radiofrequency applications at this site (red dots) did not eliminate the premature ventricular complexes. Accurate ECG analysis revealed a maximum deflection index of 0.66, suggesting an epicardial origin of ventricular activation. Therefore, the coronary sinus was accessed and mapped and the greatest precocity (33 ms) was obtained at the distal great cardiac vein (lower, left).

point. Finally, if all previous access attempts failed to reach the location of the VT origin, epicardial access is performed.

2 Approaching the epicardium

An epicardial access procedure should ideally be performed before systemic anticoagulation to avoid complications derived from puncturing the heart. However, depending on operator skill, experience and confidence, epicardial access can be performed after endocardial mapping/

ablation or it can be delayed. In our laboratory it is common practice to introduce a thin guidewire for epicardial access when an epicardial VT is suspected and then to give anticoagulation for endocardial mapping purposes if no complications have occurred. Only in a few cases is direct epicardial mapping and ablation performed (see "Recommendations on choosing the epicardial approach").

The overall efficacy of epicardial ablation depends on the approach strategy and the prevalence of epicardial circuits. For instance, in the study by Sosa *et al.*,[2] ablation efficacy in ischemic patients was less than 40% when epicardial mapping and ablation was attempted first (even when selecting patients with inferior MI). Efficacy cannot be higher because the prevalence of epicardial circuits is not higher. In contrast, as in our study in patients with incessant VTs,[3] when endocardial ablation is attempted first and epicardial ablation is only performed in case of endocardial ablation failure, epicardial ablation efficacy increases to approximately 80% because true epicardial VTs are selected.

2.1 Transthoracic epicardial access

After proper asepsis of the subxiphoid area, an epidural needle with Tuohy bevel (Perican, Braun, Germany) is introduced at an angle of 30-45° toward the left scapula, depending on the mapping region of interest. The patient is under deep sedation with midazolam and fentanyl, with intra-arterial (radial) pressure monitoring. The region most frequently reached is located at the medial third of the RV free wall. Guided by fluoroscopy, the needle is advanced close to the cardiac silhouette under fluoroscopic guidance until the beating heart movement is felt. To demonstrate the location of the needle tip, small amounts of contrast media (50% dilution with saline) are injected. If the needle is outside the pericardial space, the contrast accumulates in the mediastinum. However, when the needle tip is inside this space, the contrast medium surrounds the cardiac silhouette as a thin layer. At this moment, a floppy tip guidewire is advanced through the needle until it surrounds the cardiac silhouette, to ensure that is not placed inside the cardiac cavities (see figure 3).

2.2 Epicardial mapping and ablation

An 8-French introducer is advanced, the guidewire removed and an externally irrigated-tip RF ablation catheter advanced for mapping and ablation. A deflectable sheath is often used to facilitate mapping and obtain a stable position with good tissue contact. In the absence of pericardial adhesions, the ablation catheter is easily moved. No irrigation is necessary for mapping inside the pericardial sac. Radiofrequency application parameters are similar to those used for endocardial ablation (40-50 W, 45° C temperature limit, 30 mL/min irrigation). The amount of liquid infused should be taken into account and removed periodically (see figure 4).

2.3 Coronary arteries and epicardial fat

Even when the epicardial surface can be easily accessed, effective energy delivery adjacent to the coronary vessels may not be possible in some cases or may be dangerous in others. An experimental study demonstrated that epicardial ablation with irrigated catheters produces larg-

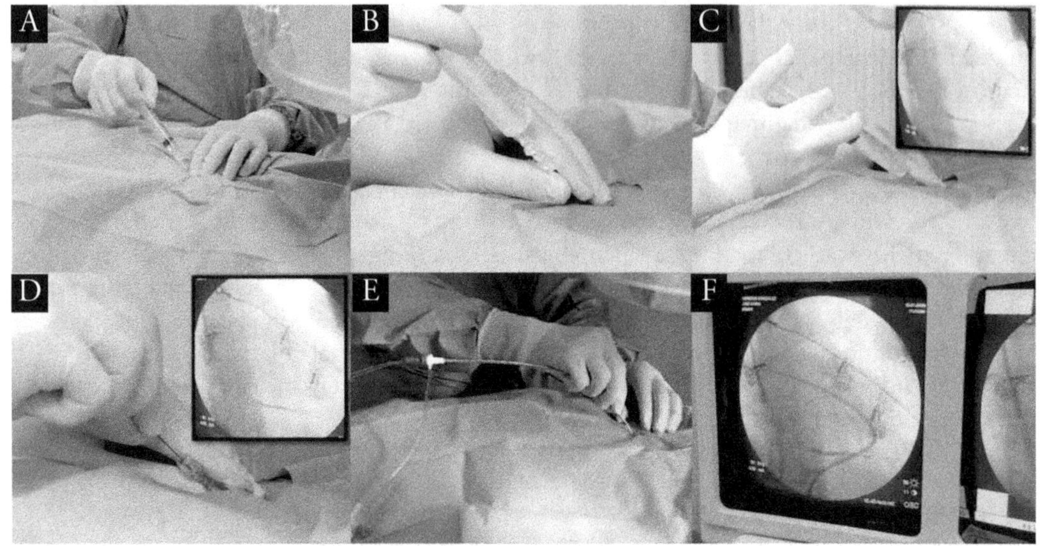

Figure 3. Transthoracic epicardial access (see text).
A. Injection of local anesthesia; B. Introducing the needle at a 45º angle; C. Contrast injection
while visualizing the cardiac silhouette; D. Introduction of the guidewire; E. An 8-French introducer
is advanced; F. Visualization of the introducer inside the pericardial sac.

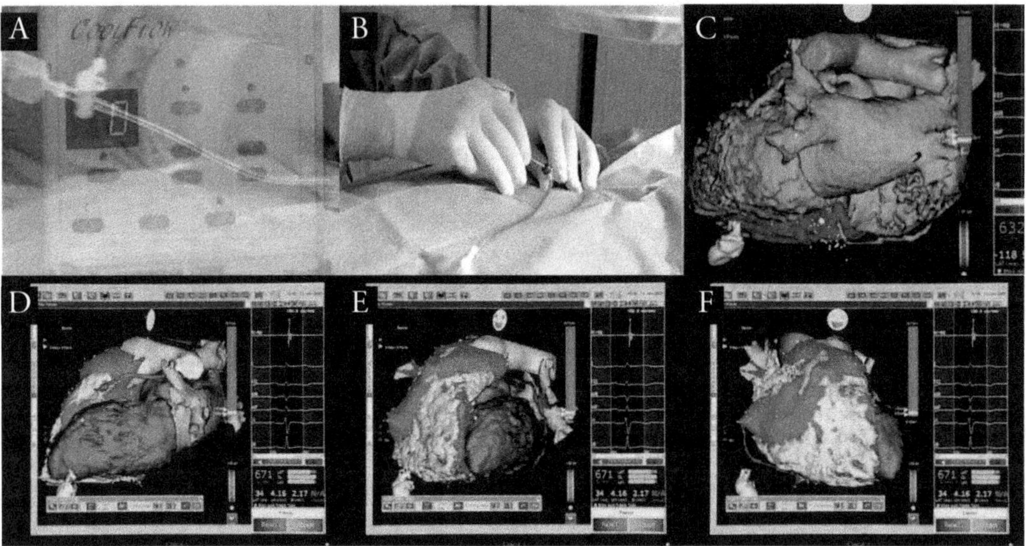

Figure 4. Epicardial mapping and ablation (see text).
A, B. After a small quantity of liquid is drained, the RF catheter is advanced without irrigation;
C. A 3D reconstruction of the cardiac chambers and coronary arteries created by integrating
a CT image with the 3D electroanatomical map. The pericardium has been reached by posterior access
and the catheter tip is visualized close to the posterior wall of the left atrium; D, E, F. The relationship
between the coronary arteries and the catheter tip can be visualized prior to RF application.

er lesions (6.7±1.7 mm) than with conventional catheters. The presence of epicardial fat prevents lesion formation with standard RF but only moderately attenuates the efficacy of cooled-tip ablation.[27] Moreover, coronary blood flow even through small vessels can cool the tissue and prevent adequate lesion formation at the subepicardium adjacent to the vessel.[28]

On the other hand, it has been demonstrated that the risk of damage during RF ablation directly over the artery is inversely proportional to vessel diameter, with little evidence of injury when the vessel diameter exceeds 0.5-1.0 mm.[29] Another study demonstrated that cryothermal ablation can cause neointimal proliferation with a probability directly proportional to lesion depth and inversely proportional to vessel diameter. The mean lesion depth was 2.7 mm. No evidence of damage was observed in coronary arteries with internal diameters greater than 0.7 mm.[30] Therefore, the larger the coronary artery, the safer the application. Finally, in ischemic cardiomyopathy, energy is delivered in scar tissue where the vessels have been previously occluded or damaged and therefore should not be expected to give rise to serious complications.

When defining the scar areas it is important to ensure that epicardial fat will not produce a fractionated electrogram. However, thick fat layers can decrease the voltage and create difficulties in interpreting the substrate maps. An epicardial fat layer <5 mm interposed between the ablation catheter and the epicardium does not modify the amplitude/duration of the bipolar epicardial electrogram or the epicardial ventricular stimulation threshold. Therefore, the presence of an epicardial fat layer <5 mm may not be enough to mimic scar tissue.[31] In general, normal epicardial electrograms demonstrate an amplitude > 0.94 mV.[32]

2.4 Coronary angiography

Damage to a coronary artery continues to be a potential and serious complication. Coronary angiography is therefore recommended to check the proximity between the target sites and vessels. This approach requires frequent coronary contrast injections in various projections. An alternative may be to integrate a preacquired computed tomography (CT) image with endocardial and epicardial 3D-EAM, providing real-time visualization of the catheter tip in relation to the epicardial coronary arteries. This approach has proven to be accurate in establishing the relationship between the catheter tip and the major coronary arteries[33] and is frequently used in our laboratory (see figure 4).

2.5 Complications

Although epicardial mapping and ablation is a relatively safe procedure, a high level of operator skill is required and serious complications can occur. Right ventricular puncture without hemopericardium can be observed in 10-20% of patients. Hemopericardium is reported to occur in around 20% of patients and does not preclude continuing the procedure in most cases. Hemoperitoneum has been described as a possible complication resulting from the puncture of diaphragmatic vessels and requires surgery. Transient thoracic discomfort after the procedure can be easily managed with anti-inflammatory medication. Pacing can identify the course of the phrenic nerve and various strategies can be used to avoid injury by separating it from the epicardial surface (balloon catheter or the creation of an artificial hydropneumopericardium). Coronary artery injury is rare (<1%) and may present acutely or several weeks after the procedure. Acute occlusion appears to require coronary stenting.[34]

3   When to change to the epicardium

3.1   After a previous failed ablation procedure

It is commonly accepted that a failed endocardial ablation procedure is sufficient reason to attempt epicardial ablation. In this regard we analyzed the efficacy of epicardial RF ablation in a series of patients with incessant VT and a previous failed ablation.[3] Epicardial ablation effectively terminated the VT in all except one patient. The success rate of the epicardial approach was 85%, giving a total catheter ablation success rate of 95%. Therefore, a prior failed endocardial ablation procedure guarantees a high success rate when using the epicardial approach by selecting truly epicardial VTs.

3.2   When there is no access to the left ventricular cavity

Patients with a thrombus in the LV or mechanical mitral and aortic valve prostheses might have VTs that are not amenable to ablation from the endocardium, such as all VTs for which the mechanism involves the subendocardium and Purkinje system (e.g., bundle branch reentry VTs, fascicular VTs, papillary muscle VTs, or ventricular arrhythmias triggered by premature ventricular beats arising from the Purkinje fibers). These arrhythmias share several common distinctive features that show up on the ECG during VT as a rapid initial deflection of the QRS complex and usually also as a short QRS duration. At the very least, therefore, careful ECG analysis during VT is advisable before deciding upon an epicardial approach in this subset of patients.

3.3   Electrocardiogram suggesting an epicardial origin

The epicardial origin of the ventricular activation during sinus rhythm and during VT can be recognized on the ECG because the initial part of the QRS complex is prolonged and resembles a pseudodelta wave.[4] The duration of this pseudodelta wave on the surface ECG matches the duration of the transmural activation time. The duration intervals and cut-off values for the pseudodelta wave and for intrinsicoid deflection in V2 identified an epicardial origin of VTs with high sensitivity and specificity (see table 1). These morphological and metric criteria are only applicable to VTs with an RBBB-like configuration; VTs with an LBBB-like configuration were not included in this study because they commonly originate in the interventricular septum and may be unsuitable for epicardial ablation.[4] Figure 5 shows an example of an epicardial VT.

Other ECG criteria that identify the epicardial origin of VTs have been described (see table 1). These include the MDI, which is also based on the concept of quantifying the slowed initial precordial QRS activation of the epicardial LV outflow tract VTs.[5] A delayed shortest precordial MDI ≥0.55 identified epicardial VT remote from the AOSV with a high level of discrimination (see figure 4). Another morphological criterion has been reported to predict the epicardial origin of VTs in non-ischemic cardiomyopathy: the presence of an initial Q-wave during VT in leads that reflect local ventricular activation.[6]

To maintain similar sensitivity and specificity, the criteria should be applied to the population (cardiomyopathy and type of VT) for which they were described. In our laboratory, careful ECG analysis during VT is the first step to identify the mapping area of interest and screen for indications for an epicardial approach. A summary of the ECG criteria is shown in table 1.

ECG criteria	Main limitations
Berruezo *et al.*:[4] — Pseudodelta wave ≥34 ms — Intrinsicoid deflection V2 ≥85 ms — Shortest RS complex ≥121 ms	LBBB-like VTs excluded
Bazan *et al.*:[6] — Initial Q wave in leads that reflect local ventricular activation	Not useful if prior myocardial infarction or baseline Q-waves
Daniels *et al.*:[5] — Precordial maximum deflection index	Applicable only in LVOT VTs

Table 1. ECG criteria that can help in identifying the epicardial origin of the ventricular activation.

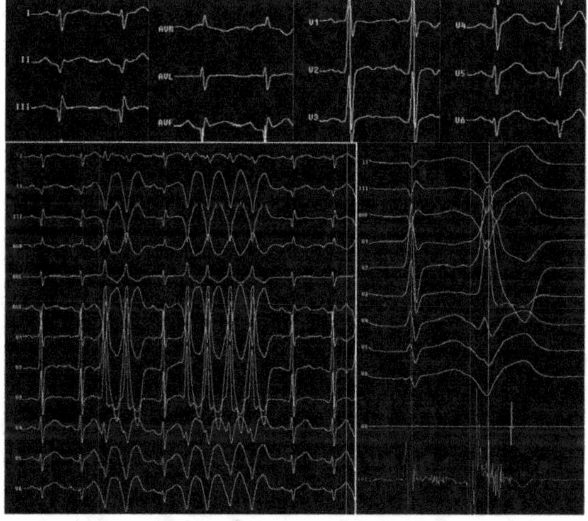

Figure 5. Epicardial reentrant VT associated with a small left ventricular aneurysm. A patient with normal coronary arteries, a small inferolateral aneurysm and preserved left ventricular ejection fraction, was admitted because of an incessant VT.
A. A 12-leads surface ECG during sinus rhythm showed small inferior Q-waves; B. Intermittent runs of non-sustained VT with a QRS complex morphology suggesting that the ventricular activation starts inferior, lateral and near the apex; C. A more accurate analysis suggests that the VT originates at the epicardium by the presence of a pseudodelta wave. Distal bipolar electrogram of the ablation catheter at the location of the effective RF application showed a fractionated diastolic electrogram.

3.4 *Imaging techniques suggesting an epicardial ventricular tachycardia*

Critical anatomic substrates that sustain VTs, even in cases of a focal origin, show different degrees of fibrosis/scarring.[35] Most VTs in patients with structural heart disease are scar-related myocardial reentries. Identification of scar tissue by CE-CMR has been proven to match the histology of the MI, to be related to the inducibility of sustained VT, to have prognostic value for long-term total mortality and to correlate with 3D voltage maps. Scar identification and characterization could help to regionalize the mapping areas of interest, estimate scar extent, and analyze in 3D the complexity of scarring and the endocardial versus epicardial involvement of the ventricular wall. Taken together, this would contribute valuable additional information to that obtained with 3D electroanatomical maps. However, imaging techniques have not yet been shown to positively influence VT ablation outcomes.

Contrast-enhanced cardiovascular magnetic resonance analysis has shown that the distribution pattern of scar tissue across the thickness of the LV wall can be useful in differentiating between endocardial and epicardial VTs.[36,37] The presence of isolated epicardial Hyperenhacement (HE) on the ablation segment had very high sensitivity and specificity in predicting an epicardial VT origin.[37] This suggests that a preprocedural CE-CMR could be useful to determine whether an epicardial or endocardial approach is needed. In addition, image integration between the EA mapping system and CE-CMR scar depiction[38] can help to precisely locate the scar on each segment and facilitate the procedure.

The most important counterindication to the use of CE-CMR scar identification and integration to determine VT ablation targets is in patients with an implanted ICD. Although CT techniques would not have this limitation, the reproducibility and true sensitivity of CE-MDCT in visualizing scarred myocardium is still unclear and PET-CT has less spatial accuracy than CE-CMR.

3.5 *Endocardial electrograms in epicardial ventricular tachycardias*

When an accurate ECG analysis is not possible and imaging techniques are not an option, endocardial mapping or mapping in the coronary sinus can provide clues to whether an epicardial approach should be attempted.

In patients with structural heart disease, scars are the substrate for VTs and these scars can be identified by electrogram abnormalities. Therefore, the absence of endocardial electrogram abnormalities on an electroanatomical map during sinus rhythm at the zone of interest could suggest scars located deep in the ventricular wall or at the epicardium.[39] This situation is observed in non-ischemic cardiomyopathy.

In a case of VTs suspected of originating from the basal area of the LV, mapping the coronary sinus and the proximal part of its branches may also facilitate distinguishing between endocardial and epicardial VTs. Finally, a late VT interruption during RF application with persistent inducibility could also suggest that the VT circuit is located deep in the myocardium or at the epicardium.

4   Recommendations on choosing the epicardial approach

In order to achieve a high success rate with epicardial mapping and ablation, the decision to change to the epicardium must be based on solid evidence. Except in the case of a previous failed ablation, our laboratory usually requires the presence of at least two of the conditions described below as suggesting an epicardial origin.

Epicardial access is performed in the following situations: *1)* endocardial ablation failure; *2)* impossiblility to access the LV cavity, together with a QRS complex during VT suggestive of an epicardial origin; *3)* idiopathic LVOT VTs with a QRS suggestive of an epicardial origin and inappropriate precocity of the endocardial electrogram (30 ms), after first mapping the coronary sinus; *4)* non-idiopathic VTs with a QRS suggestive of an epicardial origin, after endocardial mapping; and *5)* non-idiopathic VTs with a QRS suggestive of an epicardial origin and CE-CMR evidence of an epicardial scar without an endocardial component in the presumed segment of origin. In addition, in non-ischemic cardiomyopathy (i.e., idiopathic dilated cardiomyopathy and ARVC/D), due to the high incidence of epicardial VT circuits, an epicardial guidewire can be placed at the beginning of the procedure prior to endocardial mapping and anticoagulation.

References

1. Sosa E, Scanavacca M, D'Avila A, *et al.* A new technique to perform epicardial mapping in the electrophysiology laboratory. J Cardiovasc Electrophysiol 1996; 7(6): 531-6.

2. Sosa E, Scanavacca M, d'Avila A, *et al.* Nonsurgical transthoracic epicardial catheter ablation to treat recurrent ventricular tachycardia occurring late after myocardial infarction. J Am Coll Cardiol 2000; 35: 1442–9.

3. Brugada J, Berruezo A, Cuesta A, *et al.* Nonsurgical transthoracic epicardial radiofrequency ablation: an alternative in incessant ventricular tachycardia. J Am Coll Cardiol 2003; 41(11): 2036-43.

4. Berruezo A, Mont L, Nava S, *et al.* Electrocardiographic recognition of the epicardial origin of ventricular tachycardias. Circulation 2004; 109(15): 1842-7.

5. Daniels DV, Lu YY, Morton JB, *et al.* Idiopathic epicardial left ventricular tachycardia originating remote from the sinus of Valsalva: electrophysiological characteristics, catheter ablation, and identification from the 12-lead electrocardiogram. Circulation 2006; 113(13): 1659-66.

6. Bazan V, Gerstenfeld EP, Garcia FC, *et al.* Site-specific twelve lead ECG features to identify an epicardial origin for left ventricular tachycardia in the absence of myocardial infarction. Heart Rhythm 2007; 4(11): 1403-10.

7. Sosa E, Scanavacca M, D'Avila A, *et al.* Endocardial and epicardial ablation guided by nonsurgical transthoracic epicardial mapping to treat recurrent ventricular tachycardia. J Cardiovasc Electrophysiol 1998; 9(3): 229-39.

8. Pagé PL, Cardinal R, Shenasa M, *et al.* Surgical treatment of ventricular tachycardia. Regional cryoablation guided by computerized epicardial and endocardial mapping. Circulation 1989; 80: 124-34.

9. Kaltenbrunner W, Cardinal R, Dubuc M, *et al.* Epicardial and endocardial mapping of ventricular tachycardia in patients with myocardial infarction. Is the origin of the tachycardia always subendocardially localized? Circulation 1991; 84: 1058-71.

10. Lacroix D, Klug D, Grandmougin D, *et al.* Ventricular tachycardia originating from the posteroseptal process of the left ventricle with inferior wall healed myocardial infarction. Am J Cardiol 1999; 84: 181-6.

11. Svenson RH, Littman L, Gallagher JJ, *et al.* Termination of ventricular tachycardia with epicardial laser photocoagulation: a clinical comparison with patients undergoing successful endocardial photocoagulation alone. J Am Coll Cardiol 1990; 15: 163-70.

12. Cesario DA, Vaseghi M, Boyle NG, *et al.* Value of high-density endocardial and epicardial mapping for catheter ablation of hemodynamically unstable ventricular tachycardia. Heart Rhythm 2006; 3: 1-10.

13. Lee JT, Ideker RE, Reimer KA. Myocardial infarct size and location in relation to the coronary vascular bed at risk in man. Circulation 1981; 64: 526-34.

14. Sosa E, Scanavacca M, d'Avila A, *et al.* Nonsurgical transthoracic epicardial catheter ablation to treat recurrent ventricular tachycardia occurring late after myocardial infarction. J Am Coll Cardiol 2000; 35: 1442-9.

15. Brugada J, Berruezo A, Cuesta A, *et al.* Nonsurgical transthoracic epicardial radiofrequency ablation. An alternative in incessant ventricular tachycardia. J Am Coll Cardiol 2003; 41: 2036-43.

16. Soejima K, Stevenson WG, Sapp JL, *et al.* Endocardial and epicardial radiofrequency ablation of ventricular tachycardia associated with dilated cardiomyopathy. The importance of low-voltage scars. J Am Coll Cardiol 2004; 43: 1834-42.

17. Hsia HH, Callans DJ, Marchlinski FE. Characterization of endocardial electrophysiological substrate in patients with nonischemic cardiomyopathy and monomorphic ventricular tachycardia. Circulation 2003; 108: 704-10.

18. Nava A, Thiene G, Canciani B, *et al.* Familial occurrence of right ventricular dysplasia: a study involving nine families. J Am Coll Cardiol 1989; 12: 1222–28.

19. Corrado D, Basso C, Thiene G. Arrhythmogenic right ventricular cardio-myopathy: diagnosis, prognosis, and treatment. Heart 2000; 83: 588–95.

20. Corrado D, Basso C, Leoni L, *et al.* Three-dimensional electroanatomic voltage mapping increases accuracy of diagnosing arrhythmogenic right ventricular cardiomyopathy/dysplasia. Circulation 2005; 111: 3042–50.

21. Corrado D, Basso C, Leoni L, *et al.* Three-dimensional electroanatomical voltage mapping and histologic evaluation of myocardial substrate in right ventricular outflow tract tachycardia. J Am Coll Cardiol 2008; 51: 731–39.

22. Basso C, Thiene G, Corrado D, *et al.* Arrhythmogenic right ventricular cardiomyopathy: dysplasia, dystrophy or myocarditis? Circulation 1996; 94: 983–91.

23. Corrado D, Basso C, Thiene G, *et al.* Spectrum of clinicopathologic manifestations of arrhythmogenic right ventricular cardiomyopathy/dysplasia: a multicenter study. J Am Coll Cardiol 1997; 30: 1512–20.

24. Dalal D, Jain R, Tandri H, *et al.* Long-term efficacy of catheter ablation of ventricular tachycardia in patients with arrhythmogenic right ventricular dysplasia/cardiomyopathy. J Am Coll Cardiol 2007; 50: 432–40.

25. Garcia FC, Bazan V, Zado ES, *et al.* Epicardial substrate and outcome with epicardial ablation of ventricular tachycardia in arrhythmogenic right ventricular cardiomyopathy/dysplasia. Circulation 2009; 120: 366-75.

26. Tanner H, Hindricks G, Schirdewahn P, *et al.* Outflow tract tachycardia with R/S transition in lead V3. Six different anatomic approaches for successful ablation. J Am Coll Cardiol 2005; 45: 418-23.

27. D'Avila A, Houghtaling C, Gutierrez P, *et al.* Catheter ablation of ventricular epicardial tissue: a comparison between standard and cooled-tip radiofrequency energy. Circulation 2004; 109: 2363–9.

28. Fuller IA, Wood MA. Intramural coronary vasculature prevents transmural radiofrequency lesion formation: implications for linear ablation. Circulation 2003; 107: 1797–803.

29. D'Avila A, Gutierrez P, Scanavacca M, *et al.* Effects of radiofrequency pulses delivered in the vicinity of the coronary arteries: implications for nonsurgical transthoracic epicardial catheter ablation to treat ventricular tachycardia. Pacing Clin Electrophysiol 2002; 25: 1488–95.

30. Lustgarten DL, Bell S, Hardin N, *et al.* Safety and efficacy of epicardial cryoablation in a canine model. Heart Rhythm 2005; 2: 82–90.

31. D'Avila A. Epicardial catheter ablation of ventricular tachycardia. Heart Rhythm 2008; 5: S73-5.

32. Cano O, Hutchinson M, Lin D, *et al.* Electroanatomical substrate and ablation outcome for suspected epicardial ventricular tachycardia in left ventricular nonischemic cardiomyopathy. J Am Coll Cardiol 2009; 54: 799-808.

33. Zeppenfeld K, Tops LF, Bax JJ, *et al.* Epicardial radiofrequency catheter ablation of ventricular tachycardia in the vicinity of coronary arteries is facilitated by fusion of 3-dimensional electroanatomical mapping with multislice computed tomography. Circulation 2006; 114: e51-2.

34. Roberts-Thomson KC, Steven D, Seiler J, *et al.* Coronary artery injury due to catheter ablation in adults: presentations and outcomes. Circulation 2009; 120: 1465-73.

35. Pogwidz SM, *et al.* Mechanisms underlying spontaneous and induced ventricular arrhythmias in patients with idiopathic dilated cardiomyopathy. Circulation 1998; 98: 2404-14.

36. Bogun FM, Desjardins B, Good E, *et al.* Delayed-enhanced magnetic resonance imaging in nonischemic cardiomyopathy. Utility for identifying the ventricular arrhythmia substrate. J Am Coll Cardiol 2009; 53: 1138-45.

37. Berruezo A, Ortiz JT, Guasch E, *et al.* Usefulness of contrast enhanced cardiac magnetic resonance to identify the epicardial origin of ventricular tachycardias. Heart Rhythm 2009; 6: S224.

38. Desjardins B, Crawford T, Good E, *et al.* Infarct architecture and characteristics on delayed enhanced magnetic resonance imaging and electroanatomic mapping in patients with postinfarction ventricular arrhythmia. Heart Rhythm 2009; 6: 644-51.

39. Berruezo A, Boussy T, Ortiz JT, *et al.* Endocardial electrograms in epicardially ablated ventricular tachycardias. Heart Rhythm 2009; 6: S303.

Chapter 5. Ventricular outflow tract tachycardias: tips and tricks for successful ablation

E. Wissner, K.H. Kuck, F. Ouyang

[1] **Staff Physician**
II Medizinische Abteilung
Asklepios Klinik St. Georg
Hamburg, Germany

[2] **Department Head**
II Medizinische Abteilung
Asklepios Klinik St. Georg
Hamburg, Germany

[3] **Director-Cardiac Electrophysiology Laboratory**
II Medizinische Abteilung
Asklepios Klinik St. Georg
Hamburg, Germany

Address for correspondence:
II Medizinische Abteilung
Asklepios Klinik St. Georg
Dr. Karl-Heinz Kuck
k.kuck@asklepios.com

Introduction

Tachyarrhythmias emanating from the outflow tract (OT) are the most common subtype of idiopathic ventricular tachycardia. Analysis of the 12-lead ECG provides important clues to diagnose the anatomical site of origin (SOO). If an ablative approach is warranted, activation or pace mapping are utilized to facilitate accurate localization of tachycardia origin. Most OT tachycardias can be successfully ablated in the right ventricular OT (RVOT). If no suitable site for ablation is detected along the RVOT, alternative sites such as the aortic root need to be investigated. In general, ablation for OT tachycardia is highly successful with a low rate of recurrence.

1 Clinical characteristics

Among patients referred for evaluation of ventricular tachycardia, 10% present with ventricular tachycardia in the absence of overt structural heart disease.[1] More than 70 to 80% of idiopathic ventricular tachycardias emanate from the RVOT.[1] Occasionally, OT tachycardias may originate from the left ventricular OT (LVOT) or above the semilunar valves. Patients usually present in their third to fifth decade. RVOT tachycardia is twice as common in women, while LVOT tachycardia has a comparable prevalence between both genders.[2] Patients commonly report palpitations exacerbated by exercise, stress and caffeine. Alternatively, OT tachycardia may be suppressed by exercise and only arise during the recovery phase or at times of rest in a repetitive monomorphic pattern. In general, patients present with salvos of non-sustained ventricular OT tachycardia. In women, hormonal flux during the premenstrual period or menopause can trigger OT tachycardia.[3] In general, tachycardia from the OT shows a benign course. Although the development of cardiomyopathy induced by OT tachycardia or frequent ventricular ectopy is uncommon, depressed ventricular function may normalize following successful ablation within the RVOT.[4,5] In the presence of multifocal ventricular ectopy or pleomorphic ventricular tachycardia from the OT, occult structural heart disease such as arrhythmogenic right ventricular dysplasia, must be excluded. Rarely, ectopy from the OT can trigger ventricular fibrillation and may be distinguished from benign ventricular ectopy by a markedly shorter coupling interval to the preceding QRS complex.[6]

2   Arrhythmia mechanisms and medical treatment

Calcium-dependent triggered activity mediated through cyclic adenosine monophosphate resulting in delayed afterdepolarizations represents the predominant mechanism for the initiation of OT tachycardia.[7] In one-third of patients programmed stimulation (burst pacing) may facilitate arrhythmia induction. Furthermore, triggered activity is exacerbated by sympathetic stimulation such as during catecholamine surge or isoproterenol infusion. Drugs that suppress sympathetic surge are used for the medical treatment of OT arrhythmias. Beta-blockers and calcium channel blockers are first-line agents; however, class IC (flecainide) or III (sotalol) antiarrhythmic drugs may be used alternatively. The efficacy of arrhythmia suppression should be judged clinically during exercise testing or 24-hour ECG monitoring. An electrophysiology study for this purpose is not indicated.

3   Indications and contraindications for an ablative approach

An ablative approach is recommended in patients with severely symptomatic ventricular ectopy or tachycardia or if antiarrhythmic drug therapy remains ineffective, is poorly tolerated or not favored by the patient. In addition, catheter ablation is indicated if left ventricular dysfunction develops secondary to OT tachycardia. Contraindications to catheter ablation are the presence of mobile left ventricular thrombus, asymptomatic ventricular ectopy or nonsustained tachycardia or if OT tachycardia is due to reversible causes.

4   Anatomy of the outflow tract region

Before embarking on an ablative approach, a thorough review of the anatomic intricacies of the OT region is warranted (see figure 1). The OT may be divided into right and left, as well as sub- and supravalvar regions. The pulmonary and aortic valve planes are positioned perpendicular to each other, whereas the level of the pulmonary valve annulus lies superior to the aortic valve. The RVOT is located anteriorly to the LVOT and describes a leftward and posteriorly directed course beyond the pulmonary valve plane. By strict anatomical means the RVOT is to the left of the LVOT, a fact crucial for correct mapping and ablation of OT tachycardia.[8]

The LVOT is directed rightward and anteriorly at the aortic valve level. Because of its central location the aortic valve is anatomically connected to the ventricles, the mitral and tricuspid valve, as well as to the atrial appendages. The left coronary cusp (LCC) forms the most superior, the right coronary cusp (RCC) the most anterior and the noncoronary cusp (NCC) the most inferior point at the junction between LVOT and aorta. The LCC and RCC are in

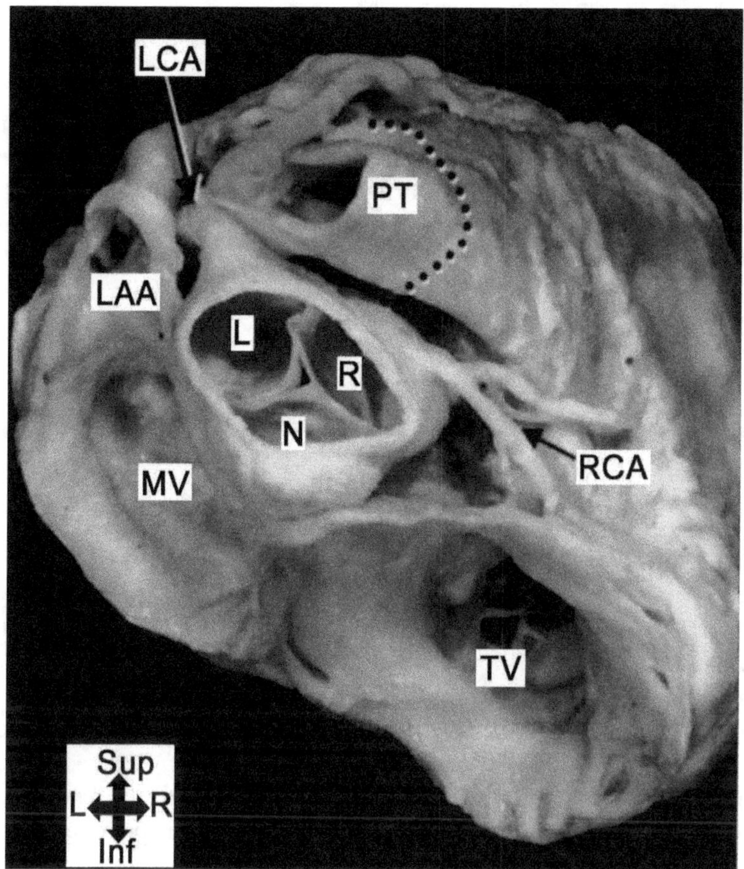

Figure 1. Transverse view of the outflow tract at the level of the aortic valve. Note the central location of the aortic root and the position of the RVOT in relation to the aortic root. The left main coronary artery courses in immediate vicinity to the posterior wall of the RVOT, while the LCC and RCC lie in apposition to the septal portion of the RVOT. The NCC is adjacent to the interatrial and interventricular septum and posterior to the LCC and RCC.
LAA = left atrial appendage; MV = mitral valve; TV = tricuspid valve; RCA = right coronary artery; L = left coronary cusp; R = right coronary cusp; N = noncoronary cusp; PT = pulmonary trunk; LCA = left main coronary artery (from reference 11).

close proximity to the septal portion of the RVOT, while the NCC borders at the membranous portion of the interventricular and interatrial septum. A catheter positioned across the tricuspid valve at the commissure between septal and anterior leaflet will record a His bundle potential just inferiorly to the junction of the RCC and NCC. The LCC and NCC lie opposite the anterior mitral valve leaflet representing an area of fibrous continuity. Rarely, muscular extensions expand into the region of the aortomitral continuity. The left main coronary artery courses in close proximity to the posterior RVOT. The coronary ostia are positioned approximately 15 mm cranial from the nadir of the coronary cusps. Crescent-like myocardial fibers can extend beyond the pulmonary and aortic valve plane and may generate a source for OT tachycardia.[9,10]

5   Sites of tachycardia origin

In general, tachycardia emanates from the RVOT inferior to the pulmonary valve, typically from the anteroseptal region of the RVOT. Rarely, focal activity may originate from the supravalvar area with discrete potentials recorded from the pulmonary artery.[12] The site of tachycardia origin along the LVOT is commonly localized supravalvular at the LCC or RCC.[11] Rarely, tachycardia originates from the NCC.[11,13,14] In our laboratory, a total of 42 patients presented between 1999 and 2007 with ventricular tachycardia originating from the aortic cusps. The LCC was the most common site of origin in 25 (60%) patients, followed by the RCC in 16 (38%) and the NCC in one (2%) patient. Similar results were reported in a recent study by Yamada *et al.*[14] An epicardial SOO localized to the great cardiac vein or the anterior interventricular vein is found in a minority of patients.[15] OT tachycardia originating from the mitral or tricuspid annulus will not be covered in this chapter.

6   The role of the 12-lead electrogram in the diagnosis and localization of OT tachycardia

The 12-lead electrogram (ECG) is invaluable in the diagnosis of ventricular tachycardia originating from the OT. Characteristic ECG patterns are consistently seen because tachycardia arises from a focal site within healthy myocardium. The physician should verify proper surface ECG lead positioning, since minor positional variation may result in false interpretation of the ECG. Anticipating the SOO facilitates preparation for an appropriate mapping strategy. If activation mapping is utilized, the 12-lead ECG will help to limit the region of interest, thus preventing excessive mapping at unsuccessful ablation sites. In the presence of rare ventricular ectopy or noninducible OT tachycardia, the 12-lead ECG can serve as a template for pace mapping.

6.1   *General considerations regarding electrocardiographic interpretation of OT tachycardias*

Ventricular tachycardias originating from the OT typically demonstrate left bundle branch block morphology with inferiorly directed frontal QRS axis (see figure 2). Without referring to complex ECG algorithms, general observations on the 12-lead ECG can aid in defining the SOO. A wide and notched QRS complex in the inferior leads implies that local activation initiates from the lateral RVOT spreading sequentially towards the left myocardium. Conversely, a septal SOO results in simultaneous activation of right and left ventricular musculature causing a relatively narrow QRS complex. A posterior SOO will cause electrical forces to move towards the anterior chest wall resulting in positive polarity of the QRS complex in lead I. Negative polarity in lead I indicates an anterior SOO. Caudal sites produce an isoelectric or positive QRS complex in lead aVL while a negative QRS complex is anticipated at cranial sites. Late precordial transition (R/S ratio >1 by lead V3 or V4) is seen in RVOT tachycardia. Early precordial transition by lead V1 or V2 is expected if tachycardia originates from the aortic root since its anatomic position is posterior to the RVOT. More detailed ECG analysis can facilitate differentiation between specific SOO.

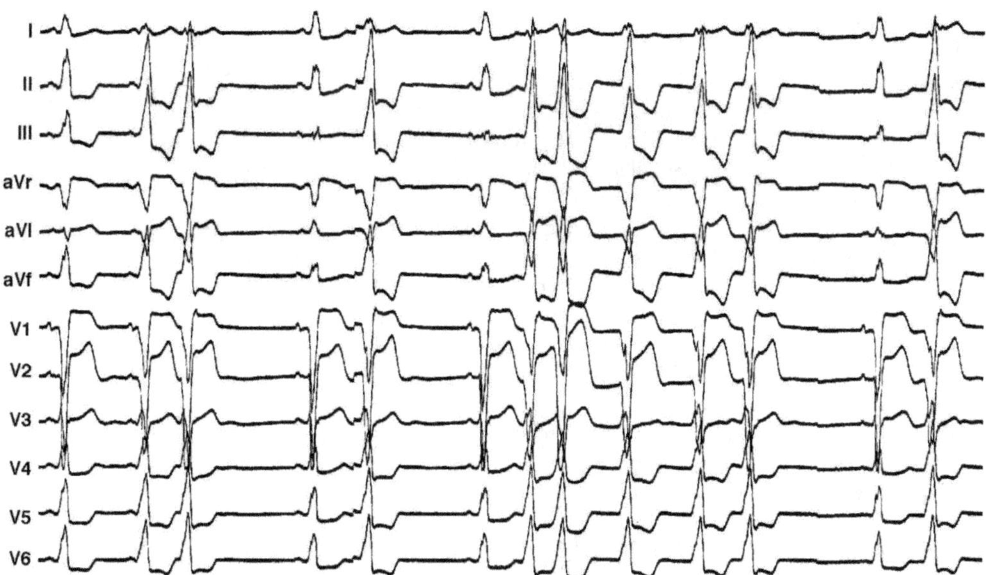

Figure 2. Non-sustained ventricular tachycardia originating from the RVOT with left bundle branch block morphology, inferior axis and precordial transition in lead V4 (see text for details).

6.1.1 ECG Criteria for detailed localization of RVOT tachycardia

Several authors have proposed detailed ECG criteria to accurately diagnose the SOO of RVOT tachycardia.[15-17] A summary is presented in table 1.

6.1.2 ECG criteria for the differentiation of aortic root from RVOT tachycardia

Ouyang *et al.* described two unique surface ECG criteria that were able to distinguish LCC from RVOT tachycardia.[11] Analyzing lead V1 or V2, an R-wave duration ≥50% of the total QRS duration and an R/S amplitude ratio ≥30% strongly favored an SOO from the LCC. In addition, the presence of an S-wave in lead I differentiates aortic root from RVOT origin.[17]

6.1.3 Specific ECG algorithms for the diagnosis of OT tachycardia from the aortic cusps

In order to discriminate OT tachycardias originating from the individual aortic cusps additional ECG criteria were developed (see table 2). Because of the infrequency of OT tachycardia emanating from the NCC, consistent ECG criteria have yet to be reported.

6.1.4 Specific ECG algorithms for the diagnosis of supravalvar and epicardial OT tachycardias

The pulmonary artery may be the origin of supravalvar OT tachycardia in 8-15% of idiopathic left bundle branch block morphology ventricular tachycardias. The focal SOO is common-

Site of origin	Suggested ECG criteria
Free wall	QRS duration ≥140 ms[15] Long QRS duration in lead II[16] QRS notching in leads II, III and aVF[15,16] Smaller QRS amplitude in leads II, III and aVF[16] Late precordial transition in V4[15,16] S-wave in lead V2 >3,0 mV[17]
Septal wall	Narrow QRS complex <140 ms[15] Shorter QRS duration in lead II[16] Precordial transition in lead V3[15,16] S-wave in V2 ≤3.0 mV[17]
Anterior wall	Negative or isoelectric QRS complex in lead I[15]
Anterior leftward	Negative QRS complex in lead I[16]
Posterior wall	Positive QRS complex in lead I[15]
Posterior rightward	Positive QRS complex in lead I[16]
Caudal	Negative QRS complex in lead aVL[15]
Cranial	Positive or isoelectric QRS complex in lead aVL[15]

Table 1. ECG criteria suggestive of a specific site of origin within the RVOT.

Site of origin	Suggested ECG criteria
LCC	Analyzing lead V1 or V2, an R-wave duration ≥ 50% of the total QRS duration and an R/S amplitude ratio ≥ 30%[11] Early precordial transition by lead V2 and an R-wave amplitude ratio of >0.9 in lead III/II[14] Multiphasic M or W pattern in lead V1[18]
LCC/RCC commissure	QRS pattern in leads V1 to V3[19] QS morphology in lead V1 with notching of the descending limb of the QS complex[20]
RCC	QS or QR pattern in lead V1 with overall negative QRS vector[18]

Table 2. ECG criteria suggestive of a specific site of origin from the aortic root.

ly within 1.5 cm of the level of the pulmonary valve. Large amplitude R-waves (>2.0 mV) in the inferior leads and early precordial transition may be seen on the 12-lead ECG.[12]

An epicardial focus should be suspected if mapping at typical sites demonstrates suboptimal results. Hallmark of an epicardial origin is slow initial conduction in the precordial leads.

The maximum deflection index is defined as the shortest QRS onset to maximal precordial deflection divided by the QRS complex duration. A ratio of ≥ 0.55 was 100% sensitive and 99% specific for an epicardial SOO.[21]

7 General considerations for a successful mapping strategy

Standard setup during mapping of ventricular OT tachycardia should include recording of a His bundle potential and right ventricular signal. The coronary sinus catheter should be advanced distally to allow recording of ventricular activation in or near the great cardiac vein. In the absence of spontaneous ventricular ectopy or tachycardia, programmed stimulation, burst pacing and infusion of isoproterenol should be performed. Care should be taken so as not to bump the focal SOO resulting in transient mechanical block and non-inducibility of tachycardia. Activation mapping is the preferred mapping strategy in the presence of sustained tachycardia or frequent clinical ventricular ectopy. The use of a three-dimensional mapping system permits local activation to be rendered on a virtual anatomic map and may facilitate successful mapping and ablation.[1] Initial mapping commences in the RVOT since the majority of OT tachycardias originate from this region. If unsuccessful, mapping needs to be extended to alternative sites including the region above the pulmonary valve, the area near the His bundle, distal coronary sinus and the aortic cusps.

7.1 Activation mapping

During activation mapping the earliest bipolar activity measured at the peak absolute amplitude and a local unipolar QS pattern are most reliable in identifying the focal site of origin. Earliest local ventricular activation recorded on the mapping catheter should precede the onset of the surface QRS complex by 10 to 60 ms.[1] Inaccuracy of activation mapping results from local activity spreading rapidly across normal myocardium, covering an area of 3.0 ± 1.6 cm^2 during the first 10 ms.[22] A unipolar QS pattern with rapid intrinsic deflection demonstrates a high sensitivity for successful ablation sites, but may also be recorded at unsuccessful sites up to 11 mm from the SOO.[23-25] If mapping in the RVOT is unsuccessful, the pulmonary artery should be explored. Discrete potentials recorded from the pulmonary artery or the aorta should alert the operator to a supravalvar site of origin. If earliest ventricular activation is recorded on the His catheter, a focal site originating from the RCC or NCC should be suspected.[14] In patients with an epicardial SOO, initial mapping should be performed from within the coronary sinus at the level of the great cardiac vein or anterior interventricular vein. If unsuccessful, mapping should proceed via a percutaneous pericardial access.[21]

7.2 Pace mapping

Pace mapping is used in the presence of rare ventricular ectopy or if OT tachycardia remains non-inducible. A preprocedural recording of the clinical tachycardia or ventricular ectopy serves as a template during pace mapping. Pace mapping is performed at the tachycardia cycle length or at a cycle length identical to the coupling interval of ventricular ectopy. Pacing at faster cycle lengths or shorter coupling intervals will result in rate-dependent changes in QRS morphology.[26] The

QRS morphology of the first beat of successive VT should be compared with the paced QRS morphology produced by single extra-stimulation.[27] The ideal pace map results in an identical QRS pattern in all 12 surface ECG leads (12/12 match). Pacing should be performed at minimal output so as not to capture remote myocardial tissue resulting in fusion of the QRS complex. Despite these precautions, pace mapping is limited by its poor spatial resolution. A perfect pace map might be seen at a distance of up to 1.8 cm^2 from the actual SOO within the RVOT.[28] Due to tiny muscle bundles connecting the aortic root and RVOT, pace mapping along the aortic cups may require high output pacing and is less likely to reproduce the true VT morphology.

8   Catheter ablation of OT tachycardia

Antiarrhythmic medication should be discontinued five half-lives prior to the planned ablation procedure in order to increase the likelihood of spontaneous or inducible arrhythmia. Deep sedation may result in noninduciblity of OT tachycardia and should be avoided if possible.

8.1   Intraprocedural imaging

During ablation of RVOT tachycardia correct catheter tip position at the target site should be verified by fluoroscopic imaging. If ablation is performed within the aortic cusps in close proximity to the coronary arteries additional imaging tools are commonly used. Intracardiac echocardiography allows visualization of catheter tip and surrounding structures, but requires addi-

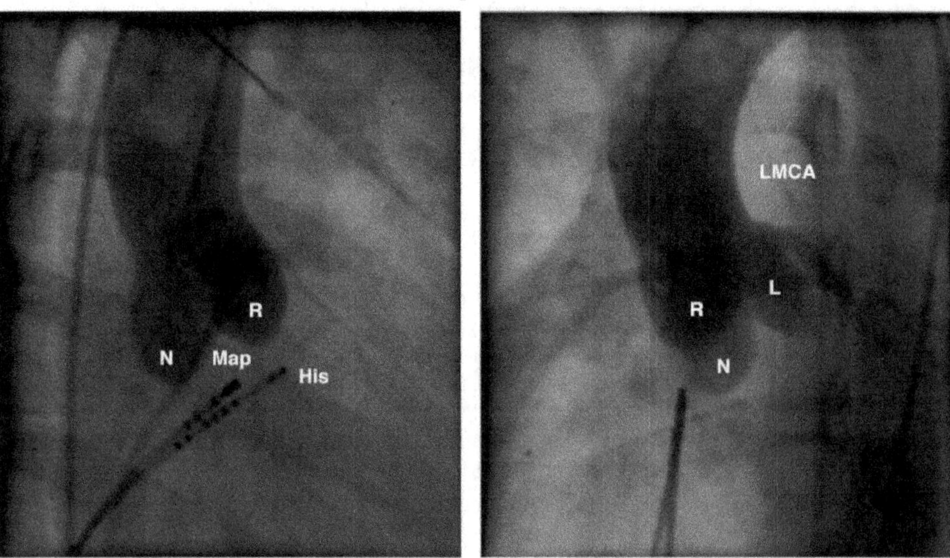

Figure 3. Angiogram of the aortic root in right anterior oblique 30° and left anterior oblique 40° projection (a pig-tail catheter is visible in the aortic root).
Map = mapping catheter; N = non-coronary cusp; R = right coronary cusp;
His = His bundle recording catheter; L = left coronary cusp; LMCA = left main coronary artery.

tional expertise in its use and interpretation. Aortic root angiography or selective coronary catheterization will allow proper visualization of aortic cusps and left and right coronary ostia (see figure 3). When targeting an SOO within the LCC or RCC, placing a 5F Judkins catheter within the ostium of the respective coronary artery will serve as anatomic marker and protection in case of dislodgement of the ablation catheter.

8.2 Catheter choice and energy settings

Ablation within the RVOT is performed using a conventional solid tip catheter. Since OT tachycardia commonly originates from healthy myocardial tissue, use of an irrigated tip catheter is generally not warranted. Termination is expected to occur within 10 seconds of radiofrequency current energy delivery, otherwise remapping of the area of interest should be performed. During ablation within the RVOT the maximum temperature is set at 55 ºC. Power should be set at 20 W, carefully titrating to a maximum of 40 W. If the SOO is located within the aortic cusps, ablation is performed utilizing a solid tip catheter, a maximum temperature of 55 ºC. and power delivery initially set at 20 W titrating to a maximum of 30 W.

8.3 Specific intracardiac findings at successful ablation sites

8.3.1 RVOT

The local bipolar recording at the successful ablation site may demonstrate presystolic high frequency, low-voltage signals and should precede the onset of the surface QRS complex by 10 to 60 ms.

8.3.2 Pulmonary artery

Discrete potentials preceding the QRS complex during ventricular tachycardia and following the QRS complex in SR may be recorded.[29] Furthermore, a local ventricular electrogram of less than 1.0 mV can be seen at the successful ablation site.[12]

8.3.3 Aortic cusps

The focal SOO within the LCC is usually 6.8 to 20 mm below the ostium of the left main coronary artery and ablation should not be performed if the catheter is positioned within 6.4 mm from the coronary ostium. The successful ablation site will demonstrate a high amplitude ventricular signal concurrent with the surface QRS complex, preceded by a low amplitude presystolic or late diastolic potential by 28-154 ms.[11] This characteristic pattern reverses during sinus rhythm. The unipolar recording will demonstrate a late negative intrinsic deflection concurrent with the second ventricular component recorded on the bipolar signal (see figure 4). The focal SOO within the RCC is commonly located 7-15 mm anterior of the ostium of the right coronary artery. In contrast to an LCC origin there is an earlier local ventricular activation to surface QRS onset of less than 15 ms recorded on the His catheter. The local bipolar electrogram demonstrates only a presystolic potential preceding the onset of the sur-

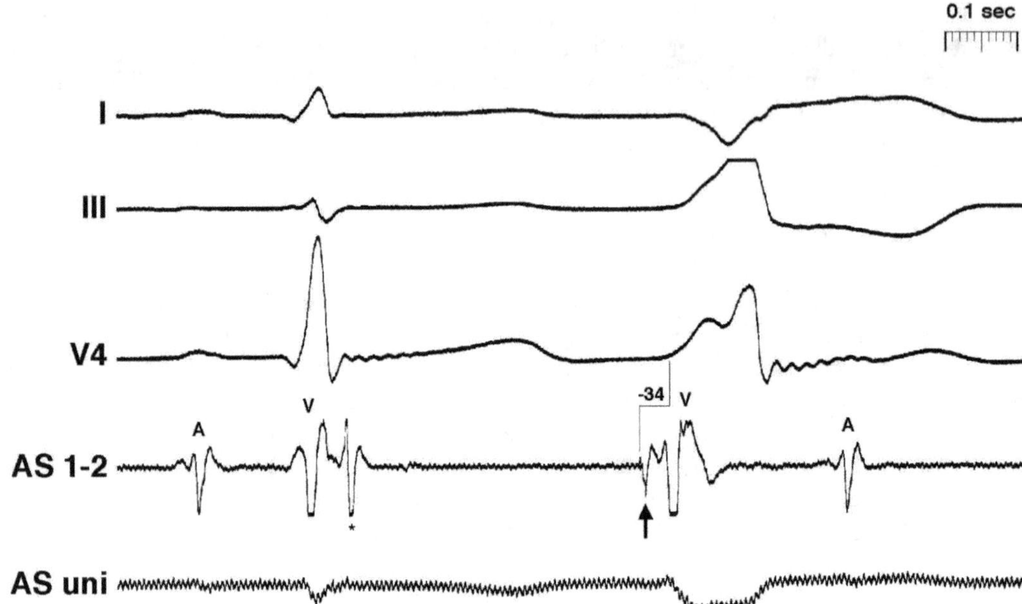

Figure 4. Recording of surface lead I, III and V4 during a spontaneous PVC. At the site of successful ablation in a patient with ventricular ectopy originating from the LCC, a low amplitude presystolic potential (arrow) preceding the surface QRS complex by 34 ms is seen in the bipolar recording (AS 1-2). This pattern reverses during sinus rhythm (asterisk). The unipolar signal (AS uni) demonstrates a negative intrinsic deflection coincident with the second component on the bipolar recording.

face QRS complex by 21-45 ms. Finally, a large atrial and relatively small ventricular signal is recorded at the successful ablation site within the NCC, while the local ventricular activation to surface QRS onset recorded on the His catheter is earlier compared to an LCC SOO.[14]

8.4   Complications

Complications typically occur at structures in close anatomical proximity to the site of ablation. Along the posterior RVOT, ablation may result in damage to the left main coronary artery.[8] The distance from the RVOT to the left main coronary artery is 4.1±1.9 mm, to the RCA 4.3±1.9 mm, and to the LAD 2.0±0.6 mm.[30] Other risks include cardiac perforation resulting in tamponade, damage to the His bundle, thromboembolism or air embolism which is of particular concern if ablation is performed within the aortic cusps and injury to the aortic valve during retrograde mapping and ablation.

9   Procedural outcome following catheter ablation of OT tachycardias

No randomized trials have evaluated the success rate of ablation of ventricular OT tachycardia. According to non-randomized studies, the acute success rate for ablation of RVOT tachy-

> - In the presence of multifocal ventricular ectopy or pleomorphic ventricular tachycardia from the OT, occult structural heart disease such as arrhythmogenic right ventricular dysplasia, must be excluded
> - In strict anatomical terms the RVOT is left to the LVOT
> - If the earliest local ventricular electrogram to surface QRS complex is noted at the His bundle recording site, mapping within the aortic root is warranted
> - Ablation at the posterior RVOT (level pulmonary valve plane above aortic valve annulus) may result in damage to the left main coronary artery
> - Do not ablate within 6.4 mm. of the coronary ostium
> - The most common cause of procedural failure is non-inducibility of ventricular ectopy or tachycardia

Table 3. Tips and tricks for successful ablation.

cardia generally exceeds 80% with a low recurrence rate of 5%.[1] Small case series reported on the success rate of ablation of OT tachycardia emanating from sites other than the RVOT. The combined success rates were generally greater than 95% with a low risk for complications.[1] However, ablation was performed at high-volume centers, therefore high success and low complication rates may not reflect those of less experienced centers. Some tips for successful ablation are shown in table 3.

References

1. Aliot EM, Stevenson WG, Almendral-Garrote JM, *et al.* EHRA/HRS Expert Consensus on Catheter Ablation of Ventricular Arrhythmias: developed in a partnership with the European Heart Rhythm Association (EHRA), a Registered Branch of the European Society of Cardiology (ESC), and the Heart Rhythm Society (HRS); in collaboration with the American College of Cardiology (ACC) and the American Heart Association (AHA). Europace 2009; 11(6): 771-817.

2. Nakagawa M, Takahashi N, Nobe S, *et al.* Gender differences in various types of idiopathic ventricular tachycardia. J Cardiovasc Electrophysiol 2002; 13(7): 633-8.

3. Marchlinski FE, Deely MP, Zado ES. Sex-specific triggers for right ventricular outflow tract tachycardia. Am Heart J 2000; 139(6): 1009-13.

4. Yarlagadda RK, Iwai S, Stein KM, *et al.* Reversal of cardiomyopathy in patients with repetitive monomorphic ventricular ectopy originating from the right ventricular outflow tract. Circulation 2005 23; 112(8): 1092-7.

5. Grimm W, Menz V, Hoffmann J, *et al.* Reversal of tachycardia induced cardiomyopathy following ablation of repetitive monomorphic right ventricular outflow tract tachycardia. Pacing Clin Electrophysiol 2001; 24(2): 166-71.

6. Viskin S, Rosso R, Rogowski O, *et al.* The "short-coupled" variant of right ventricular outflow ventricular tachycardia: a not-so-benign form of benign ventricular tachycardia? J Cardiovasc Electrophysiol 2005; 16(8): 912-6.

7. Lerman BB, Belardinelli L, West GA, *et al.* Adenosine-sensitive ventricular tachycardia: evidence suggesting cyclic AMP-mediated triggered activity. Circulation 1986; 74(2): 270-80.

8. Suleiman M, Asirvatham SJ. Ablation above the semilunar valves: when, why, and how? Part I. Heart Rhythm 2008; 5(10): 1485-92.

9. Yamada T, Litovsky SH, Kay GN. The left ventricular ostium: an anatomic concept relevant to idiopathic ventricular arrhythmias. Circ Arrhythm Electrophysiol 2008; 1(5): 396-404.

10. Anderson RH. Clinical anatomy of the aortic root. Heart 2000; 84(6): 670-3.

11. Ouyang F, Fotuhi P, Ho SY, *et al.* Repetitive monomorphic ventricular tachycardia originating from the aortic sinus cusp: electrocardiographic characterization for guiding catheter ablation. J Am Coll Cardiol 2002; 39(3): 500-8.

12. Sekiguchi Y, Aonuma K, Takahashi A, *et al.* Electrocardiographic and electrophysiologic characteristics of ventricular tachycardia originating within the pulmonary artery. J Am Coll Cardiol 2005; 45(6): 887-95.

13. Kanagaratnam L, Tomassoni G, Schweikert R, *et al.* Ventricular tachycardias arising from the aortic sinus of valsalva: an under-recognized variant of left outflow tract ventricular tachycardia. J Am Coll Cardiol 2001; 37(5): 1408-14.

14. Yamada T, McElderry HT, Doppalapudi H, *et al.* Idiopathic ventricular arrhythmias originating from the

aortic root prevalence, electrocardiographic and electrophysiologic characteristics, and results of radiofrequency catheter ablation. J Am Coll Cardiol 2008; 52(2): 139-47.

15. Joshi S, Wilber DJ. Ablation of idiopathic right ventricular outflow tract tachycardia: current perspectives. J Cardiovasc Electrophysiol 2005; 16 Suppl 1: S52-8.

16. Dixit S, Gerstenfeld EP, Callans DJ, *et al.* Electrocardiographic patterns of superior right ventricular outflow tract tachycardias: distinguishing septal and free-wall sites of origin. J Cardiovasc Electrophysiol 2003; 14(1): 1-7.

17. Ito S, Tada H, Naito S, *et al.* Development and validation of an ECG algorithm for identifying the optimal ablation site for idiopathic ventricular outflow tract tachycardia. J Cardiovasc Electrophysiol 2003; 14(12): 1280-6.

18. Lin D, Ilkhanoff L, Gerstenfeld E, *et al.* Twelve-lead electrocardiographic characteristics of the aortic cusp region guided by intracardiac echocardiography and electroanatomic mapping. Heart Rhythm 2008; 5(5): 663-9.

19. Yamada T, Yoshida N, Murakami Y, *et al.* Electrocardiographic characteristics of ventricular arrhythmias originating from the junction of the left and right coronary sinuses of Valsalva in the aorta: the activation pattern as a rationale for the electrocardiographic characteristics. Heart Rhythm 2008; 5(2): 184-92.

20. Bala R, Garcia F, Hutchinson M, *et al.* Electrocardiographic and electrophysiologic features of ventricular arrhythmias originating from the right/left coronary cusp commissure. Heart Rhythm 2009; 7(3): 312-22.

21. Daniels DV, Lu YY, Morton JB, *et al.* Idiopathic epicardial left ventricular tachycardia originating remote from the sinus of Valsalva: electrophysiological characteristics, catheter ablation, and identification from the 12-lead electrocardiogram. Circulation 2006; 113(13): 1659-66.

22. Azegami K, Wilber DJ, Arruda M, *et al.* Spatial resolution of pacemapping and activation mapping in patients with idiopathic right ventricular outflow tract tachycardia. J Cardiovasc Electrophysiol 2005; 16(8): 823-9.

23. Man KC, Daoud EG, Knight BP, *et al.* Accuracy of the unipolar electrogram for identification of the site of origin of ventricular activation. J Cardiovasc Electrophysiol 1997; 8(9): 974-9.

24. Soejima Y, Aonuma K, Iesaka Y, *et al.* Ventricular unipolar potential in radiofrequency catheter ablation of idiopathic non-reentrant ventricular outflow tachycardia. Jpn Heart J 2004; 45(5): 749-60.

25. Stevenson WG, Soejima K. Recording techniques for clinical electrophysiology. J Cardiovasc Electrophysiol 2005; 16(9): 1017-22.

26. Goyal R, Harvey M, Daoud EG, *et al.* Effect of coupling interval and pacing cycle length on morphology of paced ventricular complexes. Implications for pace mapping. Circulation 1996; 94(11): 2843-9.

27. Kamakura S, Shimizu W, Matsuo K, *et al.* Localization of optimal ablation site of idiopathic ventricular tachycardia from right and left ventricular outflow tract by body surface ECG. Circulation 1998; 98(15): 1525-33.

28. Bogun F, Taj M, Ting M, *et al.* Spatial resolution of pace mapping of idiopathic ventricular tachycardia/ectopy originating in the right ventricular outflow tract. Heart Rhythm 2008; 5(3): 339-44.

29. Timmermans C, Rodriguez LM, Crijns HJ, *et al.* Idiopathic left bundle-branch block-shaped ventricular tachycardia may originate above the pulmonary valve. Circulation 2003; 108(16): 1960-7.

30. Vaseghi M, Cesario DA, Mahajan A, *et al.* Catheter ablation of right ventricular outflow tract tachycardia: value of defining coronary anatomy. J Cardiovasc Electrophysiol 2006; 17(6): 632-7.

Chapter 6. Ablation of atrial fibrillation: who, when and how?

M. Nadal, L. Mont

Thorax Institute, Hospital Clínic
University of Barcelona
Institut d'Investigació Biomèdica
August Pi i Sunyer (IDIBAPS)

Address for correspondence:
Thorax Institute
Hospital Clinic, University of Barcelona
Dr. Lluís Mont
lmont@clinic.ub.es

Atrial fibrillation (AF) is the most frequent sustained cardiac arrhythmia, and catheter ablation has evolved in the last decade from a nearly experimental and uncertain procedure to a routine and well-established procedure. Due to the efficacy and positive effect on quality of life,[1-2] together with the relatively low rate of complications, the indications for catheter ablation have expanded rapidly. Technological advances have helped operators to perform the procedure with a more detailed anatomical approach, reducing radiation exposure and lowering the required time for both left atrium (LA) mapping and pulmonary vein (PV) ablation. All efforts are now focused on obtaining the safest and most efficient strategy.

1   Indications for AF ablation: "who"

Symptomatic AF refractory or intolerant to antiarrhythmic medication remains the only well-established indication for AF ablation as described in the consensus statement from the Heart Rhythm Society (indication class IIb with level of evidence C).[3] However, on top of this broad indication, a high preprocedural probability of success seems a reasonable requirement, together with a satisfactory risk/benefit ratio. Preprocedural predictors of AF recurrence after circumferential pulmonary vein ablation (CPVA) might be useful for selecting candidates and avoiding unsuccessful procedures. Up to now, the most powerful and independent preprocedural predictors of recurrences after AF ablation are *left atrial size* and *persistent* or *long-standing AF*.[4-7]

Whether or not to ablate long-standing persistent AF patients is debated in another chapter. However, it is important to acknowledge here that ablation success decreases in persistent and long-standing AF overall, although there are significant differences among the published series, depending on patient selection, operator experience, technical aspects and methodology for AF recurrence monitoring in the follow-up.[4,6,7] Efficacy ranges from 50% to 70% or higher after several procedures. Therefore, although not as successful as in paroxysmal AF, ablation is a good option in most patients with persistent AF.

It is crucial to attempt to identify the AF etiology in every patient, not only because it may influence the success of the procedure, but also because it can help in designing the associated therapy.

- *Hypertension* allows us to classify patients into four subgroups with increasing probabilities of recurrence, from <15% in those with LAD ≤45 mm without hypertension to ~50% in hypertensive patients with LAD >45 mm (see figure 1).[4]
- On the other hand, it is conceivable that strict treatment with antihypertensive agents may decrease recurrences in the long term.
- *Obstructive sleep apnea (OSA) patients.* Some studies have shown a consistent and strong association between OSA and ablation outcomes, suggesting OSA as an independent predictor of ablation failure. However, most of them are retrospective studies or analyzed OSA based on Berlin Questionnaire results as an estimation of risk[8-10]. In a prospective study,[11] OSA seems to be the strongest predictive factor for AF ablation failure (see figure 2). Additional prospective studies are required to analyze the potential role of Continuous Positive Pressure in decreasing recurrences.
- The etiological role of long-term *endurance sport* in AF has been increasingly recognized.[12] CPVA in AF in that population seems to be as effective as in non-endurance sport related lone AF.[13]
- *Advanced age* is in itself an etiological factor for AF. Due to the aging of the population, the number of people suffering from AF is rapidly increasing. The addition of frequent comorbidities such as hypertension, diabetes, ischemic heart disease or valve diseases gives the elderly an especially high risk for thromboembolism, which forces us to focus all our efforts to prevent embolic events.[14] Nevertheless, almost all of the published AF ablation trials have been performed with patients at a mean age of <60 years. The small amount

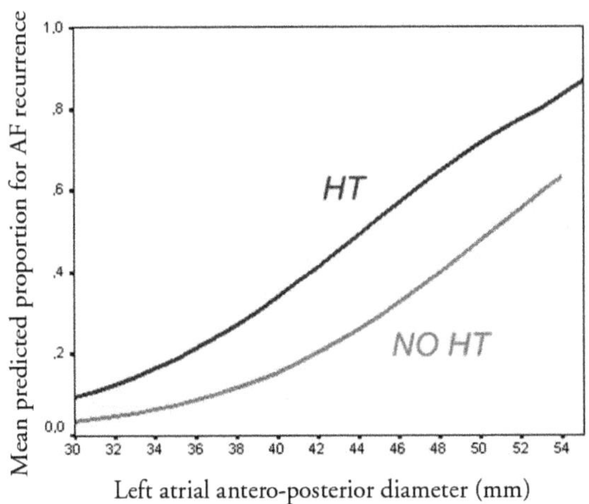

Figure 1. The mean predicted proportion of patients with atrial fibrillation (AF) recurrence after ablation procedure, related to anteroposterior left atrial diameter (expressed in millimetres) and to the presence of hypertension. Reference 4.
HT = hypertension.

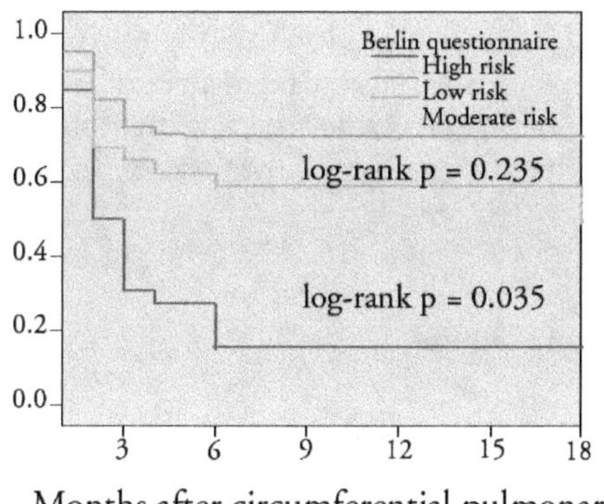

Months after circumferential pulmonary
vein ablation

Figure 2. Kaplan-Meier curves for long-term freedom from recurrent arrhythmias after AF ablation based on OSA risk score group (low risk for OSA, moderate risk for OSA and high risk for OSA). Reference 11.

of data published about elderly patients seems to conclude that AF ablation might be as effective and safe as in younger patients.[15-17] Some studies have specifically analyzed ablation outcomes in elderly patients. The Corrado group reviewed a series of 175 consecutive patients over 75 years of age who underwent AF ablation, showing 73% maintaining sinus rhythm with a single procedure, without significant complications. Zado *et al.* divided the patients into three age groups: <65 years (n = 948), 65-75 years (n = 185) and >75 years (n = 32), without observing significant differences in AF control (89%, 84%, and 86%, respectively; p = NS). A more recent study demonstrated consistent results in octogenarian patients, despite the small number of enrolled patients (n = 35).

- *AF ablation in heart failure patients.* Pharmacological trials and studies of various ablation strategies (such as AFFIRM and AF-CHF) failed to show a benefit of rhythm control for a low left ventricular ejection fraction (LVEF) population.[18-20] In the AF-CHF trial, 1,376 patients with severe systolic dysfunction were randomized to rhythm and rate-control strategies. No differences in cardiovascular death were observed between the two groups and new hospitalizations were more frequently required in the rhythm-control group due to AF and bradyarrhythmia, which probably reflects the need for repeated cardioversion and antiarrhythmic therapy adjustment. Whether AF ablation may lead to an increase in survival remains to be proven. However, some small studies have recognized the benefits of ablative therapy in this population. A recent non-randomized study[20] compared 94 patients with impaired ejection fraction (EF) and 283 patients with normal EF, observing that 73% of patients with impaired EF were free of AF recurrences at 14 ± 6 months, compared with 87% of patients with preserved EF (p = 0.03), which suggests that pulmonary vein isolation might be a feasible therapeutic option in these patients. A case-control study (1:1) with 72 patients found no differences in the probability of AF recurrences in patients with depressed versus normal LVEF.[21] In that study, LA diameter seemed to be the only variable correlated to recurrence and after 6 months of follow-up, the low EF group showed a significant increase in EF. AF ablation may have a significant benefit in patients with impaired EF, mainly when systolic dysfunction is secondary to AF (tachycardiomyopathy), but further studies are still required.

- *Severe limitations to AF ablation.* Ablation should probably be discouraged or at least carefully balanced in patients with highly enlarged atrium (anteroposterior diameter >50 mm) and long-standing AF of 5 years. Other special situations that have been associated with poor results include rheumatic mitral valve disease and hypertrophic cardiomyopathy with enlarged atrium.[22,23]

2   Timing for AF ablation: "when"

AF ablation consensus recommends catheter ablation in symptomatic AF refractory or intolerant to at least one class I or III antiarrhythmic medication.[3] Once the pharmacological therapy has failed in the attempt to maintain sinus rhythm, ablation strategy should be encouraged without delay, since the longer the AF duration, the larger the left atrial remodelling will be and the lower the success of any therapeutic strategy intended to maintain sinus rhythm.[24] In some clinical situations, it could be appropriate to perform catheter ablation of AF as a first line therapy:

- In patients who can expect a great benefit, such as highly symptomatic patients with congestive heart failure and/or depressed ejection fraction.[20]
- In highly symptomatic patients with a high probability of success who are reluctant to take antiarrhythmic drug therapy.

3   Ablation technique: "how"

The choice between segmental ostial ablation and antral ablation requires a short history lesson. A progressive understanding of the mechanisms of AF explains the different catheter ablation strategies that have been used since Swartz and colleagues recreated Maze-I lesion in a small series of patients using an RF catheter ablation procedure.[25] One of the major steps was the recognition by Haïssaguerre *et al.* of the ectopic "triggers" that precipitate AF.[26] On the other hand, another important step was the creation of large antral lesions to modify the substrate as initially described by Pappone *et al.*[27] The most commonly employed ablation strategy today is probably a blend of both these ablation techniques that involves the electrical isolation of the PVs, together with an antral ablation that probably has an impact on both the trigger and the substrate of AF.[28] These encircling lesions reduce the available area for circulating wavelets needed to perpetuate AF; they eliminate triggers and perhaps denervate the atrium by ablating autonomic ganglia.[29]

4   The use of navigating systems and image merging

The regular use of 3D navigating systems certainly facilitates the ablation procedure by giving a 3D virtual image of the atrium. It allows us to follow ablation lines, since the location of the ablation catheter is related to anatomy and not only to the 2D x-ray image (see figure 3).[30-31] On the other hand, the possibility to merge the 3D image obtained with the catheters with the previous MRI or CT scan image may uncover pulmonary vein abnormalities or complex anatomy.

However, these systems still have important limitations. A careful technique should be used to map and to merge the images, to ensure good concordance between the shell and real anato-

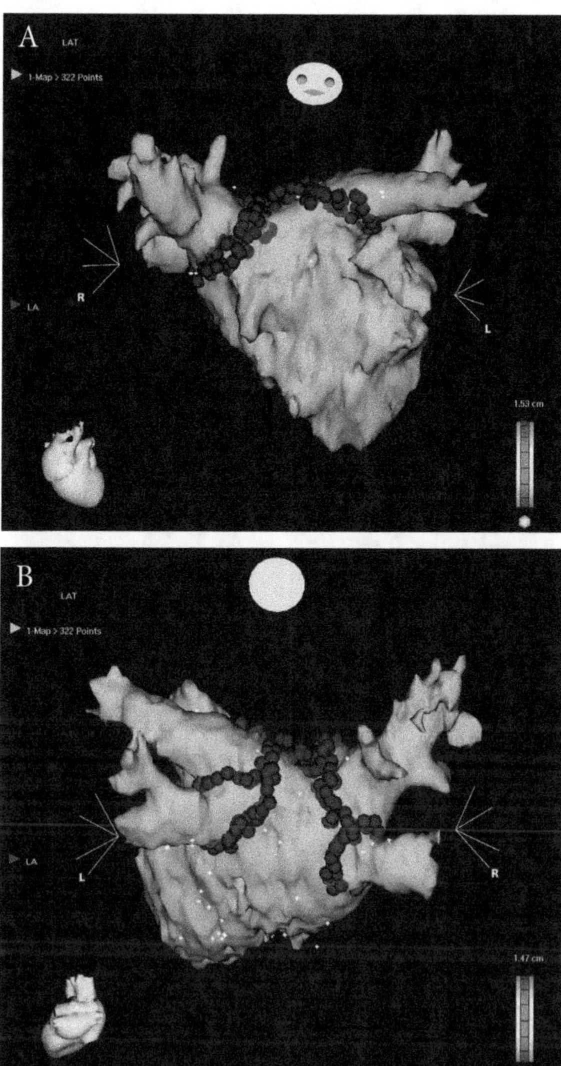

Figure 3. Left atrium images reconstructed from the 3D non-fluoroscopic mapping system (CARTO) once circumferential and roof line ablation lesions are performed. Anteroposterior (A) and posteroanterior views (B).

my. Furthermore, patient movement or impedance changes during the procedure may cause the obtained shell to move, and the map should then be repeated. Testing the position of the catheter in relation to PV or appendage reference positions during the procedure is mandatory.

5   LA additional linear lesions

Other strategies have been used to improve outcomes. Linear lesions in the LA have been performed, most commonly the LA roof line connecting the superior aspects of the left and right upper PV isolation lesions, and the mitral isthmus line, between the mitral valve and the left inferior PV. These additional lines were initially described to eliminate macro reentrant tachycardias around the PV isolation lines.[32] However, ablation lines are now used mainly as an additional strategy in patients with persistent AF to eliminate sources of AF that arise on the posterior wall of the left atrium, and to reduce the incidence of LA macro reentrant AT.[33] Some studies have demonstrated a benefit derived from performing additional lines in the LA,[32,34] but if these lines are applied, complete conduction block should be demonstrated to avoid residual gaps that may perpetuate macro reentrant tachycardias. Complete block is not easily achieved, particularly at the mitral isthmus, where it might be necessary to complete the ablation line within the coronary sinus. Although it has been suggested that the LA posterior wall contains potential triggers and may support sustained AF, a recent randomized study failed to demonstrate any additional benefit of posterior wall isolation.[35]

6 Complex fractionated atrial electrograms: electrogram-guided atrial fibrillation ablation

In patients with persistent and long-standing persistent AF, ostial PV isolation alone may not be sufficient, because extensive atrial fibrosis increases the number of AF drivers and shifts their location away from the PV/ostial regions.[36] Complex fractionated atrial electrograms (CFAEs) might define areas related to underlying fibrosis or slow conduction, suggested by Nademanee *et al.* as potential targets for ablation.[37] Alternatively, however, they may represent only areas of wavelet collision. CFAEs are described as low-voltage electrograms (0.05 to 0.25 mV) with highly fractionated potentials or with a very short cycle length (120 ms).[38] However, the concept of CFAE definition and the role of CFAE ablation is still under debate. Oral *et al.* enrolled 100 patients with chronic AF and performed RF ablation of extensive CFAE areas until AF terminated or all identified CFAEs were eliminated; however, only 57% of patients remained free of arrhythmia recurrence without antiarrhythmic drugs, >40% of them after a second ablation, which represents a modest short-term efficacy.[39] In a subsequent study, they enrolled 100 patients with long-standing persistent AF who remained in AF after antral pulmonary vein isolation (APVI), randomized to CFAE ablation or no further ablation.[40] In this study, up to 2 hours of additional CFAE ablation after APVI did not improve clinical outcomes, measured as sinus rhythm at 10±3 months of follow-up (34% versus 36%, respectively, p = 0.84). CFAE ablation may be considered, if PV isolation is judged insufficient, as an additional strategy in long-standing persistent AF, but further studies are needed to document its usefulness.

7 Complications

Catheter ablation is one of the most laborious electrophysiological procedures, and although complication rates have been decreasing with the operators[3] learning curve and technical improvement, major complications are still present in 6% of patients, based on the outcomes presented by a worldwide survey on the methods, efficacy and safety of catheter ablation of AF,[41] published in 2005.

Most of the complications appear during or immediately after the procedure, and only some of them will be detected during follow up. Cardiac tamponade is the most common potentially life-threatening complication of PV ablation, occurring in up to 6% of procedures, depend-

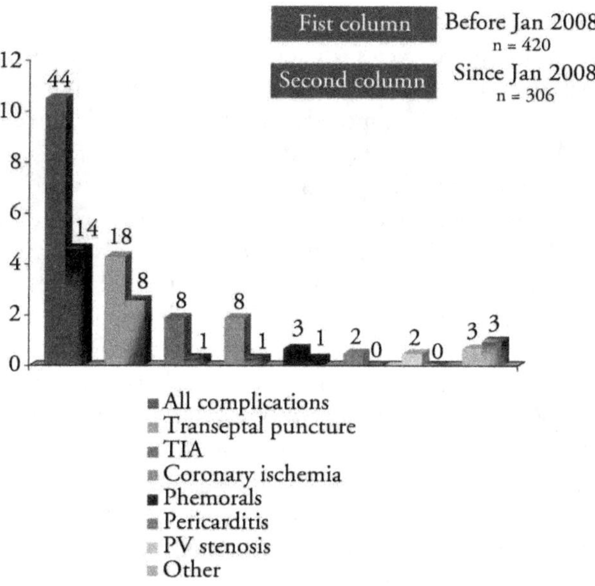

Figure 4. Periprocedural complications in PV ablation procedures. Differences between the procedures performed before and after January 2008. Reference 48.

ing on proper systemic anticoagulation and the operator's technical skills, especially with respect to transeptal punctures, catheter manipulation and avoiding cardiac perforation during ablation. The most common problems are pulmonary vein stenosis and vascular and thromboembolism complications, with incidence rates varying from 0% to 38%, 13% and 7%, respectively. Most of these are strictly related to methodology and individual experience, and other potential complications are very uncommon.

In our series, the implementation of a standardized protocol of anticoagulation and conscious sedation, in addition to operator experience, has made possible a reduction in total significant complications from 10.5% to 4.6% (see figure 4).

8   New ablation tools

Progressive technical improvement and standardization of the procedure have helped operators to improve ablation outcomes, reducing the radiation burden with non-fluoroscopic navigation systems, the duration of the procedure, and of course, complications. Cooled tip ablation catheters and multielectrode circular mapping catheters are typically used,[42] and mapping with a circular catheter to ensure PV isolation seems to ensure better results.[43] New tools may facilitate the ablation procedures:

- *Remote robotic navigation systems* may improve catheter manipulation and ensure better contact, and the process may be automated to create previously designed lesions. Finally, it reduces the x-ray burden for both operator and patient.[44] However, despite initial high expectations, in their present form, the systems have severe limitations. For example, when remote magnetic navigation is used in conjunction with electroanatomical mapping, the accuracy of the lesions depends on the correctness of the shell, which, as previously discussed, still has some inaccuracies. In addition, PV isolation often has to be completed manually. Finally, its cost-effectiveness has not been carefully evaluated.

- *Cryoballoon ablation* has been proposed as a faster and simpler method of PV isolation.[45,46] It consists of a balloon that is inflated at the ostium of the PV, where thermic injury is applied. Although the system has proven efficacious in achieving PV isolation, it has some technical limitations, since the balloon has to adapt to the anatomy of each patient and it cannot be used in the left main artery. Furthermore, there is a clear risk of phrenic paralysis when isolating the right superior pulmonary vein, and there is a potential for PV rupture if excessive pressure is applied. Prospective randomized studies are needed to demonstrate the superiority of this technique as compared to RF ablation.

- *Duty cycled RF ablation* has been proposed as an alternative approach to AF ablation.[47] The possibility to apply energy through multiple electrodes at the PV antrum may achieve isolation faster and more safely, avoiding the need for detailed electroanatomical reconstruction. Specific catheters have been designed to ensure CFAE ablation at the septal level and other regions of the left atrium. Further randomized comparative studies will show whether this new approach has advantages over the traditional RF ablation systems.

8   Periprocedural anticoagulation and other considerations

Although different substantial anticoagulation strategies are used, there is a consensus among Task Force members that patients with persistent AF who are in AF at the time of ablation should receive a transesophageal echocardiography to screen for thrombus, regardless of anticoagulation prior to ablation, to reduce periprocedural embolization (typically due to sheath-related thrombi), as well as heparin infusion during the procedure to achieve and maintain an ACT of at least 300 seconds. Finally, after catheter ablation and sheath removal, anticoagulation should be reinitiated within 4 to 6 hours and maintained for at least 2 months. Decisions regarding discontinuation of anticoagulation therapy must be based on the patient risk factors for stroke (CHADS score). Continuous irrigation systems and careful manipulation of the sheaths, especially during removal, are imperative to avoid thrombus formation and embolization, as well as the introduction of air into the transeptal sheath through the infusion line. Finally, with the exception of high-risk patients, in agreement with the Task Force Consensus, intravenous conscious sedation is usually preferred, although the choice is determined by the institution.[3] In our center, a standardized protocol of conscious sedation and anticoagulation has been helpful to reduce procedural complications.[48]

Conclusions

The evolving indications for AF catheter ablation and the growing prevalence of AF in our population are generating increased demand for experienced centers to perform AF ablation procedures. Electrophysiologists should develop their technical skills; the evolving technology will help trainees to achieve the best outcomes with the minimal risks. All recognized factors, whether technical or patient-related, such as age, hypertension, type of AF and LA size, as well as the risks and potential benefits of the procedure, must be weighed carefully to choose the best therapeutic strategy for each selected patient.

References

1. Jais P, Cauchemez B, Macle L, *et al.* Catheter ablation versus antiarrhythmic drugs for atrial fibrillation: The A4 Study. Circulation 2008; 118: 2498-505.

2. Pappone C, Augello G, Sala S, *et al.* A randomized trial of circumferential pulmonary vein ablation versus antiarrhythmic drug therapy in paroxysmal atrial fibrillation: the APAF Study. J Am Coll Cardiol 2006; 48: 2340-47.

3. HRS/EHRA/ECAS Expert Consensus Statement on Catheter and Surgical Ablation of Atrial Fibrillation: Recommendations for Personnel, Policy, Procedures and Follow-up: Calkins H, Brugada J, Packer DL, *et al.* Europace 2007; 9: 335-79.

4. Berruezo A, Tamborero D, Mont L, *et al.* Pre-procedural predictors of atrial fibrillation recurrence after circumferential pulmonary vein ablation. Eur Heart J 2007; 28: 836-41.

5. Arya A, Hindricks G, Sommer P, *et al.* Long-term results and the predictors of outcome of catheter ablation of atrial fibrillation using steerable sheath catheter navigation after a single procedure of 674 patients. Europace 2010; 12: 173-80.

6. De Potter T, Tavernier R, Devos D, *et al.* Predictors of success after a first circumferential pulmonary vein isolation for atrial fibrillation. J Atrial Fibrillation 2009; 1: 311-20.

7. Vasamreddy CR, Lickfett L, Jayam VK, *et al.* Predictors of recurrence following catheter ablation of atrial fibrillation using an irrigated-tip ablation catheter. J Cardiovasc Electrophysiol 2004; 15: 692-97.

8. Jongnarangsin K, Chugh A, Good E, *et al.* Body mass index, obstructive sleep apnea, and outcomes of catheter ablation of atrial fibrillation. J Cardiovasc Electrophysiol 2008; 19: 668-72.

9. Chilukuri K, Dalal D, Marine JE, *et al.* Predictive value of obstructive sleep apnoea assessed by the Berlin Questionnaire for outcomes after the catheter ablation of atrial fibrillation. Europace 2009; 11: 896-901.

10. Tang RB, Dong JZ, Liu XP, *et al.* Obstructive sleep apnoea risk profile and the risk of recurrence of atrial fibrillation after catheter ablation. Europace 2009; 11: 100-05.

11. Matiello M, Berruezo A, Tamborero D, *et al.* Obstructive sleep apnoea is an independent predictor of recurrences after circumferential pulmonary vein ablation for atrial fibrillation. Europace 2010 (in press).

12. Molina L, Mont L, Marrugat J, *et al.* Long-term endurance sport practice increases the incidence of lone atrial fibrillation in men: a follow-up study. Europace 2008; 10: 618-23.

13. Calvo N, Mont Ll, Tamborero D, *et al.* Efficacy of circumferential pulmonary vein ablation of atrial fibrillation in endurance athletes. Europace 2010; 12: 30-6.

14. Wetzel U, Hindricks I, Piorkowski C. Atrial fibrillation in the elderly. Minerva Med 2009; 100: 145-50.

15. Corrado A, Patel D, Riedlbauchova L, *et al.* Efficacy, safety and outcomes of atrial fibrillation ablation in septuagenarians. J Cardiovasc Electrophysiol 2008; 19: 807-11.

16. Zado E, Callans DJ, Riley M, *et al.* Long-term clinical efficacy and risk of catheter ablation for atrial fibrillation in the elderly. J Cardiovasc Electrophysiol 2008; 19: 621-26.

17. Bunch TJ, Weiss JP, Crandall BG, *et al.* Long-term clinical efficacy and risk of catheter ablation of atrial fibrillation in octogenarians. Pacing Clin Electrophysiol 2009 (in press).

18. Van Gelder IC, Hagens VE, Bosker HA, *et al.* A comparison of rate control and rhythm control in patients with atrial fibrillation. N Engl J Med 2002; 347: 1834-840.

19. Roy D, Talajic M, Nattel S, *et al.* Rhythm control versus rate control for atrial fibrillation and heart failure. N Engl J Med 2008; 358: 2667-77.

20. Chen MS, Marrouche NF, Khaykin Y, *et al.* Pulmonary vein isolation for the treatment of atrial fibrillation in patients with impaired systolic function. J Am Coll Cardiol 2004; 43: 1004-9.

21. De Potter T, Berruezo A, Mont L, *et al.* Left ventricular systolic dysfunction by itself does not influence outcome of atrial fibrillation. Europace 2010; 12: 24-9.

22. Bunch TJ, Munger TM, Friedman PA, *et al.* Substrate and procedural predictors of outcomes after catheter ablation for atrial fibrillation in patients with hypertrophic cardiomyopathy. J Cardiovasc Electrophysiol 2008; 19: 1009-14.

23. Favad G, Le Tourneau T, Modine T, *et al.* Endocardial radiofrequency ablation during mitral valve surgery: effect on cardiac rhythm, atrial size, and function. Ann Thorac Surg 2005; 79: 1505-11.

24. Kirchhof P, Bax J, Blomstrom-Lundquist C, *et al.* Early and comprehensive management of atrial fibrillation: executive summary of the proceedings from the 2nd AFNET-EHRA consensus conference 'research perspectives in AF'. Eur Heart J 2009; 30: 2969-77c.

25. Swartz JF, Pellerseis G, Silvers J, *et al.* A catheter based curative approach to atrial fibrillation in humans. Circulation 1994; 90(Sup): 1-335.

26. Haïssaguerre M, Jaïs P, Shah P, et al. Spontaneous initiation of atrial fibrillation by ectopic beats originating in the pulmonary veins. N Engl J Med 1998; 339: 659-66.

27. Pappone C, Santinelli V. Segmental pulmonary vein isolation versus the circumferential approach: is the tide turning? Heart Rhythm 2004; 1: 326-28.

28. Lemola K, Oral H, Chugh A, *et al.* Pulmonary vein isolation as an end point for left atrial circumferential ablation of atrial fibrillation. J Am Coll Cardiol 2005; 46: 1060-66.

29. Pappone C, Oreto G, Rosanio S, *et al.* Atrial electroanatomic remodeling after circumferential radiofrequency pulmonary vein ablation: Efficacy of an anatomic approach in a large cohorte of patients with atrial fibrillation. Circulation 2001; 104: 2539-544.

30. Schreieck J, Ndrepepa G, Zrenner B, *et al.* Radiofrequency ablation of cardiac arrhythmias using a three-dimensional real time position management and mapping system. Pacing Clin Electrphysiol 2002; 25: 1699-707.

31. Sporton SC, Earley MJ, Nathan AW, *et al.* Electroanatomic versus fluoroscopic mapping for catheter ablation

procedures: a prospective randomized study. J Cardiovasc Electrophysiol 2004; 15: 310-15.

32. Pappone C, Manguso F, Vicedomini G, *et al*. Prevention of iatrogenic atrial tachycardia after ablation of atrial fibrillation: a prospective randomized study comparing circumferential pulmonary vein ablation with a modified approach. Circulation 2004; 110: 3036-42.

33. Knecth S, Hocini M, Wright M, *et al*. Left atrial linear lesions are required for successful treatment of persistent atrial fibrillation. Eur Heart J 2008; 29: 2359-66.

34. Oral H, Scharf C, Chugh A, *et al*. Catheter ablation for paroxysmal atria fibrillation: segmental pulmonary vein ostial ablation versus left atrial ablation. Circulation 2003; 108: 2355-360.

35. Tamborero D, Mont Ll, Berruezo A, *et al*. Left atrial posterior wall isolation does not improve the outcome of circumferential pulmonary vein ablation for atrial fibrillation. Circ Arrhythmia Electrophysiol 2009; 2: 35-40.

36. Oakes RS, Badger TJ, Kholmouski EG, *et al*. Detection and quantification of left atrial structural remodeling with delayed-enhancement magnetic resonance imaging in patients with atrial fibrillation. Circulation 2009; 119: 1758-67.

37. Nademanee K, McKenzie J, Kosar E, *et al*. A new approach for catheter ablation of atrial fibrillation: mapping of the electrophysiologic substrate. J Am Coll Cardiol 2004; 43: 2044-53.

38. Nademanee K. Trials and travails of electrogram-guided ablation of chronic atrial fibrillation. Circulation 2007; 115: 2592-4.

39. Oral H, Chugh A, Good E, *et al*. Radiofrequency catheter ablation of chronic atrial fibrillation guided by complex electrograms. Circulation 2007; 115: 2606-12.

40. Oral H, Chug A, Yoshida K, *et al*. Randomized Assessment of the incremental role of ablation of complex fractionated atrial electrograms after antral pulmonary vein isolation for long-standing persistent atrial fibrillation. J Am Coll Cardiol 2009; 53: 782-9.

41. Cappato R, Calkins H, Chen SA, *et al*. A worldwide survey on the methods, efficacy, and safety of catheter ablation for human atrial fibrillation. Circulation 2005; 111: 1100-5.

42. Matiello M, Mont Ll, Tamborero D, *et al*. Cooled-tip vs. 8 mm-tip catheter for circumferential pulmonary vein ablation: comparison of efficacy, safety, and lesion extension. Europace 2008; 10: 955-60.

43. Tamborero D, Mont L, Berruezo A, *et al*. Circumferential Pulmonary Vein Ablation: does the use of a circular mapping catheter improve results? A prospective randomized study (in press).

44. Schmidt B, Tilz RR, Neven K, *et al*. Remote robotic navigation and electroanatomical mapping for ablation of atrial fibrillation: considerations for navigation and impact on procedural outcome Circ Arrhythm Electrophysiol 2009; 2: 120-8.

45. Chun KR, Schmidt B, Metzner A, *et al*. The "single big cryoballoon" technique for acute pulmonary vein isolation in patients with paroxysmal atrial fibrillation: a prospective observational simple centre study. Eur Heart J 2009; 30: 699-709.

46. Siklódy CH, Minners J, Allgeier M, *et al*.Cryoballon pulmonary vein isolation guided by transesophageal echocardiography: novel aspect of an emerging ablation technique. J Cardiovasc Electrophysiol 2009;26 (in press).

47. Scharf C, Boersma L, Davies W, *et al*. Ablation of persistent atrial fibrillation using multielectrode catheters and duty-cycled radiofrequency energy. J Am Coll Cardiol 2009; 54: 1450-6.

48. Nadal M, Mont L, Berruezo A, *et al*. Factores relacionados con la reducción de las complicaciones durante la ablación de la fibrilación auricular. Rev Esp Cardiol 2009; 62, 3: 65.

Chapter 7. Ablation of left atrial flutter: how to go from a nightmare to cure

M. Wright,[1] M. Hocini,[2] P. Jaïs,[2] M. Haïssaguerre[2]

[1]St Thomas' Hospital
London, UK

[2]Hôpital Cardiologique du Haut-Lévêque
Université Victor Segalen Bordeaux II
Bordeaux-Pessac, France

Address for correspondence:
Hôpital Cardiologique du
Haut-Lévêque
Service de Rythmologie
Dr. M. Wright
Matthew.Wright@kcl.ac.uk

Introduction: the nightmare

Catheter ablation is now an established treatment modality for the most common sustained arrhythmia, atrial fibrillation (AF).[1] Although pulmonary vein isolation alone is sufficient for most patients with paroxysmal AF, for patients with persistent AF, a more extensive ablative strategy is necessary. Unfortunately, with increasing ablation of the AF substrate, a growing problem is one of secondary atrial tachycardias (AT).[1-3] During catheter ablation of persistent AF, transition to AT during the index procedure is often the indispensable step before the long-term restoration of sinus rhythm and is one of the key goals of the extensive ablation procedure.[2] In most cases patients have several different ATs and an approach that is dependent upon a 3D mapping system alone can be very time consuming. This is especially tiring for the operator after a long procedure required to terminate AF. A further problem is that of recurrent atrial tachycardia following AF ablation, which is very common with these secondary AT often being incessant and very poorly tolerated by the patient, more so than their original AF, and a proactive catheter ablation strategy rather than "wait and see" approach may be preferred.

The ablation of these ATs is particularly challenging. In this chapter our approach to these ATs is described, using conventional electrophysiological techniques, without the need for 3D mapping systems (see figure 1). The techniques described have been well established in our laboratory for a large number of patients, and using these techniques ATs can be rapidly diagnosed and successfully treated. In patients who have AT during the index procedure we aim to treat these ATs to restore sinus rhythm. In patients who experience AT within the first two months following an ablation, DC cardioversion, and antiarrhythmic drugs are tried initially to maintain sinus rhythm, or, at the very least to control the ventricular rate. Typically, after allowing the acute inflammatory response to pass and healing of lesions to complete, the patient is taken back for a repeated procedure.

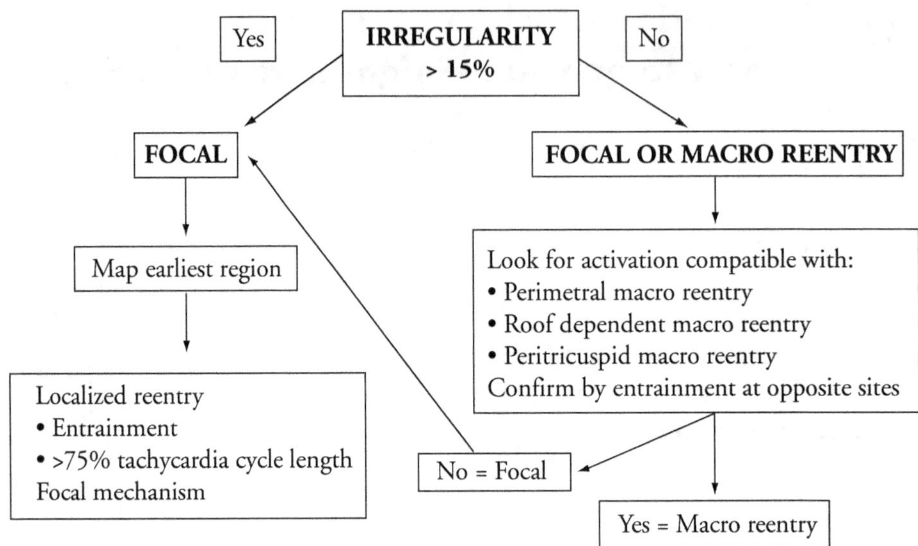

Figure 1. Diagnostic algorithm.

1   The diagnostic approach: the cure

1.2   Know thy enemy

Mechanisms of AT after prior AF ablation vary with the ablation approach taken for the treatment and type of AF (either persistent or paroxysmal). While focal origins from reconnected PVs are common after ostial PV isolation,[4-6] macro and localized reentrant AT are more frequent after a more extensive AF ablation.[2,3,7-9] However, the mapping and ablation strategy during ongoing AT remains similar whatever ablation approach was previously performed. The approach that is taken in our laboratory consists of three successive steps as follows: firstly a PV origin to the tachycardia is assessed, following this we assess for macro reentry and finally, we map for a focal origin (either focal point or localized reentry AT).

1.3   The techniques

There are two important introductory points:

- It is possible to map the direction of the activation between two segments of the left atrium simply and rapidly with the roving ablation catheter and a fixed atrial reference catheter. Although we do not routinely use 3D mapping systems, this point is critical even when using these systems, as it is of key importance to understand the direction of activation in order to correctly annotate the activation within the window of interest. Failure to do so and rely entirely upon the system without thought to local activation in relation to neighboring regions will result in erroneous maps.

- It is important to combine both activation mapping with entrainment mapping : the latter either confirms or refutes the mechanism suggested by the first. Activation mapping can be performed without fear of changing the tachycardia, which is why this is performed initially, whereas entrainment mapping can result in a change in tachycardia, which is why it is performed after the activation sequence of the atria has been deduced. In this way, even if the tachycardia is changed by the entrainment manouver, a reasonable guess can be made to the nature of the AT.

1.3.1　Step 1. Exclude cavotricuspid isthmus-dependent reentry

Cavotricuspid isthmus (CTI)-dependent reentry in the setting of markedly abnormal atrial substrate, in the context of AF ablation, rarely manifests with a typical 12-lead ECG appearance. So-called pseudo-atypical flutter can be rapidly diagnosed or excluded by mapping of the tricuspid annulus and by entrainment maneuvers on the CTI. This is performed first as the activation sequence can be quickly deduced prior to entering the left atrium, by mapping the right atrium and observation of the activation sequence of the coronary sinus.

1.3.2　Step 2. Exclude pulmonary vein-dependent AT

The pulmonary veins are an important source of AT, particularly because of their propensity to recover conduction.[10] Pulmonary vein reconduction requires reablation at the gap(s) to ensure pulmonary vein isolation for all patients, even when they are not the culprit for the presenting AT. An origin of AT from the pulmonary veins can be rapidly ruled out by placing a standard quadripolar ablation catheter into the pulmonary vein and demonstrating proximal to distal activation, indicating passive venous activation at all segments of the vein (superior, inferior, anterior and posterior). Very often even though the vein has been reconnected, it cannot maintain a 1:1 relationship with the body of the left atrium, again quickly ruling out a pulmonary vein tachycardia. If however there is a distal to proximal activation sequence in the vein, a pulmonary vein tachycardia is likely. Entrainment mapping can be used in both cases to either confirm or refute the diagnosis; however in the case of a passive activation of the pulmonary veins this would be done after activation mapping of the atrium.

Where prior ablation has only involved PV isolation, the P-wave morphology may be useful in identifying the culprit PV.[11] Isolation is performed as proximal as possible, following the same ablation line as the one performed during the initial AF ablation procedure. A circumferential mapping catheter is helpful to map the earliest activity and the presence of a reversal of polarity between two adjacent bipoles at a breakthrough site.[12] Reisolation of PVs is often quick due to the slow conduction resulting from the initial ablation procedure. While pacing maneuvers during sinus rhythm can easily distinguish PVs from far-field potentials, other methods are required during AT. Firstly, the activation sequence of PV potentials often displays bracketing on the circumferential catheter due to prior PV ablation, while that of far-field signals are generally all on time. Secondly, as PV potentials represent local myocardial activity they are usually sharper and larger than far-field potentials. Lastly, if doubt remains, far-field potentials can be unmasked by placing a recording catheter on the presumed structure responsible for the far-field activity and comparing the timing to the unknown potential. In general, far-field potentials can be recorded in the anterior part of the left PVs reflecting activation of the left atrial appendage. In the right superior PV, far-field signals can arise from the anterior part of superior vena cava or right atrium. Other far-field potentials can also be recorded from posterior or inferior LA.

If the PV is implicated in the AT, PV reisolation will lead to either restoration of sinus rhythm or transition to a further AT. Sometimes, reentrant circuits can involve gaps in the lesion sets employed to isolate the PVs. Reisolating the PVs in questions will terminate these ATs.[13,14] Even when a conducting PV is not participating in a particular AT, its reisolation may reduce potential triggers for subsequent ATs.

1.3.3   Step 3. Assessment of AT cycle length stability

We have found that assessment of AT cycle length (CL) is useful to differentiate the tachycardia mechanism.[3] We use a decapolar catheter within the coronary sinus (CS) to assess both the activation sequence and CL assessment. The use of a decapolar rather than quadripolar CS catheter facilitates the identification of a transition from one AT to another during ablation, as patients commonly have several ATs.[3] We use automated CL measurement and annotation that is available with most electrophysiology systems, alternatively ten or more cycles can be measured and the mean cycle length be deduced. The regularity of the tachycardia can be assessed using recordings from the coronary sinus or alternatively from a catheter placed within the left atrial appendage, as this is an alternative stable position with unequivocal electrograms. If the CL variability is greater than 15%, and particularly in the rare cases where the AT has a start–stop pattern, a focal AT is deemed highly likely, and mapping should focus on searching for a centrifugal source (described later). Both focal and macro reentrant AT can have a stable cycle length, with less than 15% variability, and in these cases, we initially investigate for a macro reentrant mechanism as mapping is both simple and rapid.

1.3.4   Step 4. Diagnose or exclude macroreentry (see figure 2)

The number of potential left atrial macro reentry circuits is limited to either perimitral or roof dependent (around the right or left PVs), or combinations of these. A simple combination of conventional activation and entrainment mapping is performed to determine whether the activation is consistent with one of these macro reentrant circuits.

A reference channel from the decapolar CS catheter is arbitrarily chosen based upon clarity and amplitude of the atrial signal. It is important when using the CS catheter to help with mapping that the local atrial signal is identified and the local CS potential is identified. Normally these are of the same timing, but in cases where the CS has been completely disconnected from the left atrium this is not the case. For the purpose of clarity, we shall assume that the CS has not been disconnected when explaining our method; however, if this is the case, mapping is performed in the same manner but the local left atrial signal is mapped using the ablation catheter in the left atrium. The reference channel is placed adjacent to the mapping catheter channel to clearly delineate the AT cycle length, allowing the operator to immediately know which parts (early, mid or late) of the cycle are being mapped by visual inspection and sequential electronic caliper measured delay. Inspection of the CS catheter signals will often demonstrate a consistent activation sequence (sometimes referred to as a "cascade" of activation). In the presence of a consistent CS activation sequence, either with a distal to proximal or proxi-

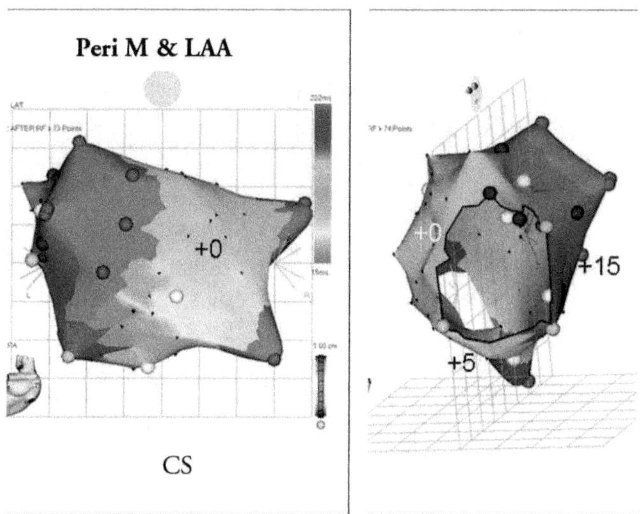

Figure 2. Diagnostic characteristics of macroreentries, localized reentries and focal tachycardias.
Values in the figures refer to PPI-TCL during pacing maneuvers.
Macroreentry: 1. Circuit involving three or more segments of the atrium; 2. >75% of the cycle length
is mapped; 3. Good PPI in three or more segments (at opposite sites).
CS = coronary sinus; LAA = left atrial appendage; Peri M = perimitral; RFD = radiofrequency, distal.

mal to distal configuration, a clockwise or counterclockwise perimitral circuit, respectively, is possible. The CS recordings only indicate posterior mitral annulus activation, and it is important to additionally determine the activation sequence of the anterior mitral annulus. This is achieved by recording lateral and septal points around the anterior mitral annulus. When the anterior annular activation is interpreted in relation to the CS activation and tachycardia CL, perimitral reentry may be suspected based on sequential circumferential activation covering the entire CL. Dragging the catheter while sequentially observing the relationship of the locally recorded signal to the reference channel enables understanding of the activation direction.

- *Mitral line*
  A mitral line is performed to disrupt a circuit around the mitral annulus or in case of persisting AF as a last resort. As such several lines can be performed, such as an anterior line from the anterior mitral annulus to a complete roof line or the isolated right superior pulmonary vein or a septal mitral isthmus line from the septal mitral annulus to the isolated right inferior pulmonary vein. However, the most commonly performed line is the lateral mitral isthmus line, from the lateral mitral annulus to the isolated left inferior pulmonary vein. For this line the coronary sinus catheter is positioned to bracket the potential linear lesion between its proximal and distal bipoles. The ablation catheter is then curved between 90° and 180° and introduced via the long sheath to the ventricular edge of the lateral mitral annulus, with an atrioventricular electrogram ratio of between 1:1 and 2:1. Ablation is then commenced and the sheath and catheter are rotated clockwise to extend the lesion posteriorly, ending at the left inferior pulmonary vein ostium. Ablation energy (35 W) is delivered for up to 120 sec at each site. The lesion is moni-

tored by observing the conduction delay between the local electrogram during pacing relative to the coronary sinus bipole immediately septal to the lesion. If the initial attempt failed to produce complete block, ablation is performed in a more lateral position, at the base of the appendage. Persisting epicardial conduction is suspected when the linear lesion resulted in an endocardial conduction delay recorded on the ablation catheter but not on the adjacent distal bipole of the coronary sinus catheter (lateral of the line). In such cases ablation needs to be performed within the coronary sinus, which is approximately 70% of the time. Ablation within the coronary sinus is performed with a flow rate of between 17-60 mL/min (maximal flow at the distal coronary sinus), a target temperature of 50 °C, and power of 20-30 W.

To assess bidirectional block of the mitral isthmus differential pacing is performed. The ablation catheter is placed just lateral to the line. Using the coronary sinus catheter, stimulation starts using the bipole just septal to the linear lesion, then the pacing site is changed to the next proximal bipole of the coronary sinus catheter without moving any of the catheters. Stimulus-to-atrial electrogram timing on either the ablation catheter or a bipole on the coronary sinus catheter that is lateral to the line, is then measured to the same point on the matching electrogram component before and after changing the pacing site. With complete block, the stimulus-to-electrogram timing is shorter after shifting the pacing site from the distal to the proximal bipole. Pacing lateral to the line through the ablation catheter demonstrates a proximal-to-distal activation sequence along the coronary sinus septal of the line, thus confirming bidirectional conduction block. In addition, widely separated local double potentials along the length of the ablation line during coronary sinus pacing septal to the line can be mapped (see figure 3).

If the activation is not sequential around the mitral annulus, perimitral reentry is excluded and roof-dependent macro reentry is mapped for. The activation wavefront on the anterior and posterior walls of the LA is assessed. The mapping catheter is positioned on the anterior wall (near mitral annulus and then near the roof) to determine the direction of activation in comparison to the previously determined reference channel (e.g., cranial to caudal or vice versa). The posterior wall is then investigated in a similar fashion. In the presence of a similar direction of activation on both walls (e.g., cranial to caudal on both the anterior and posterior wall), the roof is a bystander. If the direction of activation is opposite on the anterior and posterior wall, this rules in the possibility of roof-dependent flutter. It is unnecessarily time-consuming to localize the circuit around the right or left pulmonary veins as a complete roof line treats both possibilities (see figures 4 and 5).

- *Roof line*
  The roof line refers to a contiguous line of ablation lesions joining the right and left superior pulmonary veins. The ablation catheter is introduced into the left atrium via a long sheath to achieve stability and allow orientation of the catheter tip towards the roof of the left atrium. Ablation starts at the encircling lesion at the left superior pulmonary vein, and the sheath and catheter assembly are then rotated clockwise posteriorly and dragged towards the right superior pulmonary vein. To achieve catheter stability along the roof of the left atrium, the catheter is directed towards the left superior pulmonary vein and the sheath rotated to face the right pulmonary veins and vice versa. If this catheter and sheath position fails there are two alternative methods that can be used. A large loop can be made

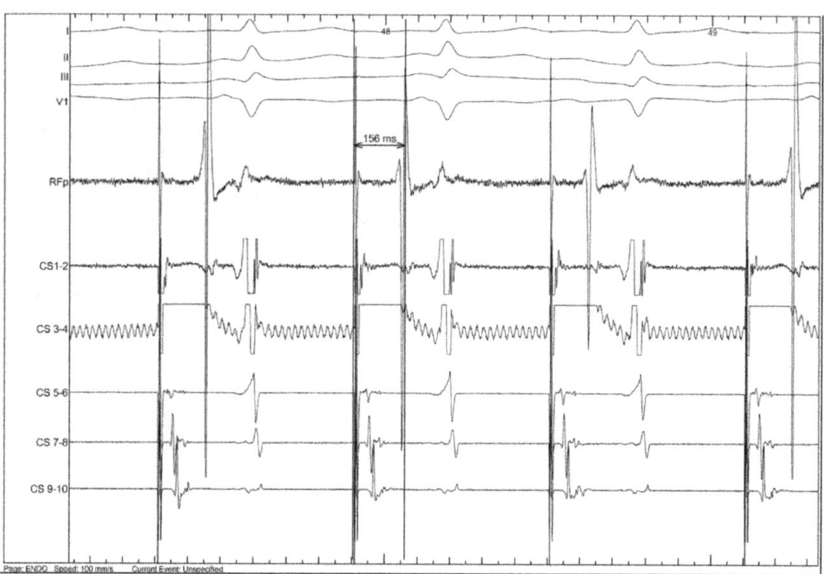

Figure 3. This example demonstrates that even when an apparently large delay is present on the mitral isthmus, block must be formally checked. When pacing proximal to the line form the distal coronary sinus a delay of 156 ms is seen. However, when pacing more proximally in the CS, the delay is longer at 176 ms, indicating that the line is incomplete. This is further demonstrated by not having a proximal to distal activation pattern in the coronary sinus when pacing anterior to the line. During ablation with distal CS pacing the delay on the line is clearly seen to jump out, eventually achieving a delay of 214 ms on the line. Pacing more proximally in the CS now results in a shorter delay, and pacing anterior to the line now results in an activation sequence in the CS that is proximal to distal.

with the catheter around the lateral, inferior, septal, walls to arrive at the roof and then the left superior pulmonary vein, ablation can then be commenced while dragging the catheter back from the left to the right superior pulmonary vein ostia. Regardless of the technique utilized, ablation is preferably performed cranially rather than posteriorly to minimize the risk of esophageal fistula. RF energy (25-30 W) is delivered for 20-120 sec at each point until the local potential is eliminated or there are double potentials. The electrophysiological endpoint of ablation was by demonstration of a complete line of block joining the two superior pulmonary veins.

Evaluation of complete linear block is performed after the restoration of sinus rhythm to allow pacing of the anterior left atrium adjacent to the line. Anterior left atrium pacing could be achieved by pacing with the proximal poles of a decapolar catheter while its distal end sits in the left atrium appendage. Alternatively, pacing can be performed by advancing the catheter to the anterior aspect of the coronary sinus. Complete linear block was defined by the following criteria: *1)* demonstration by point by point mapping of an online corridor of double potentials along the entire length of the roof during pacing of the anterior left atrium; *2)* demonstration of an activation detour circumventing the right and left pulmonary veins to activate caudocranially the posterior wall with no conduction through the left atrial roof (see figures 6 A to D).

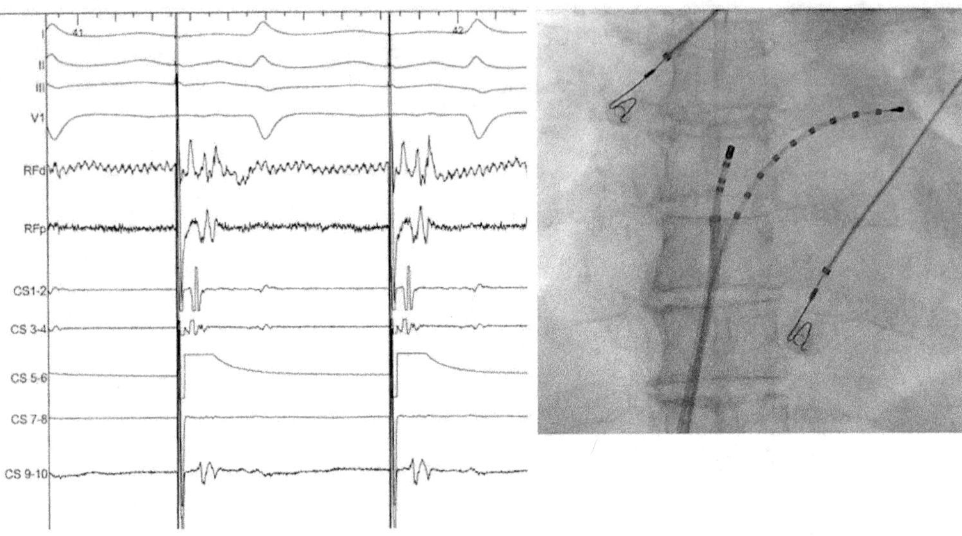

Figure 4. In this patient, a roof dependent macro reentry was successfuly terminated during a linear lesion at the LA roof. The decapolar diagnostic catheter is then placed in the left atrium (LA), with the distal tip in the left atrial appendage. Pacing at the anterior LA (bipole 5-6) and mapping using the ablation catheter shows a gap (continuous activity) in the middle of the ablation line.

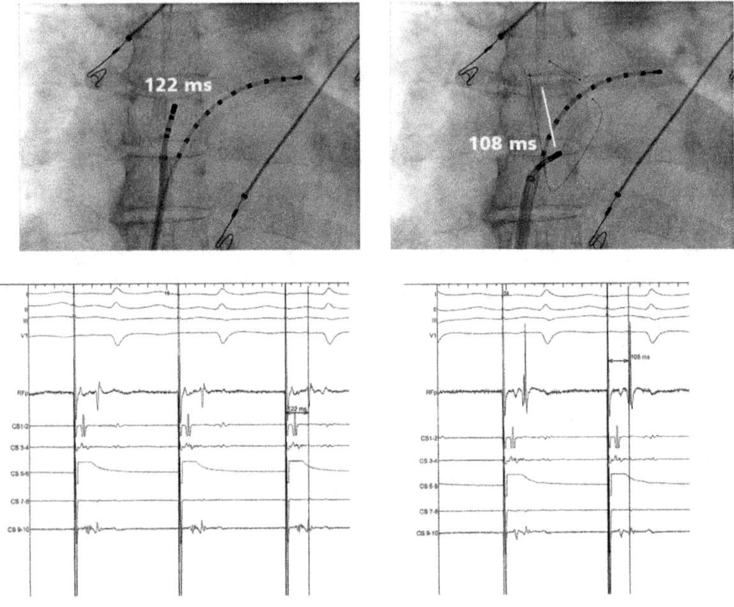

Figure 5. Ablation at the site in figure 4 resulted in a change in the local potentials suggesting a complete block. This is then demontrated (right panel) by recording an earlier activity at a lower site of the posterior LA indicating a superior activation front.

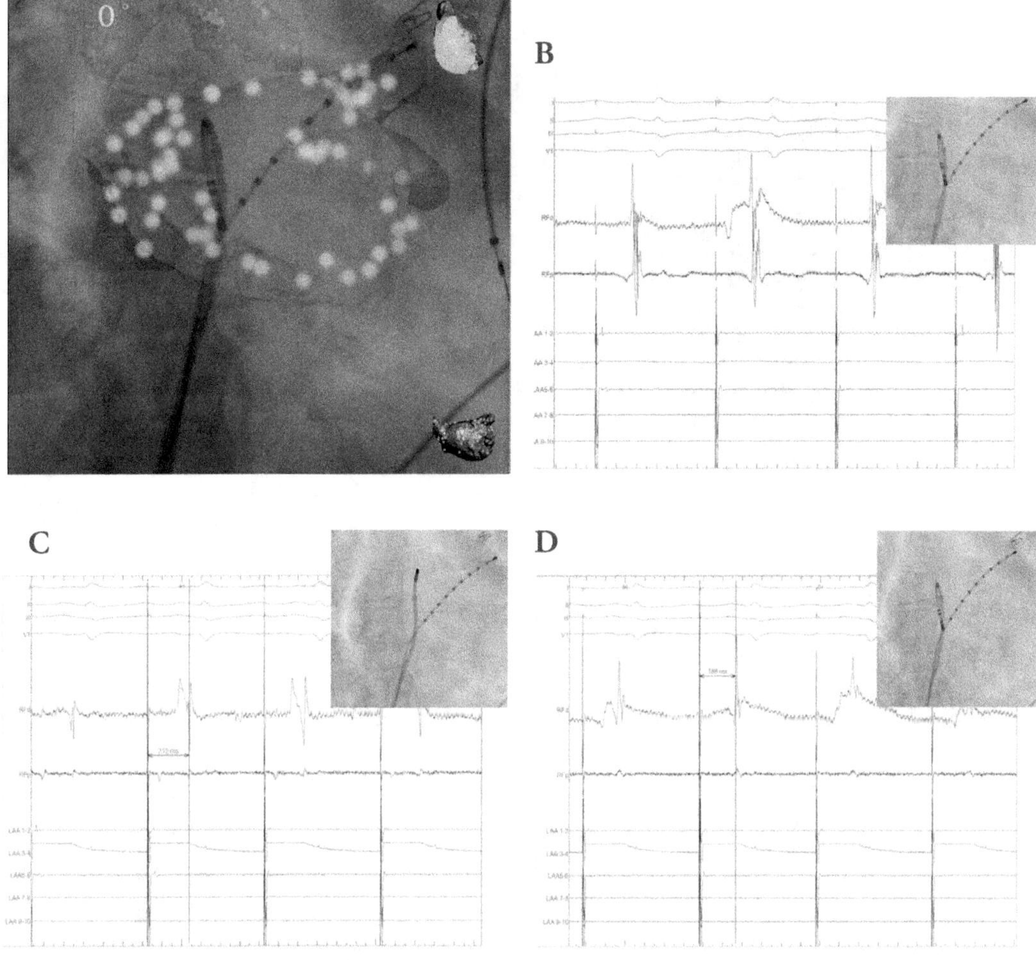

*Figure 6. This patient had a roof dependent macro reentrant atrial tachycardia. A roof line
was performed and here block of the roof line is demonstrated by observing an activation sequence that
ascends up the posterior wall. Panel A shows an overlay using rotational angiography. Panel B demonstrates
a distal to proximal sequence on the ablation catheter which is on the posterior wall, and this activation
sequence is also demonstrated by marching up and down the posterior wall
as shown in panels C (high posterior wall) and D (low posterior wall).*

Hendricks *et al.* have described the use of entrainment mapping using a 3D mapping system to give a color-coded map of the atrium to help with diagnosis of ATs,[15] with very good results, but we believe that the combination of activation and entrainment mapping is both quick and effective (see figures 7 A to J).

When a macro reentrant mechanism has been ruled out, a centrifugal AT is searched for, initially in the LA and then in the right atrium (RA). We prefer to name these "centrifugal" with the further subclassification of "focal" (see figure 8) and "localized reentry" (see figure 9) based upon their distinctive electrophysiological characteristics, which are summarized. The activation of the CS is used to guide the initial mapping to the septal side (proximal to dis-

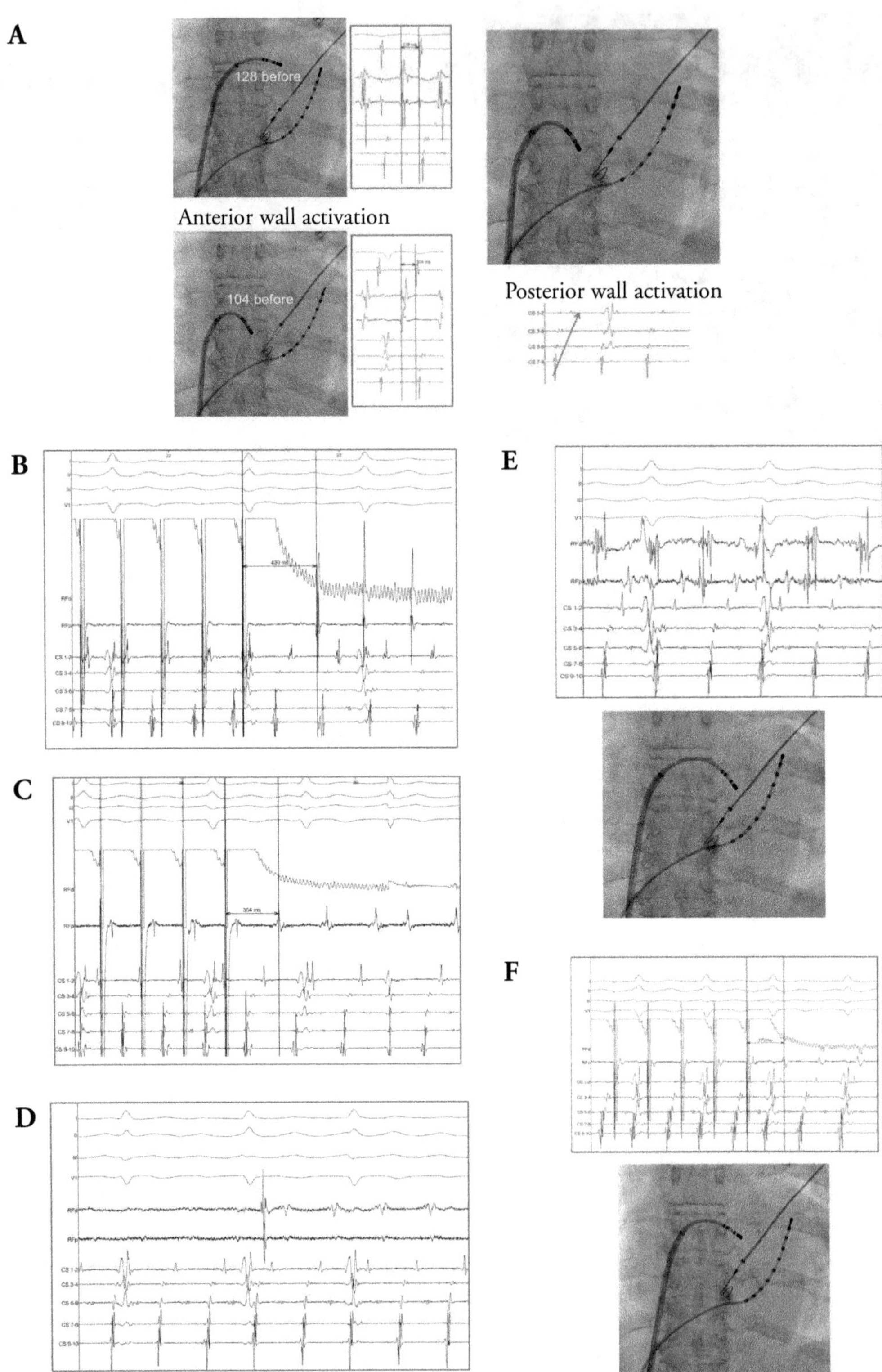

Figure 7. (See next page for description.)

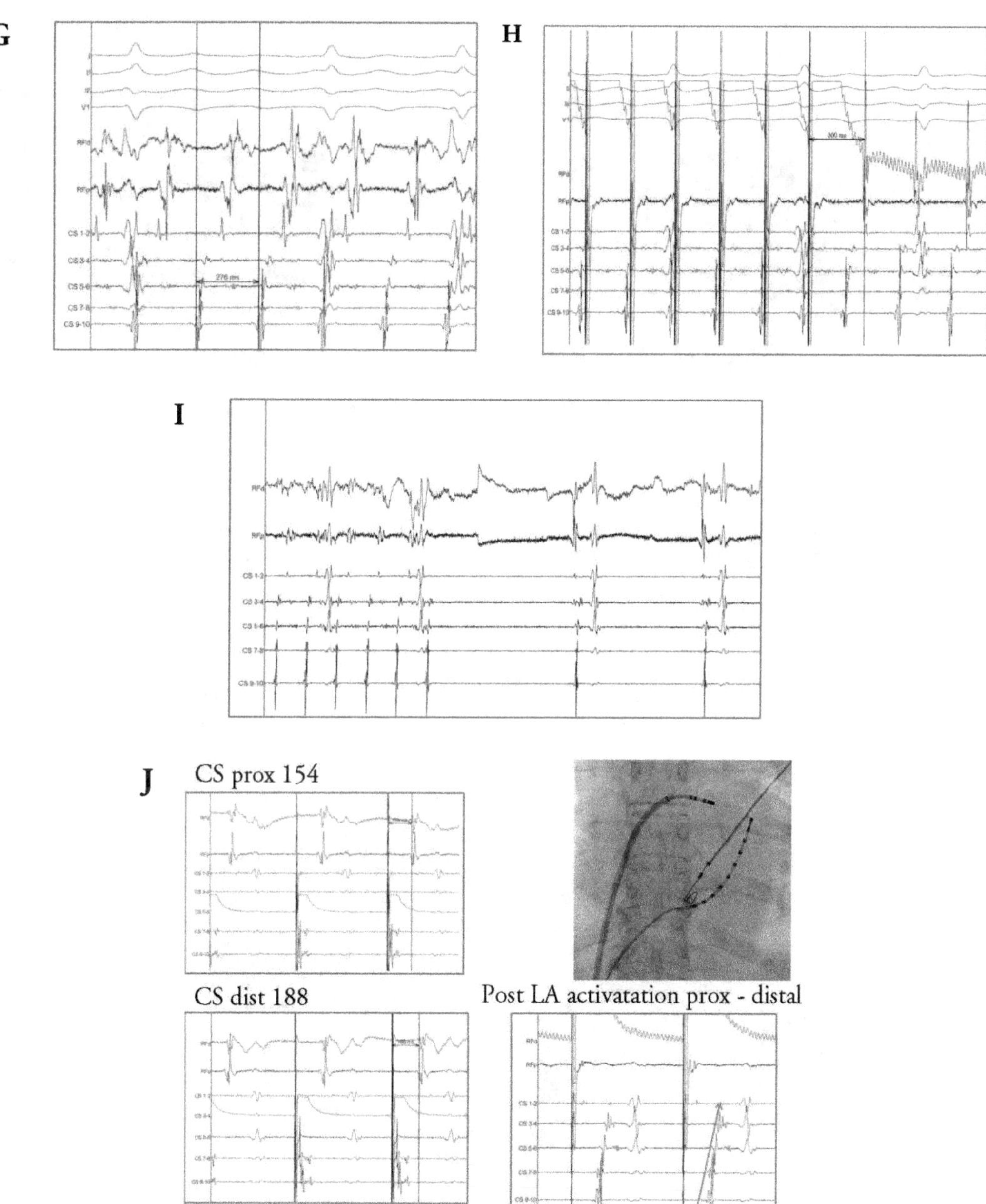

Figure 7. This case demonstrates that activation mapping alone is insufficient. In panel A the activation sequence of the left atrium is consistent with perimitral flutter. However the entrainment from the mitral isthmus is not consistent with perimitral flutter (panel B). The right superior pulmonary vein is isolated (panel C), but dissociation of this vein does not alter the tachycardia (panel D). A localized reentry circuit on the anterior left atrium is mapped (panel E) and entrainment close to this site, where capture is possible, is perfect (panel F). Following ablation of this tachycardia, the activation of the left atrium is unchanged (panel G), however, entrainment from the mitral isthmus demonstrates that this is now part of the circuit (panel H), and ablation of the mitral isthmus results in termination of tachycardia (panel I). Bidirectional block is the target for all linear lesions and is proven for the mitral isthmus in panel J.

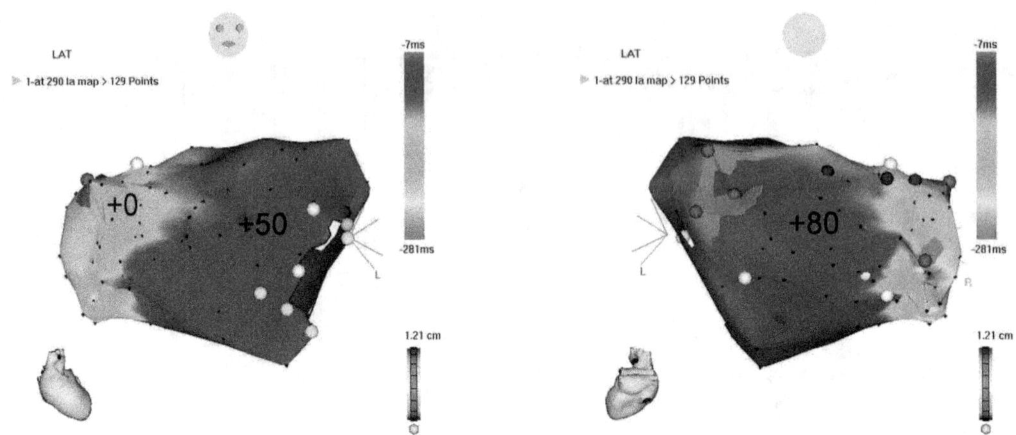

Figure 8. Focal tachycardia (Dupuy, 2b):
1. Centrifugal activation to the other segments; 2. Less than 75% of cycle length is recorded;
3. Post-pacing interval increases with the distance from the focal source.

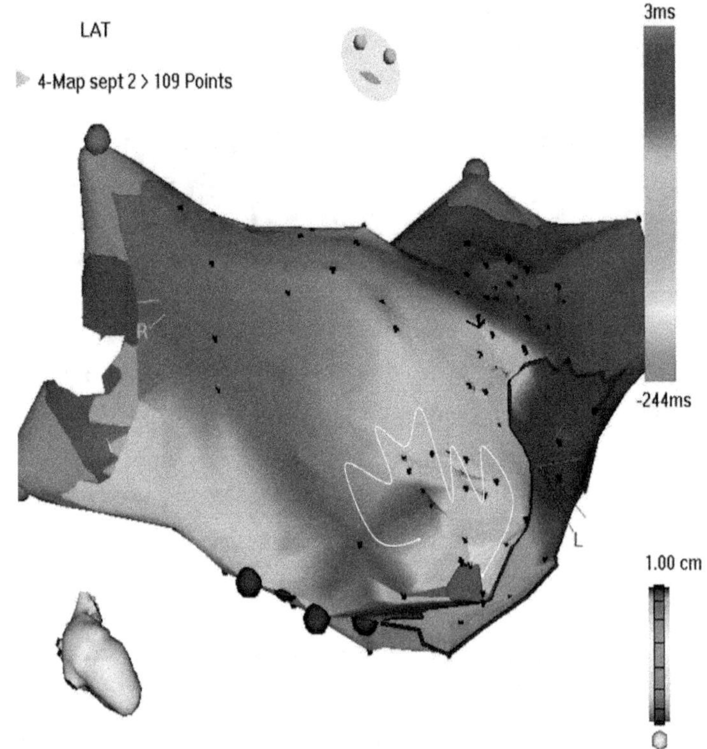

Figure 9. Localized reentries (Hessam sept, 2c):
1. Circuit limited to one (or two adjacent) LA segments: PVs, Ant, post, sept, lateral and LAA;
2. >75% of CL recorded locally; 3. Centrifugal activation to the other segments;
4. Good PPI close to the site only.

tal CS activation) or the lateral side of the LA (distal to proximal CS activation). The ablation catheter is then used to search for a region exhibiting centrifugal activation. The atrium is divided into four segments anterior, posterior, lateral and septal, and the activation in these segments is determined by comparison to the fixed reference channel. In this way we can identify a centrifugal pattern of activation (activation spreading radially) and progressively narrow the region of interest. In addition, during this mapping phase, areas showing long duration (>50% CL) fractionated potentials are noted for subsequent analysis using entrainment.

In our experience, ATs following AF ablation are quite prone to interruption or transformation, and we therefore use entrainment maneuvers sparingly in order to minimize this risk. The entrainment maneuvers are guided by the initial activation mapping and are specifically performed in two opposite left atrial segments. The opposite atrial segments usually used for perimitral reentry are septal and left isthmus sites (see figures 10 to 13). For roof-dependent reentry the opposite atrial segments are anterior and posterior wall. In the presence of a post pacing interval (PPI) exceeding the CL by more than 30 ms in either of the previously mentioned locations (two opposite atrial segments), a left atrial macro reentry is ruled out, even if the activation mapping was suggestive, leading to step 5.

1.3.5 Step 5. Identify the origin of centrifugal tachycardias

When the region of the centrifugal AT cannot be located we use the technique of repeated resetting with analysis of the post-pacing interval, initially described by Mohammed *et al.*, to progressively approach the site of origin of the tachycardia. A post-pacing interval lower or equal to

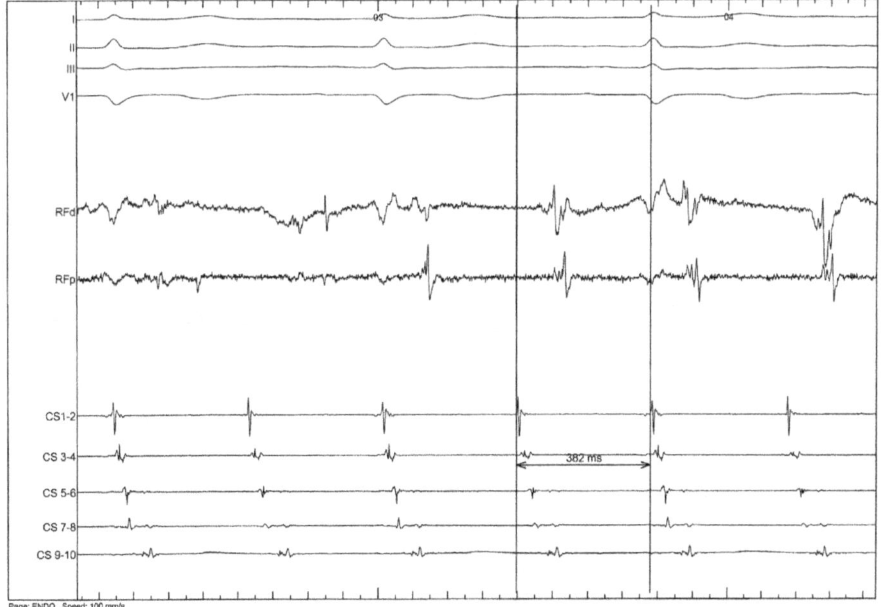

Figure 10.

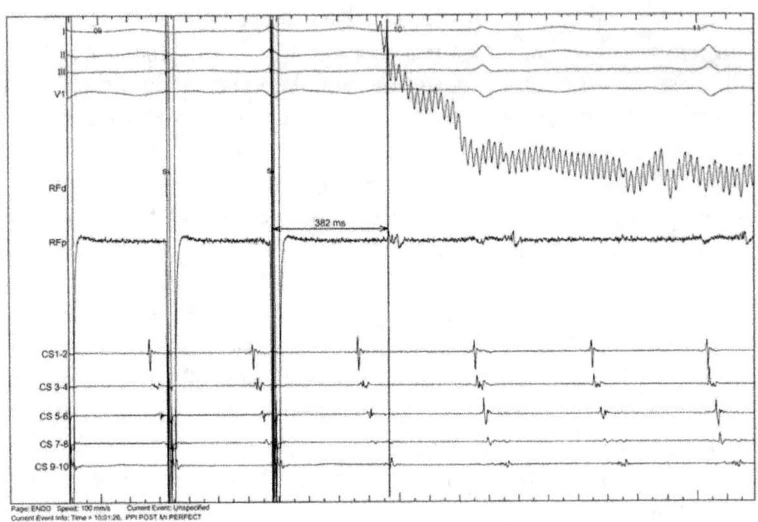

Figure 11. Post-pacing interval (PPI) from de MIG = perfect PPI.

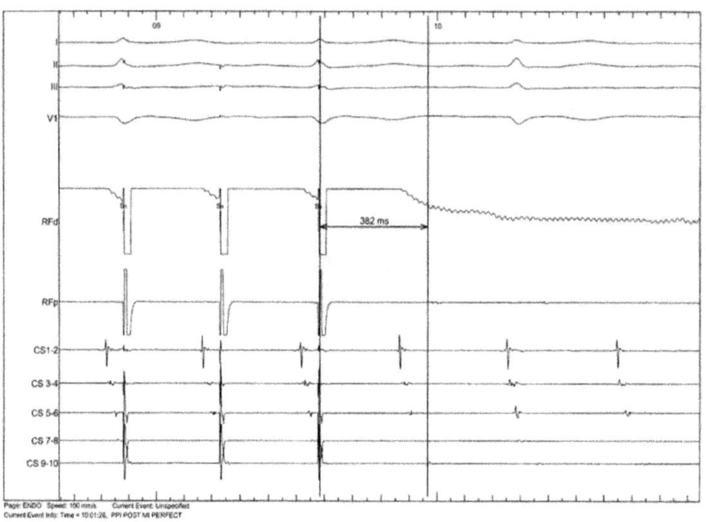

Figure 12. Post-pacing interval (PPI) from the septum = perfect PPI.

30 ms is considered as indicating the proximity of the tachycardia origin. In the presence of PPI exceeding the cycle length more than 50 ms, pacing is performed at a different segment of the atrium. Often, the site of origin of localized reentry demonstrates very low amplitude polyphasic signals and local capture is impossible even at maximal pacing output. In these cases, the PPI is measured at a slightly distant, so-called proxy site, where capture is possible. A PPI <50 ms at a proxy site is considered to indicate proximity to the tachycardia origin.

The particular characteristic of localized reentry is the recording of electrograms covering 75% of the cycle length of AT within less than 2 cm in contrast to discrete electrograms at the

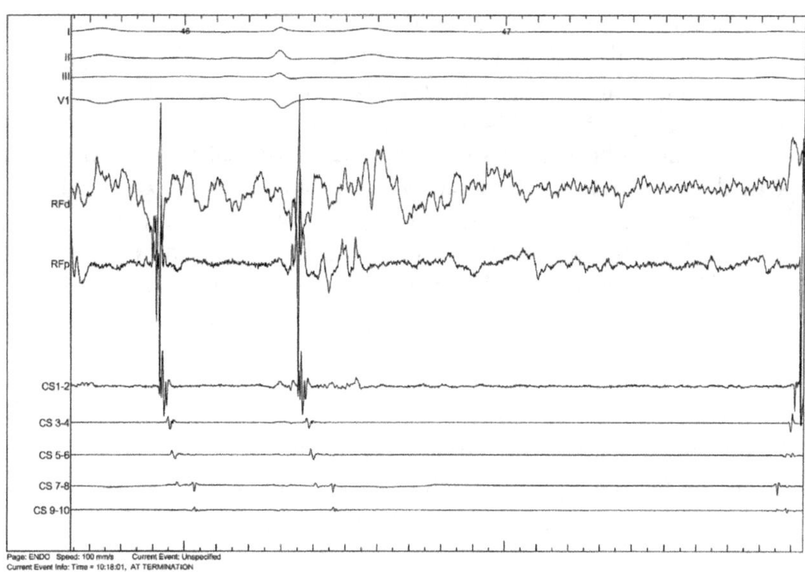

Figure 13. Termination of the flutter by ablating in CS distal.

remaining atria.[3] The characteristic electrogram at the successful ablation site is usually low amplitude and polyphasic, and therefore it can easily be misinterpreted as noise, particularly if noise is generated by irrigation flow tubing or 3D mapping systems. Ablation of these tachycardias is very successful, and when the correct site has been identified termination of tachycardia normally occurs within a few seconds.

1.4　Value of 3D electroanatomical navigation systems

3D navigation systems are used worldwide to improve the efficacy of the ablation, however, the strategy that we employ is not reliant upon the use of such systems. These systems can give a very accurate map of the left atrium and the pulmonary veins as well as help build an activation map. They allow for a reduction in the fluoroscopic time and radiation for patients and physicians. More importantly, 3D anatomical systems combined with electrogram analysis and activation mapping may help in the understanding of disorganized and organized arrhythmia.

The reason we do not routinely use 3D mapping systems is to minimize the procedure time and to focus attention on electrogram interpretation, thereby minimizing opportunity for tachycardia instability to thwart successful mapping. Furthermore, the complete understanding of 3D mapping and reconstruction of AT generally necessitate prior differentiation between focal and macro reentrant AT and incorrect annotation of activation can be misleading in the case of double or low voltage potentials, in all current systems. Therefore, in our experience, 3D navigation systems are mainly useful for the purposes of confirmation of mechanism and its illustration after the achievement of a complete understanding of the arrhythmia. The 3D electroanatomic system is based on sequential or instantaneous mapping technology allowing detailed reconstruction of chamber geometry and activation sequence. Studies have demonstrated the additional usefulness of electroanatomic mapping to construct a 3D geometry the chamber and map the location of focal or macro reentrant AT.[7] These observations have also been made in the context of post ablative AT where complex scar-related and iatrogenic AT are often present. In a recent study, Patel *et al.* showed that a strategy using non-contact mapping and a multielectrode mapping catheter allows for a rapid definition of post-ablative AT, and facilitates subsequent ablation strategy. This strategy has the advantage to collect a large amount of points within a short period of time. The authors of this study were able to create activation maps in 81% of the ATs and with an average mapping time of 8 minutes. Only one AT could not be subsequently terminated by catheter ablation. In a study by Esato *et al.*[15] an entrainment map was made using a 3D mapping system, which again in that study was helpful in ablating atrial tachycardia.

Another benefit of mapping systems is the ability to accurately archive cases, which may be interesting when patients represent with further atrial tachycardias. The accurate localization of previous lesions may be helpful in searching for likely sites of conduction recovery across lines, or zones of slow conduction. However, a caveat to this is that not all lesions marked result in actual lesions being formed as has been demonstrated by recent work utilizing MRI to assess scar burden after catheter ablation.[16]

1.4.1 *Practical algorithm for post-AF ablation AT*

We have devised a simple algorithm facilitating the AT mapping technique that we use in daily practice (see figure 1). The first step consists of assessing the cycle length variability. While a variability greater than 15% of the AT cycle length over a one minute period is suggestive of a focal origin compared to macro reentry, the converse does not hold true. The second step consists of verifying and completing PV isolation. The third step is to look for activation compatible with a perimitral or roof dependent circuit. Entrainment maneuvers at two different sites on the circuit will confirm or refute the diagnosis. If macro reentry is ruled out, a non-macro reentrant arrhythmia is suspected and mapped for. In these cases the aim of mapping is to determine the earliest region of activation. This can be facilitated by entrainment (or resetting maneuver), with the best PPI converging to the culprit region. Mapping within this region will determine whether the arrhythmia is truly focal or is localized reentry with either an early mid diastolic potential or potentials spanning all the cycle length within a 2-cm area.

A prospective cohort of 128 consecutive patients presenting 246 AT in the context of prior AF ablation has been investigated in our center[3] (see figures 14 and 15). Activation and entrainment mapping were used as described in this chapter, without the systematic use of any 3D electroanatomical navigation system. A stepwise approach to the diagnosis of each AT, evaluating successively cycle length regularity, assessing for macro reentry (mitral isthmus or roof dependent), and finally searching for a focal origin giving a centrifugal activation of the atria (either focal point AT or localized reentry). In case of extensive slow conduction or scar, entrainment maneuvers were favored. A total of 238/246 (97%) sustained AT (mean CL 284±87 ms) were successfully mapped (single AT, 51 patients; multiple AT, 77 patients) with a diagnostic time of 10±8 minutes per tachycardia. AT were macro reentrant in 109 (46%) and focal in 129 (54%). Of the latter, only 34 focal AT originated from a discrete point site fulfilling the consensus criteria while a distinct mechanism, localized reentry (AT that was neither macro reentry nor focal), was identified in 95.

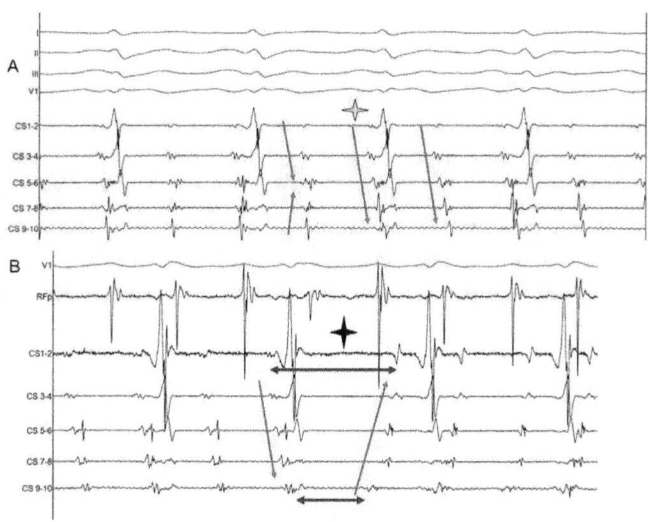

Figure 14. Panel A shows the first atrial tachycardia observed after conversion of atrial fibrilation in this patient. The initial part of the tracing shows a collision in the action of the coronary sinus (CS). The activation of the anterior and posterior segments of the left atrium (LA) were consistent with a roof dependent circuit further demonstrated by entrainment and good post-pacing interval at these segments. During ablation at the roof of the LA, a change in the CS activation is observed with a consistent distal to proximal activation (gray star). Again, the initial step is to look for a macro re-entry the most likely of wich is a perimitral circuit as the roof has just been ablated and this distal to proximal CS activation is rare in peritricuspid flutters. Conventional mapping around the mitral annulus shows a consistent activation and the ablation at the mitral isthmus is associated with a change to tachycardia number 3 (black star). A proximal to distal CS activation is now observed, consistent with a peritricuspid macroreentry, a non-macroreentrant tachycardia from the septum, the right PVs or the right atrium. Activation mapping ruled out a peritricuspid flutter and the entrainmement mapping diagnosed a localized reentry at the lateral RA.

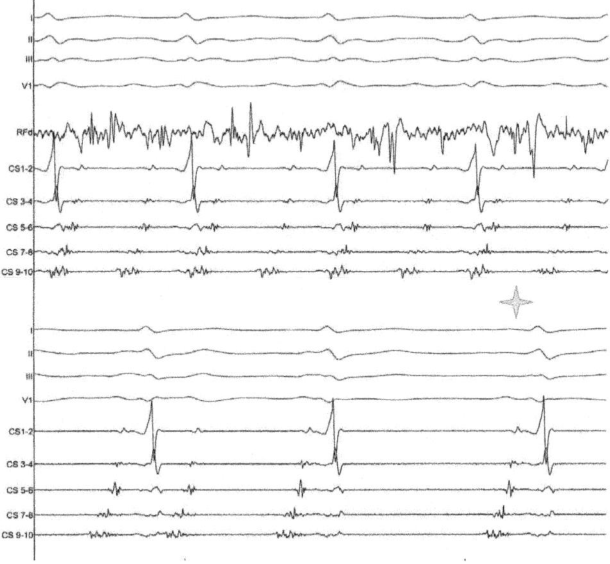

Figure 15. Ablation at the lateral right atrium.

Conclusions

Mapping and ablation of ATs has become the final frontier of AF ablation and marks the difference between clinical success and failure. In the context of prior AF ablation, focal ATs display different characteristics compared to the classically defined "focal" AT. The main difference compared to AT not encountered in the context of AF ablation resides in the increased frequency of localized reentry, which is caused by spontaneous or ablated tissue alterations creating an anchoring point. Conventional electrophysiological mapping of ATs with appropriate entrainment maneuvers, without the routine use of sophisticated 3D mapping systems, is both highly effective and efficient.

Acknowledgments

Matthew Wright acknowledges the financial support from the Department of Health via the National Institute for Health Research (NIHR) comprehensive Biomedical Research Centre award to Guy's & St Thomas' NHS Foundation Trust in partnership with King's College London and King's College Hospital NHS Foundation Trust.

References

1. Calkins H, Brugada J, Packer DL *et al.* HRS/EHRA/ECAS expert Consensus Statement on catheter and surgical ablation of atrial fibrillation: recommendations for personnel, policy, procedures and follow-up. A report of the Heart Rhythm Society (HRS) Task Force on catheter and surgical ablation of atrial fibrillation. Heart Rhythm 2007; 4: 816-61.

2. O'Neill MD, Wright M, Knecht S *et al.* Long-term follow-up of persistent atrial fibrillation ablation using termination as a procedural endpoint. Eur Heart J 2009; 30: 1105-12.

3. Jais P, Matsuo S, Knecht S *et al.* A deductive mapping strategy for atrial tachycardia following atrial fibrillation ablation: importance of localized reentry. J Cardiovasc Electrophysiol 2009; 20: 480-91.

4. Chae S, Oral H, Good E *et al.* Atrial tachycardia after circumferential pulmonary vein ablation of atrial fibrillation: mechanistic insights, results of catheter ablation, and risk factors for recurrence. J Am Coll Cardiol 2007; 50: 1781-7.

5. Ouyang F, Antz M, Ernst S *et al.* Recovered pulmonary vein conduction as a dominant factor for recurrent atrial tachyarrhythmias after complete circular isolation of the pulmonary veins : lessons from double Lasso technique. Circulation 2005; 11: 127-35.

6. Gerstenfeld EP, Callans DJ, Dixit S *et al.* Mechanisms of organized left atrial tachycardias occurring after pulmonary vein isolation. Circulation 2004; 110: 1351-7.

7. Rostock T, Drewitz I, Steven D *et al.* Characterization, mapping and catheter ablation of recurrent atrial tachycardias following stepwise ablation of long-lasting persistent atrial fibrillation. Circ Arrhythm Electrophysiol 2010.

8. Knecht S, Hocini M, Wright M *et al.* Left atrial linear lesions are required for successful treatment of persistent atrial fibrillation. Eur Heart J 2008.

9. Oral H, Chugh A, Good E *et al.* Radiofrequency catheter ablation of chronic atrial fibrillation guided by complex electrograms. Circulation 2007; 115: 2606-12.

10. Cappato R, Negroni S, Pecora D *et al.* Prospective assessment of late conduction recurrence across radiofrequency lesions producing electrical disconnection at the pulmonary vein ostium in patients with atrial fibrillation. Circulation 2003; 108: 1599-1604.

11. Kistler PM, Roberts-Thomson KC, Haqqani HM *et al.* P-wave morphology in focal atrial tachycardia: development of an algorithm to predict the anatomic site of origin. J Am Coll Cardiol 2006; 48: 1010-7.

12. Haissaguerre M, Shah DC, Jais P *et al.* Electrophysiological breakthroughs from the left atrium to the pulmonary veins. Circulation 2000; 102: 2463-5.

13. Satomi K, Bansch D, Tilz R *et al.* Left atrial and pulmonary vein macroreentrant tachycardia associat-

ed with double conduction gaps: a novel type of man-made tachycardia after circumferential pulmonary vein isolation. Heart Rhythm 2008; 5: 43-51.

14. Shah D, Sunthorn H, Burri H *et al.* Narrow, slow-conducting isthmus dependent left atrial reentry developing after ablation for atrial fibrillation: ECG characterization and elimination by focal RF ablation. J Cardiovasc Electrophysiol 2006; 17: 508-15.

15. Esato M, Hindricks G, Sommer P *et al.* Color-coded three-dimensional entrainment mapping for analysis and treatment of atrial macroreentrant tachycardia. Heart Rhythm 2009; 6: 349-58.

16. Taclas JE, Nezafat R, Wylie JV *et al.* Relationship between intended sites of RF ablation and post-procedural scar in AF patients, using late gadolinium enhancement cardiovascular magnetic resonance. Heart Rhythm 2009.

Chapter 8. Ablation of long-standing AF.
Is it wise to pursue it?

C. Pappone, V. Santinelli

Department of Arrhythmology
GVM Care and Research
Ravenna, Italy

Address for correspondence:
Department of Arrhythmology
Villa Maria Cecilia Hospital
Dr. Carlo Pappone
cpappone@gvm-vmc.it

Introduction

Catheter ablation techniques for pulmonary vein isolation (PVI) are effective in patients with paroxysmal atrial fibrillation (AF).[1-9] However, it appears inappropriate to extend the PVI technique alone from patients with paroxysmal AF to those with long-standing persistent AF (>1 year), in which several areas are characterized by disorganized atrial activity with marked regional differences.[10,11] In fact, the mechanisms underlying long-lasting persistent AF are more complex and often multifactorial. Long-standing persistent AF also includes patients with moderate-to-severe left ventricular dysfunction. Many sites within the left atrium (LA) such as the coronary sinus or the left atrial appendage show prolonged complex fractionated potentials and rapid activity while the remaining areas may be still organized.[11] Therefore, the addition of left atrial substrate modification at these sites may have a significant impact on atrial fibrillation cycle length (AFCL), which may lead to one or more organized atrial tachycardias or even to sinus rhythm, all of which may improve the outcomes of patients with long-lasting persistent AF.[10] Therefore, it is not surprising that further substrate modification not limited to PV ostia alone, as basically performed in circumferential pulmonary vein ablation (CPVA) using an electroanatomic mapping technique, has been more effective in patients with both paroxysmal and chronic AF.[2-6] This improved outcome, largely reported many years ago in patients undergoing CPVA,[2] may be explained by the fact that sequential multiple atrial sites critical for maintaining the arrhythmia are targeted for ablation. In our previous experience published in the *New England Journal of Medicine*, about 75% of patients with chronic AF, most of whom did not have enlarged atria, maintained sinus rhythm for 1 year after CPVA.[12] However, patients with long-standing AF who remain in AT/AF after a standard CPVA approach need more extensive ablation by sequentially targeting other atrial structures showing complex and disorganized activity. Currently, step-by-step linear lesions throughout the atria guided by non-inducibility are sequentially created in order to interrupt multiple reentrant wavelets usually guided by the ablation of continuous complex fractionated atrial potentials, ablation of areas with short cycle length (CL) activity, focal sources, or ablation of sites of dominant frequency. Patients with long-standing persistent AF are considered for catheter ablation if they are symptomatic and have already failed at least two conventional antiarrhythmic drugs, electrical cardioversion, or both. In many patients with long-standing persistent AF, a redo procedure is required to maintain sinus rhythm and there is no predetermined limit of the number of procedures per patient. As catheter ablation is a safe and effective treatment for patients with paroxysmal AF or persistent AF and heart failure, we perform this alternative in patients with left ventricular dysfunction in NYHA class II or higher. Preliminary results have indicated excellent long-term outcomes in almost all patients, but in many cases (about 50%) multiple procedures are required after the index ablation.[10] In our experience, this extensive ablation approach is required in patients with enlarged atria and persistent long-standing AF and consists in the sequential ablation of structures which are empirically identified by the effect of their ablation on AFCL.

1   Circumferential pulmonary vein ablation

The standard circumferential pulmonary vein ablation (CPVA) lesion set is considered as the initial ablation step in patients with long-standing persistent AF (see figure 1). The ablation procedure is usually performed using manual tip-irrigated catheters or remotely by magnetic tip-irrigated catheters. The lesion set consists of large circumferential ablation lines for performing the point-by-point tailored distal disconnection of all PV ostia, vagal denervation, as well as additional linear lesion lines with validation of the mitral isthmus line. Non-inducibility of both AF and AT at the end of the procedure is performed in all patients. Accumulating data from our laboratory indicate that in patients with paroxysmal/persistent AF without enlarged atria, standard CPVA alone is associated with an excellent outcome.[2,3,5,6,9] However, in patients with enlarged atria and long-lasting persistent AF, the addition of a left or right atrial substrate by creating more lesions in a stepwise fashion, while using minimal ablation, results in an incremental benefit by achieving a stable sinus rhythm and noninducible AF, leading to the cessation of all antiarrhythmic drugs at 1 year.

2   Endpoints of circumferential pulmonary vein ablation

2.1   *Restoration of sinus rhythm*

In our experience, the achievement of sinus rhythm is the main endpoint in patients with both paroxysmal AF and persistent AF since it is usually associated with a better clinical outcome. However, multiple steps are required to achieve sinus rhythm in patients with persistent long-standing AF (about 60% of patients are in sinus rhythm). The standard set of lesions, as performed in the CPVA approach, may be insufficient to achieve a stable sinus rhythm in patients with persistent long-lasting AF, in which case the time-consuming step-by-step addition of left atrial substrate modification using electrogram-based ablation or linear lesions is necessary. In these cases, sinus rhythm is usually restored by an intermediate step of one or multiple ATs,

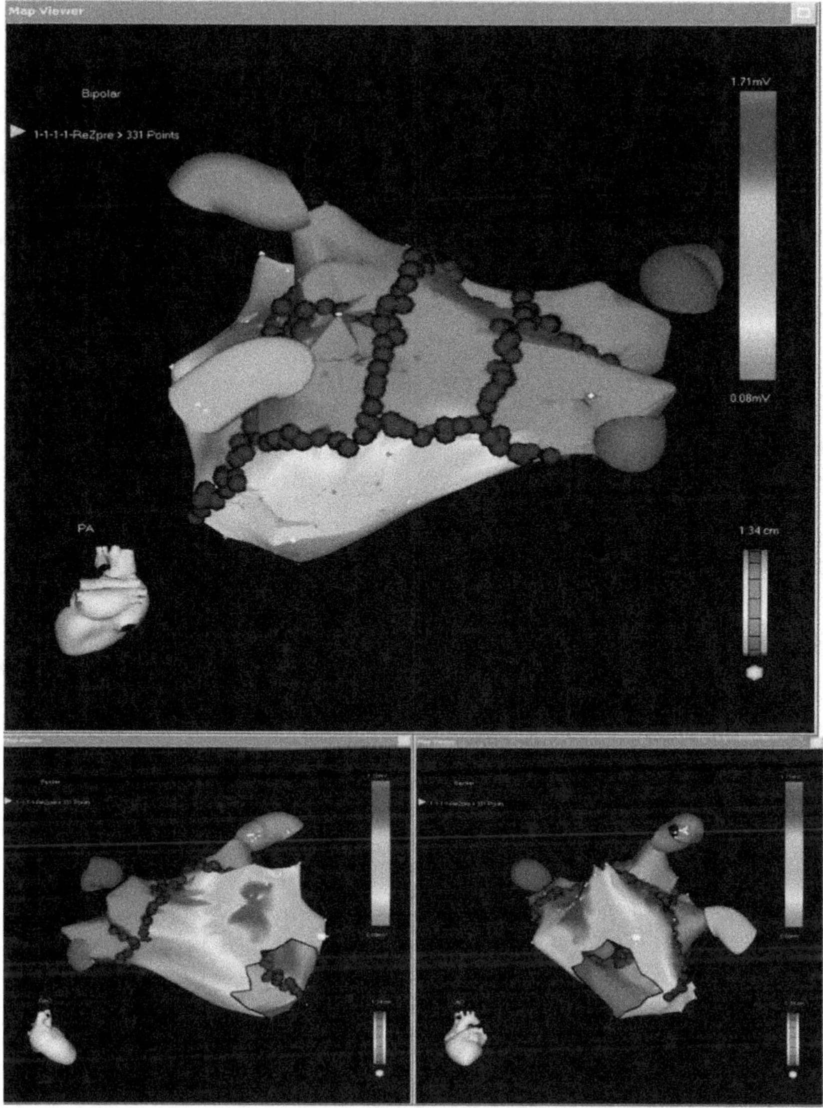

Figure 1. A voltage map of the left atrium has been generated using the CARTO system after AF termination; the red area indicates left atrial regions without electrical activity.

which are then mapped conventionally and ablated. However, all atrial regions represent potential ablation targets and distinguishing passive from active sites is time-consuming and is probably the most challenging aspect of catheter ablation in patients with long-standing AF. If sinus rhythm is still not achieved, every effort should be made to further slow and organize local atrial activity. If AF becomes an organized AT, activation mapping and entrainment are used to evaluate the circuit; and in case of transition to another AT, further activation maps are generated until sinus rhythm is restored.

2.2 *Non-inducibility*

After restoration of sinus rhythm, AF/AT inducibility is assessed by programmed extrastimuli using up to three extrastimuli at twice the diastolic threshold followed by burst atrial pacing (10-second bursts at an output of 20 mA) from the proximal coronary sinus and the right atrium (CS ostium or right atrial free wall) beginning at a CL of 350 ms and reducing by 10-ms intervals until atrial refractoriness. Sustained AT/AF is considered as inducible if the arrhythmia persists for >1 minute; induction is repeated at least three times from each site. In contrast to paroxysmal AF, where non-inducibility of AF may be achieved in most patients, in long-lasting persistent AF, AF/AT may be induced in about half of the patients at the end of the index procedure.

2.3 *Radiofrequency settings*

Radiofrequency applications are usually deployed with an open irrigated-tip catheter. The settings are usually 40 W, 40° C with an irrigation rate of 17-25 mL/min, except for ablation within the CS ablation in which the settings are 25 W, 40° C with an irrigation rate of 30-40 mL/min.

3 Step-by-step ablation in long-standing persistent atrial fibrillation

3.1 *Step 1*

In our center, standard CPVA is performed as the initial ablation step in all patients with long-lasting persistent AF.[2] Circumferential and multiple sequential linear lesions with validation, as performed in the modified CPVA,[3] are useful not only to completely disconnect PV ostia, but, particularly in patients with persistent long-lasting AF, to alter the substrate for AF by defragmentation or disrupting macroreentrant circuits capable of sustaining AF. The benefit of linear lesions is also extended to the attenuation of parasympathetic tone which plays an important role in the generation of AF by shortening the atrial refractory period.

- *PV disconnection.* Circumferential lines are aimed at the PV-atrial junction *outside* the ostia, an area considered as the antrum (see figure 1). The lesions are created to encircle the left and right PVs individually or as ipsilateral pairs in accordance with the venous anatomy and operator's preference to electrically disconnect all PVs (see figures 1 and 2). We have recently demonstrated that complete distal electrical isolation can be safely obtained by potential abatement (>90% reduction of electrogram amplitude) and an electrogram amplitude decrease of <0.1 mV around and within the encircled areas.[13] Rapid PV isolation is achieved by good catheter stability and optimal wall-contact which results in rapid attenuation of atrial electrograms during each radiofrequency (RF) energy application up to complete elimination for up to 50 sec, usually within a few seconds depending on the local effect (see figure 2). Partially ablated signals require further RF applications before moving on to the next ablation site.
- *Vagal denervation.* During the procedure we attempt to eliminate all potential vagal reflexes (see figure 3), which enhances the efficacy of the procedure regarding long-term outcome.[3]

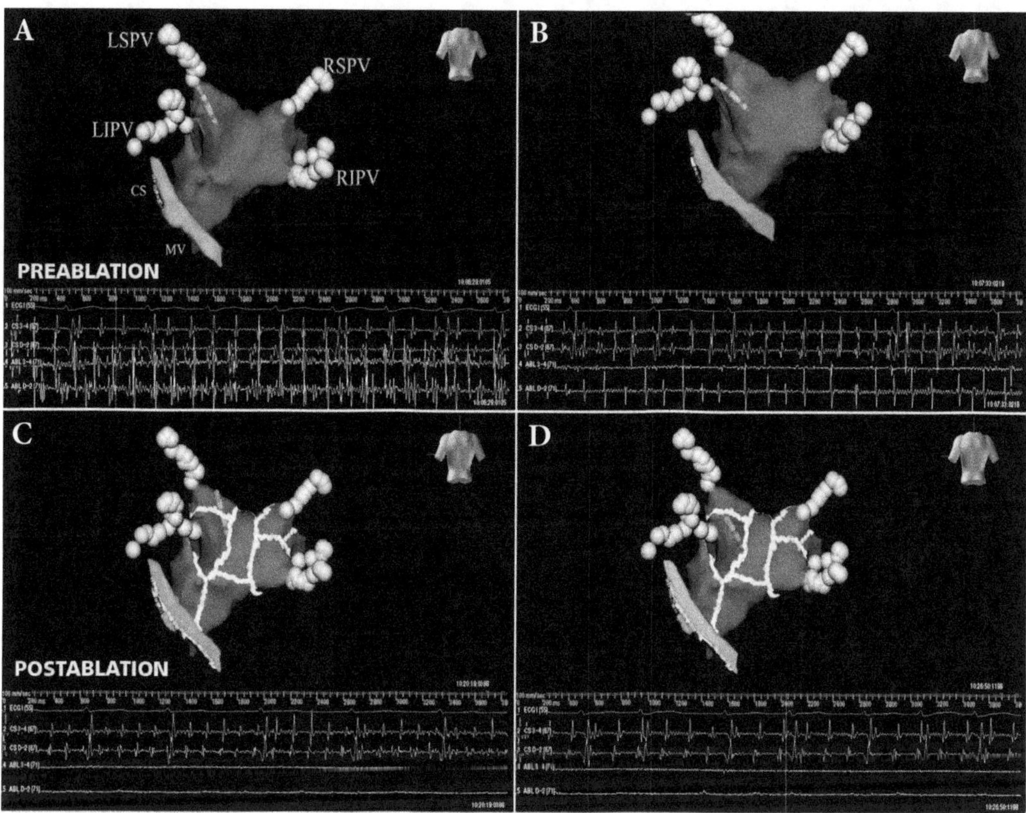

Figure 2. Complete PV isolation after CPVA. Careful mapping of the PV ostia by the ablation catheter (green tip) demonstrates the disappearance of electrical activity inside the lesion set. Note that preablation high amplitude signals in the left PVs (panels A and B) are eliminated after ablation (panels C and D).

- *Posterior and mitral isthmus ablation.* Additional ablation lines are created point-by-point along the back and roof of LA between the two sets of PVs connecting the superior and inferior PVs and the mitral valve annulus (see figures 1 and 2). The mitral isthmus line is deployed to further reduce the substrate and to prevent postablation macroreentrant left atrial tachycardias (see figure 1). Achieving a complete mitral isthmus line is an important electrophysiological endpoint and is validated during CS pacing by endocardial and coronary sinus mapping and looking for widely spaced double potentials across the line of block, and then confirmed by differential pacing.[5] The minimum double-potential interval at the mitral isthmus during CS pacing is between 80 ms and 150 ms, depending on the atrial dimensions and the extent of scarring and lesion creation.[5] Achievement of 80 ms, delay may be clinically sufficient in many patients for prevention of left atrial tachycardias, thus avoiding further and long RF applications within the CS to achieve a complete bidirectional conduction block. Ablation of the mitral isthmus may be difficult and may lead to periprocedural tamponade if "complete" mitral isthmus block is attempted.

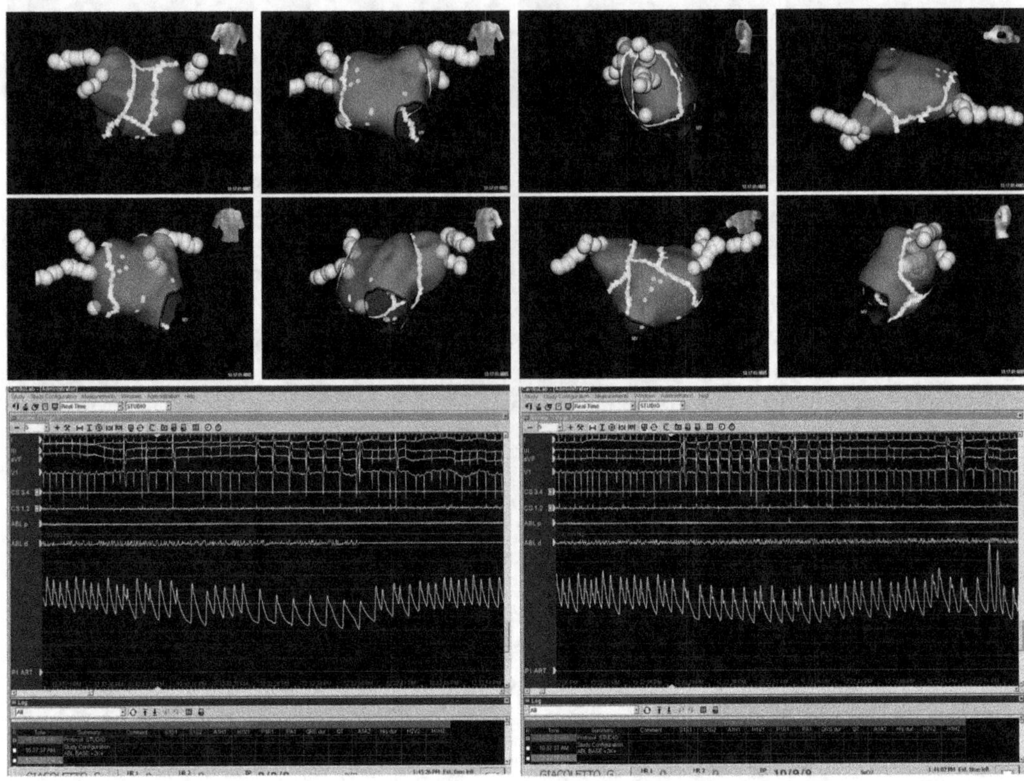

Figure 3. Vagal reflexes are elicited during RF applications; continuous
RF delivery eventually abolishes the vagal reflex.

3.2   Step 2. Endocardial coronary sinus ablation

Point-by-point ablation of the coronary sinus begins along the endocardial aspect and is usually completed from within the vessel (see figure 4). The mapping/ablation catheter is moved along the endocardium of the inferior LA after looping the catheter in such a way as to position it parallel to the coronary sinus catheter. After achieving a 270-360° loop in the left atrium, RF applications are started at the inferior LA along the posterior mitral annulus from a site adjacent to the coronary sinus ostium up to the lateral left atrium (4 o'clock in the left anterior oblique projection). The endpoint is abolition of local endocardial electrograms bordering the mitral annulus in order to prolong the CL or eliminate the sharp potentials within the coronary sinus.

3.3   Step 3. Endocardial septum ablation

Ablation of the interatrial septum is performed starting from the anterior aspect of the lesion encircling the right superior PV up to the anterior mitral annulus. Ablation is performed sequentially point-by-point with the aim of transecting areas of complex fractionated electro-

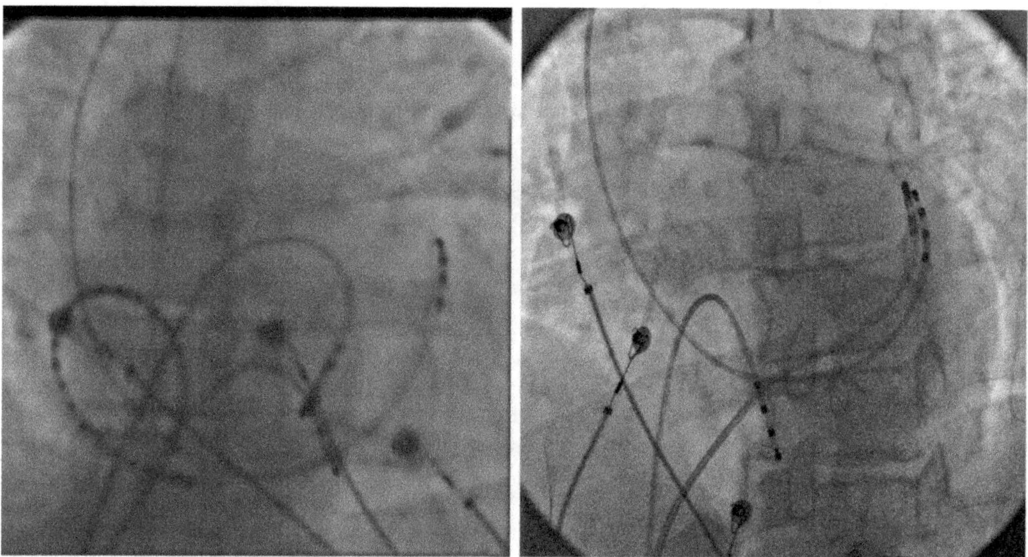

*Figure 4. Fluoroscopic images during endocardial (left panel)
and epicardial (right panel) coronary sinus ablation.*

grams. As with coronary sinus ablation, the endpoint is the abatement of local endocardial electrograms or to prolong the CL of sharp potentials in this region; complete conduction block across this lesion is not routinely assessed. During ablation of the anterior septum, areas facing the His bundle are avoided.

3.4 Step 4. Left atrial ablation

Ablation is typically performed beginning from the lesion encircling the left superior PV and is then extended to inferior and superior areas. The endpoint is elimination of local endocardial electrograms bordering the posterior, inferior and anterior left atrial appendage in an attempt to prolong the CL of sharp potentials present within the left atrial appendage; complete isolation of the left atrial appendage is intentionally avoided.

3.5 Step 5. Epicardial coronary sinus ablation

Ablation within the coronary sinus (see figure 4) is performed in case of persistent coronary sinus potentials and is usually begun distally (4 o'clock in the left anterior oblique position) and pursued along the vein up to the ostium simply by targeting local sharp potentials. Finally, additional RF applications are continued around the coronary ostium from the right atrium. Coronary sinus disconnection is validated by the dissociation or abolition of sharp potentials in its first 3 cm.

3.6 Step 6. Right atrium ablation

In our laboratory, all patients with persistent AF undergo ablation of the cavotricuspid isthmus. After ablation around the coronary sinus ostium, a linear lesion is created between the inferior vena cava and the tricuspid annulus isthmus to create a conduction block across the isthmus. Validation of bidirectional block is always done in sinus rhythm. Superior vena cava isolation is not routinely performed, but only when there is presence of an arrhythmogenic source in this vessel.

3.7 Step 7. Atrial ablation

Atrial ablation is performed at sites showing continuous electrical activity, complex fractionated potentials, sites with a gradient of activation (significant electrogram offset between the distal and proximal recording bipoles on the map electrode), or regions with a CL shorter than the mean left atrial appendage AFCL. Ablation at these sites is performed to achieve local prolongation of the CL, with synchronous activation at distal and proximal bipoles indicating passive activation of this local area. At each site, 20-60 sec of RF is delivered before moving.

4 Atrial fibrillation cycle length as a monitoring tool

A cumulative increase of AFCL leading to termination is achieved by sequentially targeting left atrial targets in a stepwise manner. Therefore, the effect of RF applications is continuously monitored by assessing potential changes of AFCL before and after each ablation step by averaging 10 consecutive cycles and at the time of AF termination. The AFCL is determined within the coronary sinus and the right and left atrial appendage. At each timepoint, annotation is manually done using online callipers at a paper speed of 100 mm/s. An individual site is considered to have a significant impact if its ablation results in AF termination or the prolongation of the AFCL (evaluated in the LAA unless specified otherwise) by 10 ms or more, when compared to the highest AFCL during the previous steps. Termination of AF is defined as a direct transition to sinus rhythm or conversion to AT. The LAA, CS and interatrial septum were identified as key areas, suggesting that their inclusion in ablation strategies to prevent recurrent paroxysmal AF after CPVA or persistent AF needs to be evaluated in order to improve the clinical outcome in these patients as well.

5 Intermediate atrial tachycardias

In many cases of long-standing AF, AF termination is followed by intermediate atrial tachycardias (see figures 6 and 7), all of which require accurate mapping (typically using Carto or NavX systems) and ablation to achieve sinus rhythm. Atrial fibrillation is defined by beat-to-beat variability in CL and morphology, while AT is defined as organized atrial activity with a stable CL, morphology, and activation sequence in both atria. Focal AT is defined by centrifugal activation from a localized region. A macroreentrant mechanism is defined by demonstrating the entire CL of activity (>70%) in a chamber with entrainment at 2 sites displaying a post-pacing interval of <20 ms longer than the tachycardia CL. When AF converts to a regular arrhythmia,

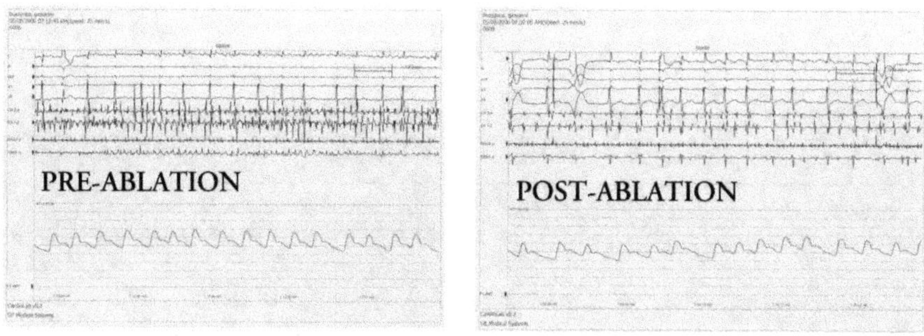

Figure 5. Atrial fibrillation cycle length is continuously monitored to evaluate the effect of RF application.

conventional activation and entrainment mapping are performed to differentiate a focal mechanism from a macroreentrant mechanism (see figure 5). In focal AT, the catheter is moved gradually in the direction of earliest activity until reaching a site showing the earliest possible activity relative to the reference electrogram in the CS or RAA or LAA; ablation at the site of earliest activity usually requires 1 min to 2 min of RF application. When a macroreentrant mechanism is diagnosed, entrainment is initially performed at the roof and the mitral isthmus to identify reentry utilizing these regions. In our experience, the prolongation of the AFCL occurs gradually with the largest increments being in the interatrial septum, CS region and LAA region and results in conversion to sinus rhythm with or without intermediate and organized tachycardia. After conversion, multiple ATs may develop, but conventional mapping techniques usually show a limited number of critical structures from which they arose. Focal ATs are frequently located at the PVs, LAA and CS regions originating at any part of their (circumferential or longitudinal) connection with the LA; some of them have narrow isthmuses with fractionation suggesting localized reentry. Macroreentrant ATs are usually perimitral or roofline and are rarely in the cavotricuspid isthmus.

6 Ablation of long-standing AF. Is it wise to pursue it?

At present, catheter ablation is effective in the treatment of all forms of AF including long-standing persistent AF. However, following the stepwise procedure, many patients may experience episodes of atrial tachycardia, most of which are due to macroreentry or microreentry arising from incomplete linear lesions. Microreentry or localized reentry is defined as the circuit being contained within an area <2 cm, and which can be easily eliminated by ablation. Therefore, the development of postablation ATs represents a future challenge to electrophysiologists and requires better mapping tools with improved ablation technologies and alternative sources of energy to RF energy. Selective areas which are actively participating in AF generation in a patient must be accurately identified to minimize the amount of ablation. Important measures need to be taken to prevent potential complications; in particular, the power used for ablation should be limited inside the CS, isolating the LAA should be avoided and continuous RF applications should be shortened (20 sec) in the same point on the posterior wall to minimize the complication rate, despite creating complete lesions. This strategy may be the main reason for the absence of major complications. In addition, ablation at some sites may be avoided or possibly minimized without compromising efficacy, for example, by SVC ablation or extensive CS abla-

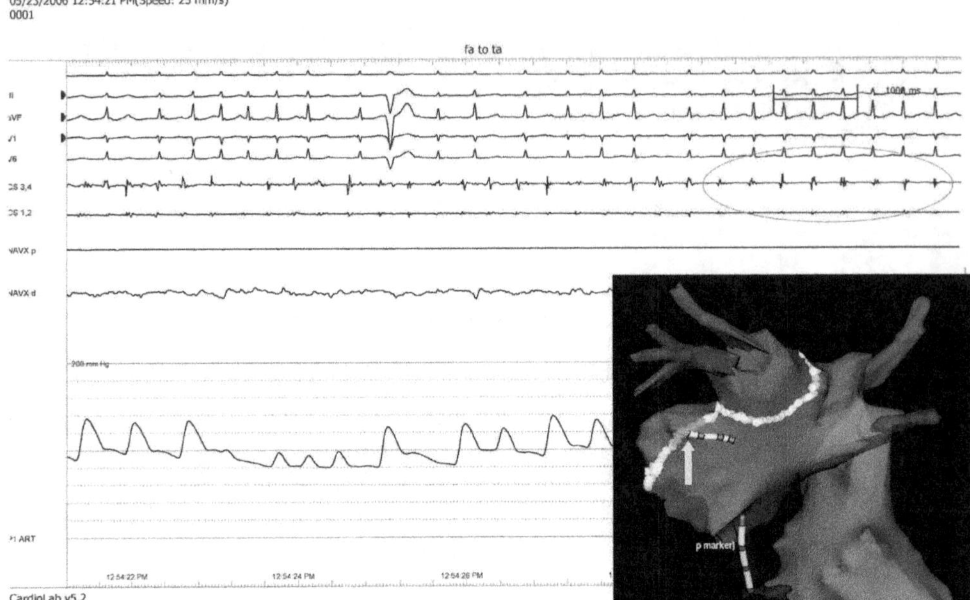

Figure 6. Ablation of the left atrial isthmus results in organized left atrial electrical activity, which is associated with a simultaneous increase of AF cycle length.

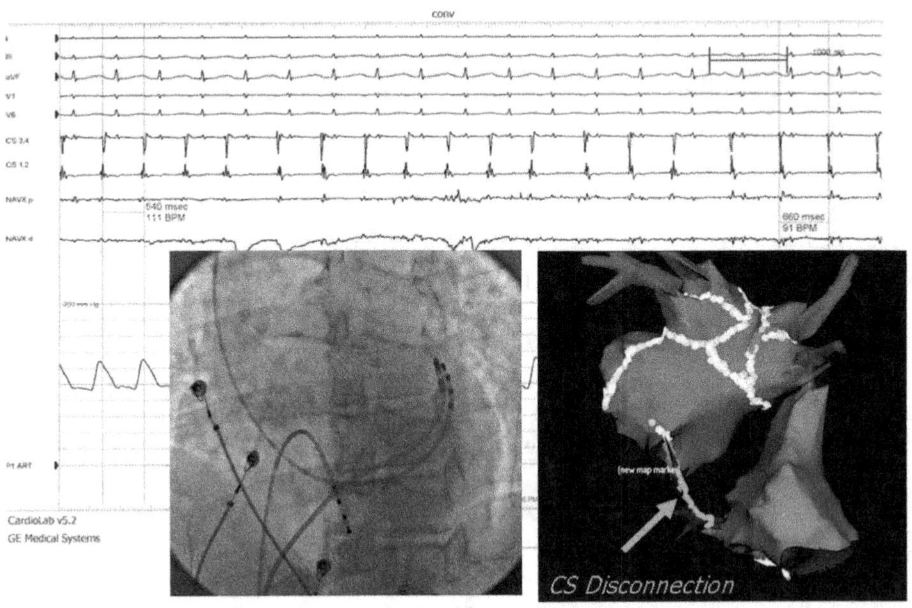

Figure 7. During RF application within the coronary sinus (CS disconnection), sinus rhythm is restored. A left lateral oblique projection is shown on the left of the figure. Note that the ablation catheter is parallel to the catheter inside the coronary sinus. RF application begins distally.

tion to produce disconnection. In our experience, despite the large amount of energy delivery required to cure AF, the procedure is well tolerated and associated with an acceptable risk-benefit ratio. In any case, further studies are needed to identify the atrial regions that can be spared ablation due to not being involved in the AF process in a particular individual or because they play an important role in ventricular filling. Initially, most patients undergoing AF ablation were affected by paroxysmal AF and many of them did not have an enlarged left atrium. The excellent results obtained in such a selected patient population have encouraged electrophysiologists to include patients with persistent AF, and recently even patients with long-lasting persistent AF and enlarged left atria have been included. As a result, many patients with enlarged atria and persistent long-lasting AF are referred for potential ablation of their arrhythmia. In our laboratory, and using this approach, the termination of AF and maintenance of sinus rhythm occurs in almost all patients after two procedures with an unprecedented rate of elimination of chronic AF by catheter ablation. In line with our data, Haissaguerre *et al.* have recently described an ablation method targeting multiple LA sites to cure long-lasting persistent AF.[10]

Conclusions

We believe that in well-established electrophysiological centers, the catheter ablation of long-standing persistent AF can be safely and effectively performed using a stepwise approach and which currently focuses on organizing left atrial activity by the mapping and ablation of intermediate atrial tachycardias. Preliminary findings from our laboratory provide evidence for conducting future larger studies to confirm the high efficacy of such an approach. Despite the encouraging initial results in patients with persistent long-standing AF, it may be reasonable to pursue a strategy of early catheter ablation in patients with AF who are at risk of rapidly progressing to persistent AF in order to prevent the symptomatic or asymptomatic transition from paroxysmal to persistent AF, which is associated with a higher risk of morbidity and mortality.[14]

References

1. Haissaguerre M, Jais P, Shah DC, *et al.* Spontaneous initiation of atrial fibrillation by ectopic beats originating in the pulmonary veins. N Engl J Med 1998; 339: 659-66.
2. Pappone C, Oreto G, Rosanio S, *et al.* Atrial electroanatomic remodeling after circumferential radiofrequency pulmonary vein ablation: efficacy of an anatomic approach in a large cohort of patients with atrial fibrillation. Circulation 2001; 104: 2539-2544.
3. Pappone C, Manguso F, Vicedomini G, *et al.* Prevention of iatrogenic atrial tachycardia after ablation of atrial fibrillation: a prospective randomized study comparing circumferential pulmonary vein ablation with a modified approach. Circulation 2004; 110: 3036-3042.
4. Ouyang F, Bansch D, Ernst S, *et al.* Complete isolation of left atrium surrounding the pulmonary veins: new insights from the double-Lasso technique in paroxysmal atrial fibrillation. Circulation 2004; 110: 2090-6.

5. Pappone C, Santinelli V, Manguso F, *et al.* Pulmonary vein denervation enhances long-term benefit after circumferential ablation for paroxysmal atrial fibrillation. Circulation 2004; 109: 327–34.
6. Pappone C, Rosanio S, Augello G, *et al.* Mortality, morbidity, and quality of life after circumferential pulmonary vein ablation for atrial fibrillation: outcomes from a controlled nonrandomized long-term study. J Am Coll Cardiol 2003; 42:185-97.
7. Wazni OM, Marrouche NF, Martin DO, *et al.* Radiofrequency ablation vs antiarrhythmic drugs as first-line treatment of symptomatic atrial fibrillation: a randomized trial. JAMA 2005; 293: 2634-40.
8. Stabile G, Bertaglia E, Senatore G, *et al.* Catheter ablation treatment in patients with drugrefractory atrial fibrillation: a prospective, multi-centre, randomized, controlled study (Catheter Ablation For The Cure Of Atrial Fibrillation Study). Eur Heart J 2006; 27: 216.

9. Pappone C, Augello G, Sala S, *et al.* A randomized trial of circumferential pulmonary vein ablation versus antiarrhythmic drug therapy in paroxysmal atrial fibrillation: the APAF Study. J Am Coll Cardiol 2006; 48: 2340-7.

10. Haissaguerre M, Sanders P, Hocini M, *et al.* Catheter ablation of long-lasting persistent atrial fibrillation: critical structures for termination. J Cardiovasc Electrophysiol 2005; 11: 1125-37.

11. Nademanee K, McKenzie J, Kosar E, *et al.* A new approach for catheter ablation of atrial fibrillation: mapping of the electrophysiologic substrate. J Am Coll Cardiol 2004; 43: 2044-53.

12. Oral H, Pappone C, Chugh A, *et al..* Circumferential pulmonary-vein ablation for chronic atrial fibrillation. N Engl J Med 2006; 354: 934-94.

13. Augello G, Augello G, Vicedomini G, *et al.* Pulmonary vein isolation after circumferential pulmonary vein ablation: comparison between Lasso and three-dimensional electroanatomical assessment of complete electrical disconnection. Heart Rhythm 2009; 6(12): 1706-13.

14. Pappone C, Radinovic A, Manguso F, *et al.* Progression of atrial fibrillation in patients with a first-detected episode. A long-term prospective follow-up study. J Am Coll Cardiol 2007; 49: 25A(Suppl A).

Chapter 9. Understanding and ablating typical atrial flutter

F.G. Cosio, A. Pastor, A. Núñez

Cardiology Service and Arrhythmia Unit
Hospital Universitario de Getafe
Madrid, Spain

Address for correspondence:
Hospital Universitario de Getafe
Head Cardiology Service
Dr. Francisco G. Cosio
fgarciacosio.hugf@salud.madrid.org

Introduction

Typical atrial flutter (AFL) is caused by a large reentrant circuit supported by normal anatomic structures of the right atrium (RA). A unique combination of fixed obstacles and functional barriers related to myocardial bundles helps create a large posterior obstacle that makes the activation rotate around the tricuspid ring (TR). The cavotricuspid isthmus (CTI) is the key passage in the low RA and the target for ablation, with well-defined procedural endpoints. We will focus the following discussion on the description of the main electrophysiological (EP) landmarks that guide the diagnosis and catheter ablation of AFL.

1   The mechanism of typical flutter

The AFL circuit is contained in the RA with passive activation of the left atrium (LA).[1,2] Activation runs superoinferiorly on the anterior and lateral RA and inferosuperiorly on the septal RA in what has been called counterclockwise (CCW) activation (left anterior oblique view) (see figures 1 and 2). The lower turning point is the CTI, a relatively narrow segment of myocardium located on the RA "floor" between the TR and the inferior vena cava (IVC). The upper turning point is in most cases the RA roof, anterior to the superior vena cava, but it can also be below the superior vena cava, across the high posterior RA.[3,4] Transverse conduction between the ascending and descending limbs of the circuit is prevented by the terminal crest (TC) and other myocardial bundles in the posterior RA, which are highly anisotropic and offer high resistance to conduction across their longitudinal axis, due to high intercellular resistance.[5] Conduction gaps through the TC may occur[4] and in some cases more than one line of block can be detected in the posterior RA,[6,7] but the CTI remains the critical isthmus of the circuit in the lower RA.

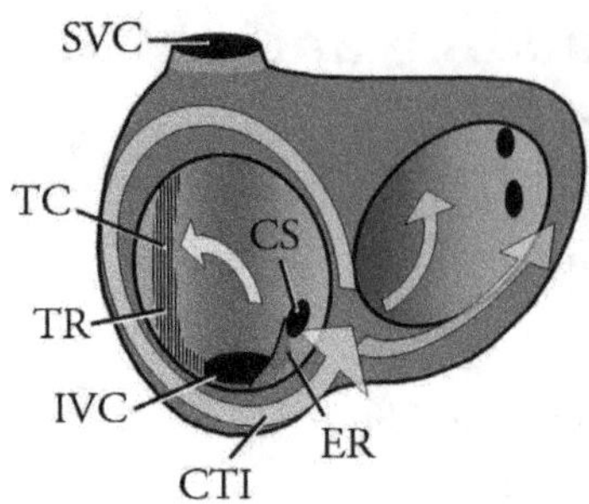

Figure 1. Schematic representation of the atria in a left anterior oblique view with disproportionately enlarged tricuspid and mitral valve orifices to show the endocardial side of the posterior walls.
CS = coronary sinus; CTI = cavo-tricuspid isthmus; ER = Eustachian ridge; IVC = inferior vena cava; SVC = superior vena cava; TC = terminal crest; TR = tricuspid ring.

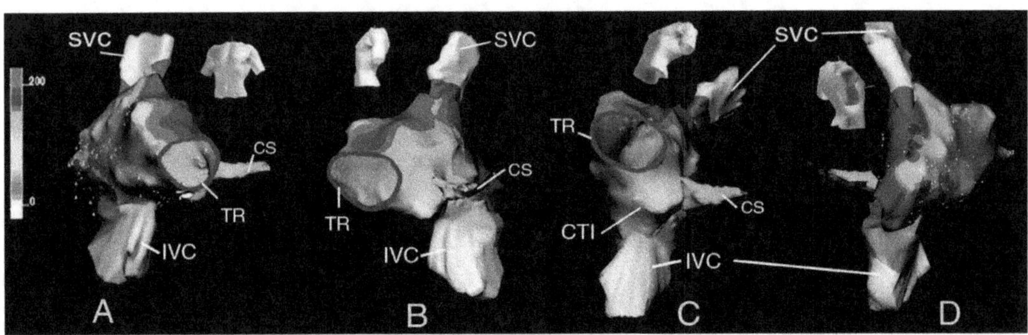

Figure 2. Electroanatomic reconstruction (NavX) of the right atrium with colour activation map in atrial flutter. The color code for activation is expressed in the bar on the left. The direction of the view is shown by the body casts. Abbreviations are as in figure 1. Note descending activation on the anterior and lateral walls (A), anteroposterior at the CTI (C) and ascending the septal wall (B). The posterolateral view (D) shows a narrow area with isochronal crowding between very late (purple) and early (red), representing block at the TC level. Brown circles mark recorded double potentials. The color map has been touched up at the RA roof to abolish the "reverse rainbow" artifact at the junction of "early" and "late" activation.
CS = coronary sinus; CTI = cavo-tricuspid isthmus; IVC = inferior vena cava; SVC = superior vena cava.

When activation rotates clockwise (CW) we talk of "reverse AFL"[8] (see figures 3 and 4). The reason for CCW activation being present in 90% of AFL is unclear, possibly related to conduction properties in the septal RA facilitating unidirectional block in the CW direction.[9] Block lines are found in the same areas as in CCW AFL and the CTI is the key inferior turning point, as in CCW AFL.

2 Mapping the flutter circuit

Atrial flutter can be easily mapped because the circuit is large and accessible. A multipolar catheter-electrode (CE) (20-24 poles, separation 2-10-2 mm) looped in the RA from the IVC

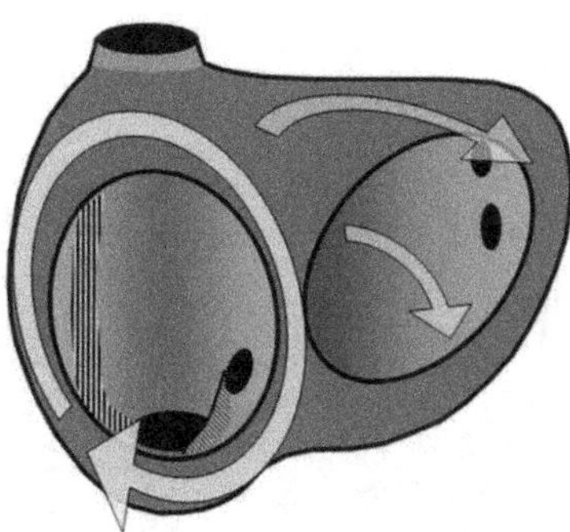

Figure 3. Schematic representation of atrial activation in reverse (clockwise) typical AFL. (See figure 1 for explanation.)

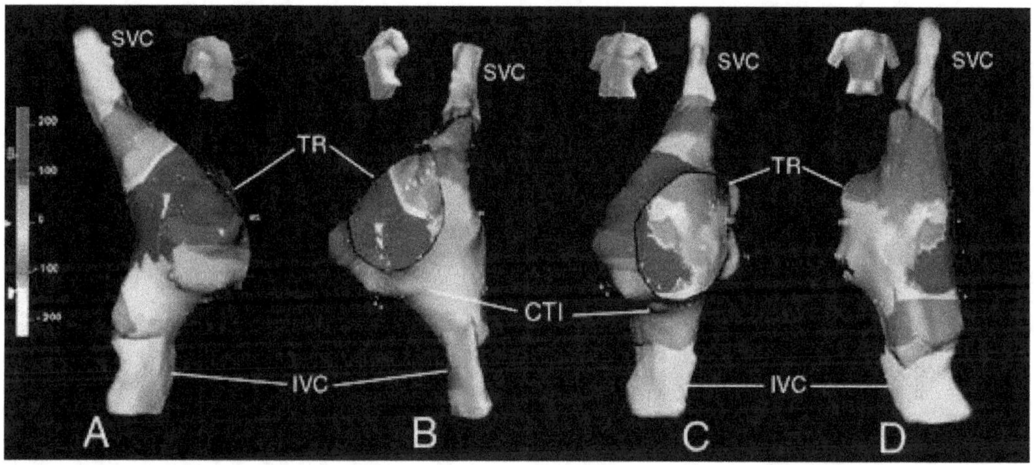

Figure 4. Electroanatomic reconstruction (NavX) of the right atrium with colour activation map in atrial flutter. The color code for activation is expressed in the bar on the left. The direction of the view is shown by the body casts. Abbreviations are as in figure 1. Note ascending activation on the anterior and lateral walls (A), descending the septal wall (B) and posteroanterior in the CTI (B). The low posterior wall is shown in C through the TR and in D in a posterior view with narrow spaces between late (blue) and early (red-orange) activation, representing conduction block. Activation may cross the upper part of the TC.

allows simultaneous recordings or pacing from the anterolateral wall, roof and septal wall, covering from 70-80% of the circuit (see figure 5A). Recordings from other areas can be obtained with a deflectable CE, or by rotating the reference CE in multipoint computerized mapping systems. This setup allows monitoring RA activation for the detection of changes during CTI ablation (see figure 6).[10] Point-by-point mapping of the CTI and other areas is done using the ablation CE. Other laboratories advance the reference CE to the CS to pace the proximal CS and record several CTI electrograms (EGM) (see figure 5B). This position limits RA recordings due to no data being received from the septal RA, and the reference CE can interfere with ablation CE positioning on the CTI.

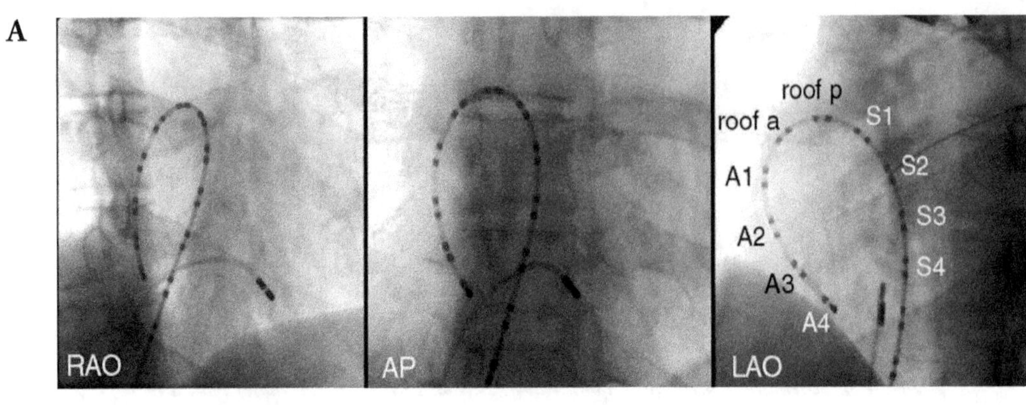

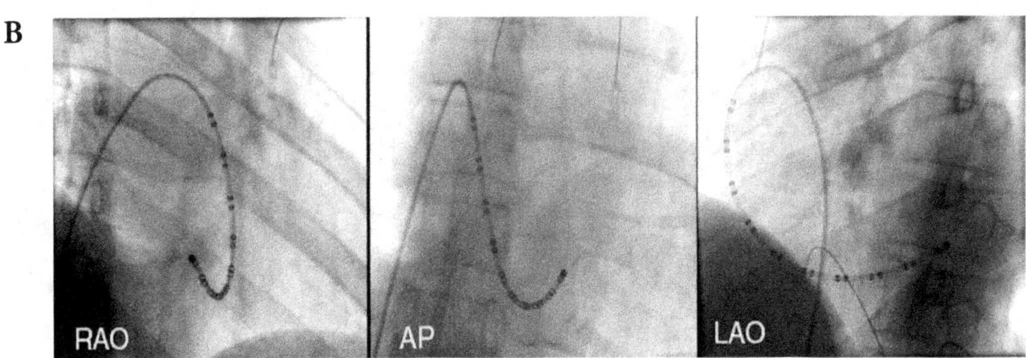

Figure 5. A. Catheter-electrode setup in our laboratory for mapping and ablation of AFL in fluoroscopic right anterior oblique (RAO), anteroposterior (AP) and left anterior oblique (LAO) views. Note that the 24-pole CE covers the lateral RA wall, the roof and the septal wall (the 4 other proximal electrodes are in the IVC). The LAO view shows the labelling that corresponds to the electrophysiological recordings. B. Fluoroscopic RAO, AP and LAO views of a 20-pole reference CE advanced into the CS for direct mapping of the CTI. For explanation see text.

A multiple EGM display should facilitate recognition of changes in activation. At the top we display descending (high-to-low) anterior RA activation followed by the CTI, then ascending (low-to-high) septal activation, because this highlights the CTI EGM bridging activation between low anterior and low septal RA (see figures 6 and 7). The same EGM arrangement monitors CTI conduction when ablation is performed in sinus rhythm. Recordings from the posterior RA do not fill the interval between low septal and low anterior RA (see figure 8), whereas the posterolateral RA will show double potentials arranged in superoinferior rows separating descending anterior wall activation from ascending septal activation (see figure 9).[11,12] Another line of block and double potentials can be found in many cases at the Eustachian ridge, on the septal side of the CTI.[13,14]

The CTI is often designated as the "slow conduction critical isthmus" of the AFL circuit; however, not all studies have confirmed slow conduction at the CTI[15] (see figures 2 and 4) and others have found a modest decrease in conduction velocity.[16] Evidence of slow conduction,

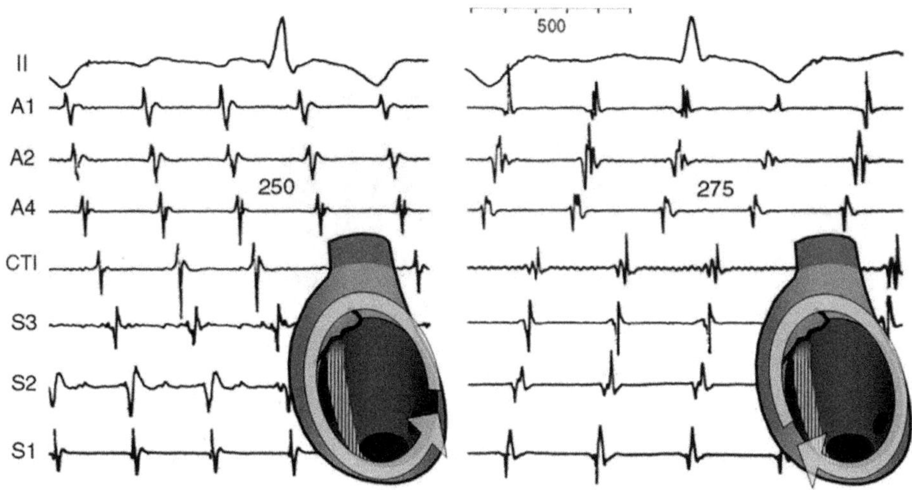

Figure 6. Simultaneous recordings from the anterior and septal RA and the CTI in a patient with both counterclockwise (left) and clockwise (right) typical AFL in the laboratory. The CTI electrogram bridges activation between low anterior and low septal RA in both instances. Figures in milliseconds (see figure 1 for abbreviations).

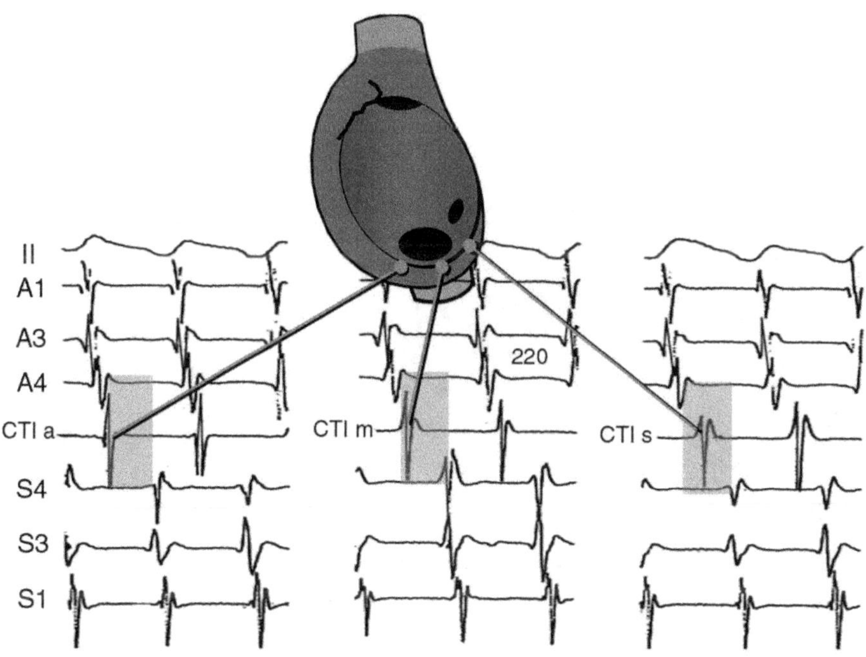

Figure 7. Mapping the CTI in the frame of multiple recordings from the anterior and septal RA. The gray window marks the interval of the AFL cycle between low anterior and low septal electrograms (EGMs), that is bridged by EGM from the anterior (a), mid- (m) and septal (s) CTI. The schema of the RA shows the CTI recording sites. Note the configuration of the AFL waves in lead II. Figures in milliseconds (see figure 1 for abbreviations).

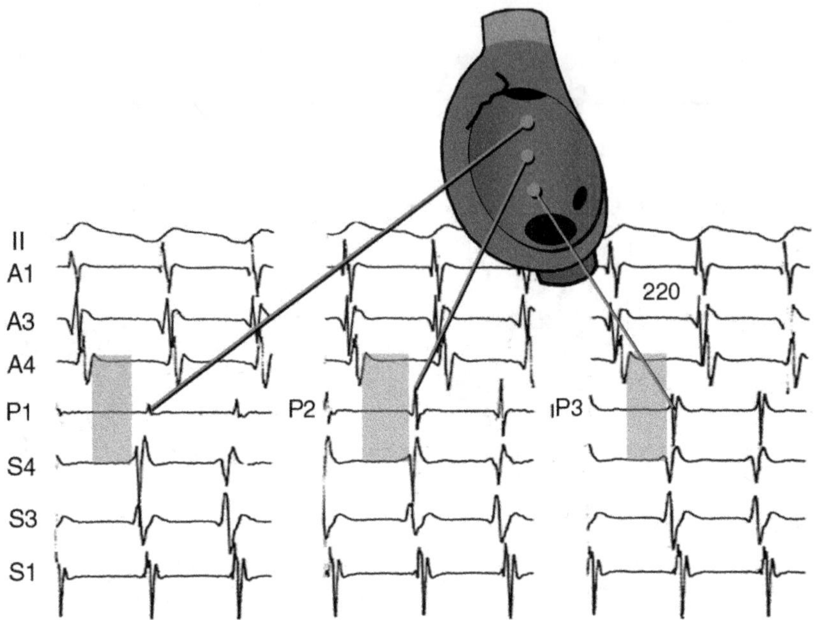

Figure 8. Mapping the posterior RA in the frame of multiple recordings from the anterior and septal RA. The schema of the RA shows the CTI recording sites. Note that all posterior RA EGM are outside the gap between low anterior and low septal RA. Figures in milliseconds (see figure 1 for abbreviations).

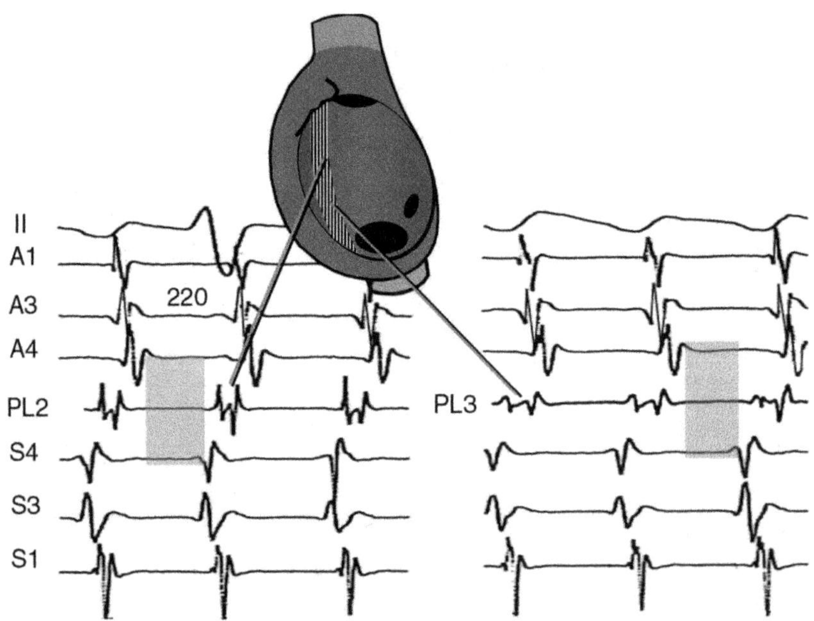

Figure 9. Mapping the posterolateral RA in the frame of multiple recordings from the anterior and septal RA. The schema of the RA shows the CTI recording sites. Note double EGM at the two recording sites. Figures in milliseconds (see figure 1 for abbreviations).

such as wide, fragmented EGM will rarely be found in the CTI before radiofrequency (RF) application (see figures 6 and 7).

3   Role of entrainment

The study of post-pacing pauses has helped to define the areas of the RA directly involved in the reentry circuit. Pacing the CTI will produce "concealed" entrainment (no fusion on the ECG) with little antidromic penetration of the circuit.[17-19] The post-pacing cycle will be ≤30 ms longer than AFL cycle length (see figures 10 and 11) confirming the role of the CTI as the critical isthmus for AFL. Some initial approaches to RF catheter ablation have used concealed entrainment to guide RF applications;[17,18] however, concealed entrainment can be produced by pacing areas of the septal and posterior RA outside the CTI[20] making it unreliable as the only guide.

4   Role of the electrocardiogram

A typical AFL pattern in a patient without a history of cardiac surgery (atriotomy) is highly predictive of a CTI-dependent AFL, making direct ablation of the CTI in sinus rhythm a sensible approach. Recognition of CCW AFL depends on leads II, III and aVF, including a negative deflection followed by a sharp upstroke making a small, positive deflection followed by a slowly descending segment leading to the next cycle (see figures 7 to 9). Reverse typical clock-

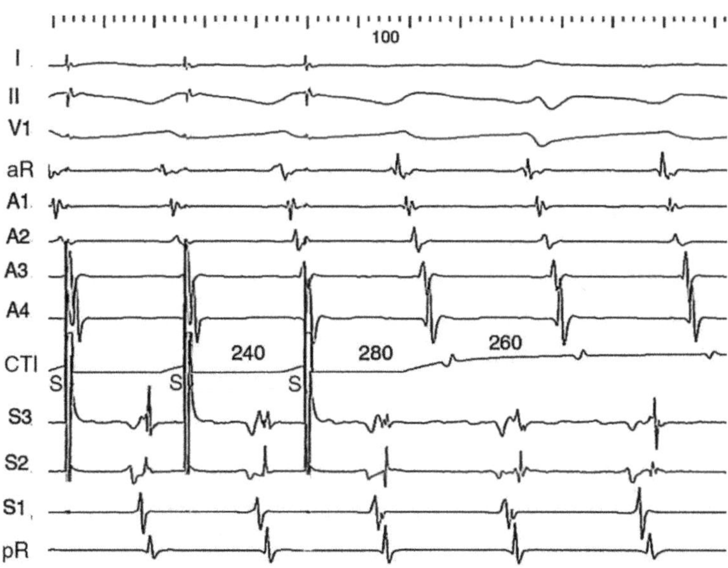

Figure 10. Entrainment of typical counterclockwise atrial flutter (AFL) from the carotricuspid isthmus (CTI). Note that during entrainment there is no change in the AFL wave in lead II and no antidromic penetration of the pacing front into the anterior wall (A1-A4 sequence unchanged). Post-pacing pause at the CTI is 20 ms longer than baseline AFL cycle length. Figures in milliseconds.

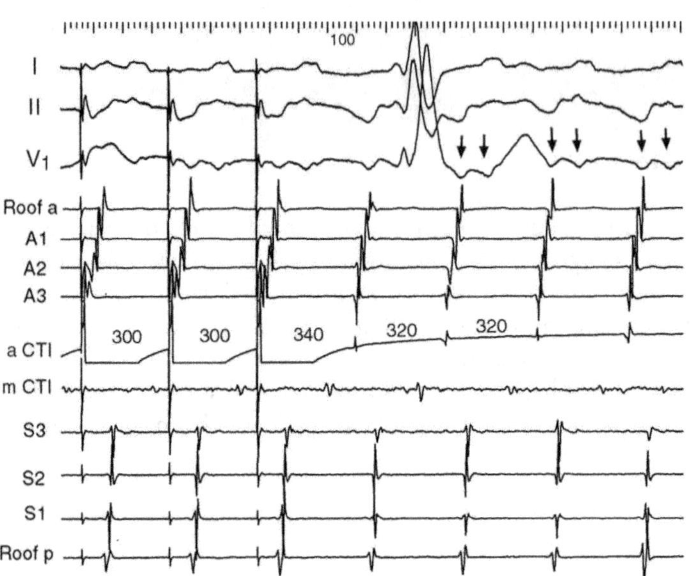

Figure 11. Entrainment of a slow typical clockwise AFL from the anterior (a) CTI. Note there is no antidromic penetration to the septal CTI or septal RA, that maintain a fully descending sequence. The return cycle is 20 milliseconds longer than spontaneous AFL cycle length.
mCTI = mid CTI. Note the broad positive deflections in II and the W-shaped wave in V1 (double arrows). Figures in milliseconds.

wise (CW) AFL is recognized by broad, positive, often notched, deflections in the inferior leads and a negative "W"-shaped wave in lead V1[21] (see figure 11).

In patients with a history or surgical atriotomy or atrial catheter ablation, a typical AFL ECG pattern is insufficient, because it may coexist or even be mimicked by other tachycardias. Mapping the arrhythmia is also essential in patients with atypical ECG patterns, which could be due to left atrial tachycardias. On the other hand, an atypical ECG pattern does not rule out a CTI-dependent circuit, particularly if atriotomy or previous ablation scars distort activation.[10]

5   Cavotricuspid isthmus ablation

Cavotricuspid isthmus ablation is performed by drawing a line of lesions across the CTI, from the TR to the IVC until bidirectional block occurs. When the CTI is smooth and thin, block can be completed with a few RF applications (2-5 min); however, in 20-30% of cases it is difficult to attain and in 5-10% the CTI is not blocked in a first procedure.[22,23] Imaging techniques may show deep recesses associated with a prominent Eustachian ridge as a cause of the difficulty.[24-26] Anatomic reconstruction with computer-assisted navigation systems helps to guide the catheter to the CTI; however, it is not enough in itself to draw an ablation line, because the CE moves along with respiration over the still anatomic cast, making accuracy less than perfect. Analysis of local EGM at the point of application is essential to guide ablation.[27,28]

6   Modes of energy application for ablation

Large (8-10 mm) or irrigated-tip CE are more effective than conventional 4-mm electrodes.[29,30] The 8-mm CEs allow more power application (60-80 W), although heating may be uneven along the electrode and tissue boiling can occur at the electrode edges, with risk of tissue disruption and perforation,[31] despite an apparently controlled temperature. For this reason, the target temperature is limited to 60 °C. Irrigated-tip CEs use a saline solution flow to decrease electrode temperature, allowing higher power delivery and more lesion depth.[30] Open-irrigation electrodes let saline flow into the bloodstream through multiple holes, whereas closed-irrigation CE recirculate the cooling solution to the catheter, avoiding fluid overload.[30] The temperature at the electrode tip can be much lower than tissue temperature and the risk of tissue boiling ("popping") exists even if the temperature limit is set to ≤50 °C.[32,33] An impedance drop of 15 ohms during RF application may reflect excessive heating.[34]

Catheter cryoablation has been applied to the CTI with similar success to RF ablation.[23] The advantages are the adherence of the catheter to the endocardium that stabilizes the catheter during application, and the lack of pain.

7   Drawing the ablation line

The ablation line starts at the low TR, at the 5 o'clock to 6 o'clock position (left anterior oblique view) (see figure 1), where a small atrial EGM and a larger ventricular EGM are recorded. We apply RF point-by-point for 60 sec in each location, then withdraw the CE toward the IVC. After each effective application the local EGM decreases in size and may become split, indicating local block; however, the line should continue toward the IVC seeking areas with a sharp EGM still bridging activation to the septal RA until the CE falls to the IVC. Sharp pain usually occurs with RF application in the IVC. An alternative approach is dragging the CE along the line, changing position every 15-30 sec in a continuous pull-back application lasting 90-150 sec until the endpoint or the IVC are reached.

When ablation is performed in AFL, the initial endpoint is AFL interruption, activation ending at the CTI (see figures 12 and 13). Before this is achieved, cycle-length prolongation may occur as a sign of prolonged conduction through the CTI (see figures 13 and 14). If the line is completed and AFL is not interrupted, the line is searched again with high-gain recordings for bridging fragmented EGM, marking conduction gaps.[28] When the CTI has deep pouches it may be necessary to bend the ablation CE sharply to reach the bottom of these recesses.[24-26] When no sharp EGM can be recorded from the CTI, sites of activation exit may be found toward the septal side of the CTI. In some cases catheter stability and firm contact with the CTI may be facilitated by long, pre-shaped guiding sheaths.

8   Precautions, complications

Moderate discomfort is common during RF application to the CTI and intravenous sedation and analgesia should be used when necessary. Severe pain occurs when RF is applied to the IVC, and is a warning sign to interrupt application. Atrioventricular block can occur when RF is applied on the septal RA and this position should be avoided.[35] Vagal reflexes

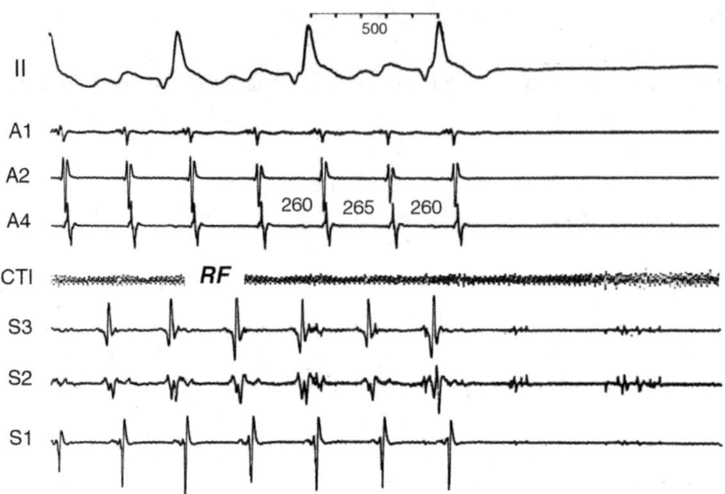

Figure 12. Interruption of counterclockwise atrial flutter (AFL) by radiofrequency (RF) application at the cavotricuspid isthmus (CTI). Note that activation sequence is interrupted at the site of application, between anterior right atrium (RA) (A4) and septal RA (S3). Figures in milliseconds.

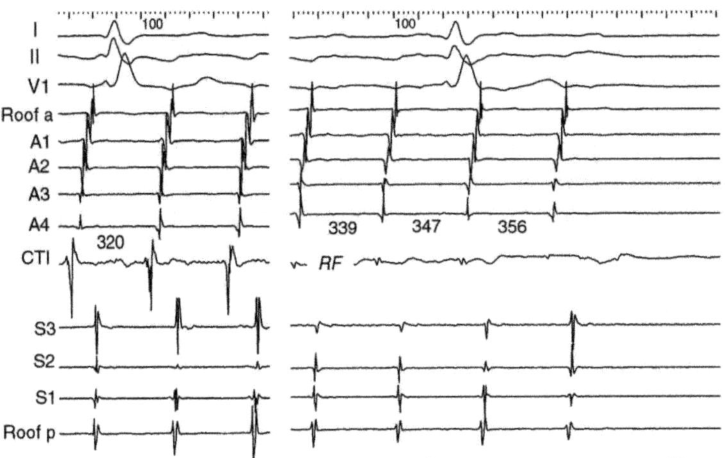

Figure 13. Interruption of clockwise AFL by RF application at the CTI (right panel). Note that the activation sequence is interrupted at the site of application, between septal RA (S3) and anterior RA (A4). The left panel shows sequence and cycle length before RF application. Note that before interruption cycle length has increased by ~30 ms. Figures in milliseconds (see figure 12 for abbreviations).

can produce atrioventricular block during an application within the CTI, often related to pain. In these instances, atropine administration allows continuation of the procedure. Cardiac tamponade has rarely been reported with the use of irrigated-tip CE, in relation to boiling sounds ("pops").[33]

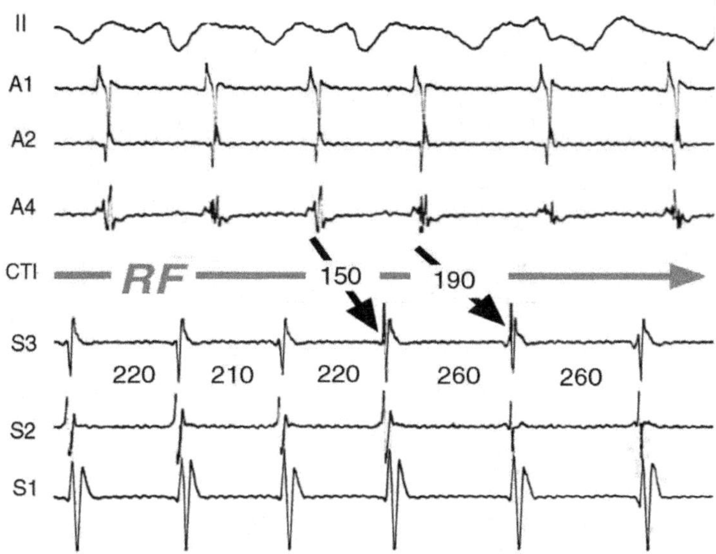

Figure 14. Cycle-length prolongation by application of radiofrequency (RF) at the CTI in counterclockwise AFL. Note that the cycle length is prolonged to the same extent as conduction through the CTI. AFL was interrupted by further RF application at the CTI. Figures in milliseconds (see figure 12 for abreviations).

9 Checking counterclockwise block

When AFL is interrupted, conduction through the CTI is still present in many cases. Counterclockwise conduction can be tested by pacing with the distal electrodes of the reference CE, while mapping the CTI with the ablation CE. When the CTI is blocked the septal RA EGMs display a descending sequence and the CTI EGM recorded on the septal CTI is later than the last septal EGM (see figure 15). A corridor of double EGMs spanning the TR to the IVC may be found; however, the first component is often not seen in recordings from the septal side of the ablation line (see figures 15 and 16).

Absolute values for transisthmus conduction have been proposed,[36,37] but these may be subject to factors such as antiarrhythmic drug effect. Unipolar recordings can help,[38] but they may be technically demanding and difficult to interpret. Counterclockwise block is best checked by differential pacing from the anterior RA[39] (see figure 16). When CTI block is present, conduction time to the septal CTI EGM decreases by moving the pacing site superiorly, whereas the opposite is true if there is slow conduction through the CTI. When a double potential is recorded at the ablation line the first component is delayed by moving the pacing site away from the CTI and double potential separation decreases (see figure 16).[39]

The ECG may help to detect CCW CTI block by a prolongation of the paced PR interval and appearance of a positive terminal P-wave deflection in lead II[40] (see figure 15). These signs, however, do not distinguish slow conduction from block and differential pacing is the ultimate test.

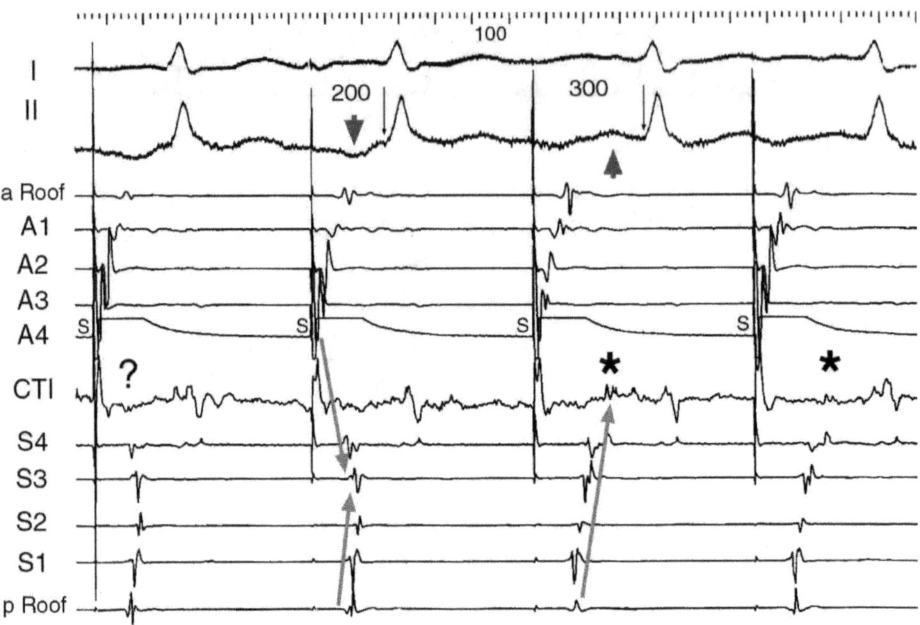

Figure 15. Development of CTI counterclockwise block during radiofrequency application, checked by pacing the low anterior wall (A4). The first two cycles show fusion of ascending and descending activation in the septal RA recordings (p Roof – S4) then activation becomes fully descending in the two last cycles. The asterisks mark a CTI potential later than low septal activation (S4) after block appears. A low voltage early potential may be present before (?). Note that the PR (S-R) interval increases and a late positive P-wave deflection appears (blue arrows). Figures in milliseconds (see figure 1 for abbreviations).

10   Checking clockwise block

Clockwise conduction may occur in the presence of signs of CCW block, and CTI block should be checked in both directions. Assessing CW CTI block can be difficult. Differential pacing can be done at different levels of the septal RA, although this direction means that CTI EGM are often difficult to interpret due to multiple deflections.[22,35] In our laboratory, we have found checking CW block by pacing at the septal CTI, close to the ablation line, to be very reliable to optimize the detection of slow conduction on anterior wall activation as a fusion pattern (see figure 17). In the presence of CW block, activation is fully descending. The long-term (>2 years) AFL recurrence rate was 3% in patients with CCW block, fulfilling this criteria for CW block (unpublished results).

When there is conduction through the TC, pacing from the CS may show fusion in anterior RA activation in the presence of CW CTI block.[41] In these cases, differential pacing on the posterior RA, close to the TC, will show the same fusion pattern, with a shorter interval between the stimulus and the anterior wall EGM. This artifact can also be avoided by pacing at the septal CTI, because this site is closer to the line of block at the CTI and further away from the TC (see figure 17).

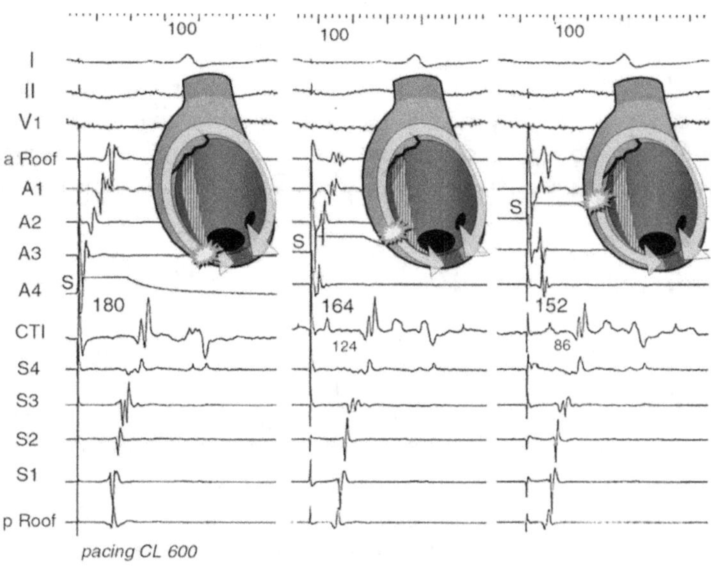

Figure 16. Differential pacing confirms counterclockwise block pacing the anterior RA at different levels, progressively further away from the CTI (A4 left panel, S3 middle panel, S2 right panel). Large figures above the CTI recording show the interval between the stimulus and the late CTI electrogram (EGM). Note that this interval decreases as the pacing site is moved away from A4 to A3 and A2. On the left panel, only the late EGM is recorded at the CTI, but in the middle and right panels an early EGM appears that becomes later as pacing is moved to A2, so that the interval between the two deflections in the CTI EGM becomes shorter (small figures). Figures in milliseconds (see figure 1 for abbreviations).

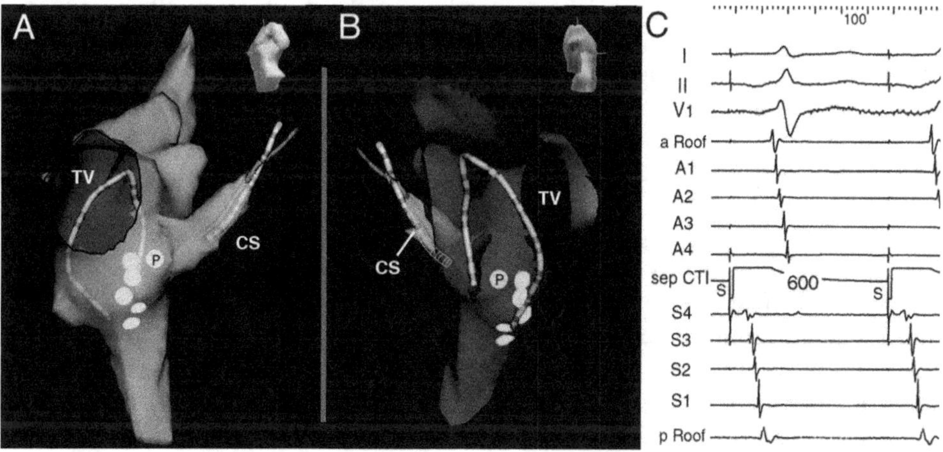

Figure 17. Testing counterclockwise CTI block by pacing the septal CTI, close to the ablation line. A shows an electroanatomic RA reconstruction (NavX) in a left anterior oblique view with caudal angulation. The red circles mark radiofrequency applications. The yellow circle (P) marks the pacing site. B shows the same anatomic area in a right lateral "endoscopic" view (the lateral RA wall has been removed) with some cranial angulation. The multipolar reference catheter and the CS reference catheter are shown. C shows EP recordings during pacing at P with ascending septal RA activation and fully descending anterior wall activation. Figures in milliseconds (see figure 1 for abbreviations).

11 Post-ablation observation time

CTI block may be transient and conduction can resume after a few seconds or a few minutes, making it necessary to confirm that bidirectional block is stable before ending the procedure.[42] Most conduction recurrences occur within 20 min to 25 min and we maintain an observation period of 30 min, pacing both sides of the CTI to detect conduction recurrence.

12 Failure despite prolonged ablation

In some cases, especially with enlarged RA, the CTI cannot be blocked or AFL interrupted despite good catheter position and highenergy RF applications. Radiofrequency applications produce edema and clots over the endocardium,[43] shielding the underlying conduction gaps. In our laboratory, we set a limit to the duration of the procedure (~3 hours) or the amount of RF applied (~25-30 min). These difficult cases can often be ablated easily in a second procedure 3-4 weeks later if there is a recurrence.

In these failed procedures it is essential to rule out a change in circuit configuration by CTI ablation, which is common in patients with surgical atriotomies, but which can also occur also without prior surgery. Close scrutiny of the ECG and the endocardial activation sequence facilitates detecting this change, and entrainment tests at the CTI will establish whether it is still an essential part of the circuit.[10]

12.1 *Long-term follow-up after cavotricuspid isthmus ablation*

When bidirectional, persistent CTI block is achieved, the prognosis regarding AFL recurrence after bidirectional CTI block is 5-10%, depending on the duration of follow-up.[25,26,29,30,35-40] Recurrences after 1 year can occur, although this is rare. In most recurrent cases, a new EP study will show conduction recurrence through the CTI and block will be attained with just a few RF applications.[28] In other cases recurrent flutter can be due to a different mechanism, such as left atrial or RA macroreentrant tachycardia not dependent on the CTI, or even focal tachycardia. The EP study of a recurrent AFL with an atypical ECG or in a patient with a history of atriotomy or atrial ablation, no matter what the ECG pattern, should rule out atypical AFL mechanisms.[10]

The main problem after AFL ablation is the progressive incidence of atrial fibrillation which is ~25-30% in the first 2 years, but that can rise above 50% in the longer term.[44-46] Atrial fibrillation is more common in patients with prior episodes of atrial fibrillation and those with an enlarged left atrium. After all, the TC and the CTI are normal anatomic landmarks and CTI ablation does not address the cause of AFL, but just an essential anatomical link in the circuit. The new challenge is to find a therapy that may arrest or revert the underlying arrhythmogenic process that may lead to atrial fibrillation in the patient.

References

1. Cosío FG, Arribas F, López-Gil M, *et al*. Atrial flutter mapping and ablation. I. Atrial flutter mapping. PACE 1996; 19: 841-53.
2. Cosío FG, Arribas F, López Gil M, *et al*. Atrial flutter mapping and ablation II. Radiofrequency ablation of atrial flutter circuits. PACE 1996; 19: 965-75.
3. Arribas F, López Gil M, Núñez A, *et al*. The upper link of the common atrial flutter circuit. PACE 1997; 20: 2924-9.
4. Shah D, Jaïs P, Haïssaguerre M, *et al*. Three-dimensional mapping of the common atrial flutter circuit in the right atrium. Circulation 1997; 96: 3904-12.
5. Spach MS, Miller WT, Geselowitz DB, *et al*. The discontinuous nature of propagation in normal canine cardiac muscle. Evidence for recurrent discontinuities of intracellular resistance that affect the membrane currents. Circ Res 1981; 48: 39-54.
6. Friedman PA, Luria D, Fenton AM, *et al*. Global right atrial mapping of human atrial flutter: the presence of posteromedial (sinus venosa region) functional block and double potentials: a study in biplane fluoroscopy and intracardiac echocardiography. Circulation 2000; 101: 1568-77.
7. Tai C-T, Huang J-L, Lee P-C, *et al*. High-resolution mapping around the crista terminalis during typical atrial flutter: New Insights into Mechanisms. J Cardiovasc Electrophysiol 2004; 15: 406-14.
8. Cosío FG, Goicolea A, López-Gil M, *et al*. Atrial endocardial mapping in the rare form of atrial flutter. Am J Cardiol 1991; 66: 715-20.
9. Cosio FG, López Gil M, Arribas F, *et al*. Mechanisms of induction of typical and reversed atrial flutter. J. Cardiovasc. Electrophysiology 1998; 9: 281-91.
10. Cosío FG, Martín-Peñato A, Pastor A, *et al*. Atypical Flutter: A Review. PACE 2003; 26: 2157-69.
11. Tai C-T, Chen S-A, Chen Y-J, *et al*. Conduction properties of the crista terminalis in patients with typical atrial flutter: basis for a line of block in the reentrant circuit. J Cardiovasc Electrophysiol 1998; 9: 811-9.
12. Cosío FG, Arribas F, Barbero JM, *et al*. Validation of double spike electrograms as markers of conduction delay or block in atrial flutter. Am J Cardiol 1988; 61: 775-80.
13. Olgin JE, Kalman JM, Fitzpatrick AP, *et al*. Role of right atrial structures as barriers to conduction during human type I atrial flutter. Activation and entrainment mapping guided by intracardiac echocardiography. Circulation, 1995; 92: 1839-48.
14. Huang J-L, Tai C-T, Liu T-Y, *et al*. High-resolution mapping around the Eustachian ridge during typical atrial flutter. J Cardiovasc Electrophysiol High-resolution mapping around the Eustachian ridge during typical atrial flutter. J Cardiovasc Electrophysiol 2006; 17: 1187-92
15. Schilling RJ, Peters NS, Goldberger J, *et al*. Characterization of the anatomy and conduction velocities of the human right atrial flutter circuit determined by non-contact mapping. J Am Coll Cardiol 2001; 38: 385-93.

16. Tai C-T, Chen S-A, Chiang CE, *et al*. Characterization of low right atrial isthmus as the slow conduction zone and pharmacological target in typical atrial flutter. Circulation 1997; 96: 2601-11.
17. Feld GK, Fleck RP, Chen PS, *et al*. Radiofrequency catheter ablation for the treatment of human type 1 atrial flutter. Identification of a critical zone in the reentrant circuit by endocardial mapping techniques. Circulation 1992; 86: 1233-40.
18. Lesh MD, Van Hare GF, Epstein LM, *et al*. Radiofrequency catheter ablation of atrial arrhythmias. Results and mechanisms. Circulation 1994; 89: 1074-89.
19. Cosío FG, López Gil M, Arribas F, *et al*. The mechanisms of entrainment of human common flutter studied with multiple endocardial recordings. Circulation 1994; 89: 2117-26.
20. Morton JB, Sanders P, Deen V, *et al*. Sensitivity and specificity of concealed entrainment for the identification of a critical isthmus in the atrium: relationship to rate, anatomic location and antidromic penetration. J Am Coll Cardiol 2002; 39: 896-906.
21. Kalman JM, Olgin JE, Saxon LA, *et al*. Electrocardiographic and electrophysiologic characterization of atypical atrial flutter in man: use of activation and entrainment mapping and implications for catheter ablation. J Cardiovasc Electrophysiol 1996; 8: 121-44.
22. Anselme F, Savouré A, Cribier A, *et al*. Catheter ablation of typical atrial flutter: a randomized comparison of 2 methods for determining complete bidirectional isthmus block. Circulation 2001; 103: 1434-39.
23. Feld GK, Daubert JP, Weiss R, *et al*. Acute and long-term efficacy and safety of catheter cryoablation of the cavotricuspid isthmus for treatment of type 1 atrial flutter. Heart Rhythm 2008; 5: 1009-14.
24. Cabrera JA, Sanchez-Quintana D, Ho SY, *et al*. The architecture of the atrial musculature between the orifice of the inferior caval vein and the tricuspid valve: The anatomy of the isthmus. J Cardiovasc Electrophys 1998; 14: 1186-95.
25. Da Costa A, Romeyer-Bouchard C, Dauphinot V *et al*. Cavotricuspid isthmus angiography predicts atrial flutter ablation efficacy in 281 patients randomized between 8 mm- and externally irrigated-tip catheter. Eur Heart J August 2006; 27: 1833-40.
26. Kirchhof P, Ozgün M, Zellerhoff S, *et al*. Diastolic isthmus length and "vertical" isthmus angulation identify patients with difficult catheter ablation of typical atrial flutter: a pre-procedural MRI study. Europace 2009; 11: 42-7.
27. Poty H, Saoudi N, Nair M, *et al*. Radiofrequency catheter ablation of atrial flutter: further insights into the various types of isthmus block: application to ablation during sinus rhythm. Circulation 1996; 94: 3204-13.
28. Shah DC, Haïssaguerre M, Jaïs P, *et al*. Simplified electrophysiologically directed catheter ablation of recurrent common atrial flutter. Circulation 1997; 96: 2505-9.

29. Marrouche NF, Schweikert R, Saliba W, *et al.* Use of different catheter ablation technologies for treatment of typical atrial flutter: acute results and long-term follow-up. PACE 2003; 26: 743-6.

30. Scavée C, Jaïs P, Hsu LF, *et al.* Prospective randomised comparison of irrigated-tip and large-tip catheter ablation of CTI-dependent atrial flutter. Eur Heart J 2004; 25: 963–9.

31. McRury ID, Whayne JG, Haines DE. Temperature measurement as a determinant of tissue heating during radiofrequency catheter ablation: an examination of electrode thermistor positioning for measurement accuracy. J Cardiovasc Electrophysiol 1995; 6: 268-78.

32. Bruce GK, Bunch TJ, Milton MA, *et al.* Discrepancies between catheter tip and tissue temperature in cooled-tip ablation: relevance to guiding left atrial ablation. Circulation 2005; 112: 954-60.

33. Hsu L-F, Jaïs P, Hocini M, *et al.* Incidence and prevention of cardiac tamponade complicating ablation for atrial fibrillation. PACE 2005; 28 (suppl 1): S106-S109.

34. Borganelli M, el-Atassi R, Leon A, *et al.* Determinants of impedance during radiofrequency catheter ablation in humans. Am J Cardiol 1992; 69: 1095-7.

35. Anselme F, Klug D, Scanu P, *et al.* Randomized comparison of two targets in typical atrial flutter ablation. Am J Cardiol 2000; 85: 1302-7.

36. Tada H, Oral H, Sticherling C, *et al.* Double potentials along the ablation line as a guide to radiofrequency ablation of typical atrial flutter. J Am Coll Cardiol 2001; 38: 750-5.

37. Oral H, Sticherling C, Tadfa H, *et al.* Role of transisthmus conduction intervals in predicting bidirectional block after ablation of typical atrial flutter. J Cardiovasc Electrophysiol 2001; 12: 169-74.

38. Villacastin J, Almendral J, Arenal A, *et al.* Usefulness of unipolar electrograms to detect isthmus block after radiofrequency ablation of typical atrial flutter. Circulation 2000; 102: 3080-5.

39. Shah D, Haïssaguerre M, Takahashi A, *et al.* Differential pacing for distinguishing block from persistent conduction through an ablation line. Circulation 2000 26; 102: 1517-22.

40. Weiss C, Willems S, Hoffmann M, *et al.* Impact of the ECG for detection of intraatrial conduction block after atrial flutter ablation. Pacing Clin Electrophysiol 1999; 22: 1457-65.

41. Scaglione M, Riccardi R, Calo L, *et al.* Typical atrial flutter ablation: conduction across the posterior region of the inferior vena cava orifice may mimic unidirectional isthmus block. J Cardiovasc Electrophysiol 2000; 11: 387-95.

42. Shah DC, Takahashi A, Jaïs P, *et al.* Tracking dynamic conduction recovery across the cavotricuspid isthmus. J Am Coll Cardiol 2000 35: 1478-84.

43. Morton JB, Sanders P, Davidson NC, *et al.* Phased-array intracardiac echocardiography for defining cavotricuspid isthmus anatomy during radiofrequency ablation of typical atrial flutter. J Cardiovasc Electrophysiol 2003; 14: 591-7.

44. Anselme F, Saoudi N, Poty H, *et al.* Radiofrequency catheter ablation of common atrial flutter: significance of palpitations and quality-of-life evaluation in patients with proven isthmus block. Circulation 1999 2; 99: 534-40.

45. Luria DM, Hodge DO, Monahan KH, *et al.* Effect of radiofrequency ablation of atrial flutter on the natural history of subsequent atrial arrhythmias. J Cardiovasc Electrophysiol 2008; 19: 1145-50.

46. Ellis K, Wazni O, Marrouche N, *et al.* Incidence of atrial fibrillation post-cavotricuspid isthmus ablation in patients with typical atrial flutter: left-atrial size as an independent predictor of atrial fibrillation recurrence. J Cardiovasc Electrophysiol 2007; 18: 799-802.

Chapter 10. Atrioventricular nodal tachycardia: a simple and fast approach to cure

P. Brugada,[1] S.A. Müller-Burri,[2] J. Brugada[3]

[1]Cardiovascular Division
UZ Brussel-VUB
Brussels, Belgium

[2]Heart Rhythm Management Centre
UZ Brussel-VUB
Brussels, Belgium

[3]Hospital Clínic, Fundació Clínic
University of Barcelona
Barcelona, Spain

Address for correspondence:
Cardiovascular Division
UZ Brussels-VUB
Dr. Pedro Brugada
pedro@brugada.org

Introduction

Atrioventricular nodal tachycardia (AVNT) is one of the most common cardiac arrhythmias.[1,2] AVNT is almost never life threatening with some exceptions: patients developing syncope because of very fast AVNT and patients with structural heart disease. However, AVNT can have a very negative impact on the quality of life of the patient. Not only because of the complaints, need of antiarrhythmic drug treatment or admission to the emergency room to terminate the arrhythmia, but also because AVNT is the most undiagnosed rhythm disturbance: AVNT occurs most commonly in young women in whom doctors underestimate the significance of paroxysmal palpitations unless an electrocardiogram (ECG) has documented the arrhythmia. Many patients with AVNT never reach the physician or the emergency room in time to have an ECG recorded during the complaints. The result can be very disastrous: the physician considers the complaints of palpitations as "functional", related to hyperventilation or anxiety disorders and the patient is irremediably placed on anti-depressive drugs. Of course these drugs have no effect at all to prevent new episodes of AVNT and a negative vicious circle between patient-doctor-medication-complaints is created that can even end with the admission of the patient into a psychiatric institution. That this is the reality is shown by the data that we collected many years ago on the diagnosis made by general practitioners in patients with proven supraventricular tachycardia. Depending upon the moment when the doctor saw the patient (during or outside the episode of arrhythmia) the diagnosis was very different (see table 1). Patients seen outside the episode of tachycardia were invariably diagnosed as suffering from hyperventilation, anxiety, sinus tachycardia or "stress". On the contrary, when the patients were seen during the arrhythmia, a diagnosis of tachycardia was suspected in the majority. Most supraventricular tachycardias are at the present time perfectly curable with catheter ablation obviating the need for unnecessary suffering and life-long antiarrhythmic drug treatment. To

Diagnosis	During tachycardia	Outside tachycardia
Arrhythmia	43 (93 %)	12 (7 %)
Hyperventilation	2	36
Sinus tachycardia	1	28
Anxiety	0	23
No abnormalites	0	78
Total	46	177

Table 1. Missing the diagnosis of tachycardia (223 patients seen by the general practitioner).

cure patients with AVNT, however, a perfectly integrated approach to diagnosis, referral and treatment is required.

In this article we describe the five clinical pathways for the rapid and effective diagnosis and cure of patients suffering from AVNT.

1 Thinking about AVNT: the "frog" sign

AVNT is a quite particular arrhythmia. It originates in the AV node and its anatomic basis is the presence of at least two (sometimes multiple) AV nodal pathways (see figure 1). Whether these dual or multiple AV nodal pathways are located within the AV node or are mere prolongations of the AV node with part of the atrium involved in the arrhythmia is still a matter of heavy electrophysiological discussion. Both hypotheses may be true, but none decreases the value of the clinical pathways discussed here. Because the AV node is located (as its name indicates) between the atria and the ventricles, and because of its anatomical small size, the reentry circuit of AVNT is one of the smallest known in the human heart. During AVNT the impulses circulating between the two AV nodal pathways result in almost simultaneous contraction of the atria and the ventricles. That means that the atria contracts against a closed AV valve resulting in reflux of the blood into the veins. For the right side of the heart, this means that blood refluxes into the superior and inferior vena cava creating a feeling of palpitations in the neck during AVNT. Our group reported detailed hemodynamic studies on the pathophysiological mechanisms involved in this reflux in the New England Journal of Medicine almost twenty years ago.[3] The reflux of blood into the neck veins creates not only a feeling of "neck palpitations" but can also be visualized. The patient has his/her neck veins kicking like a frog: the "frog" sign.

One of the essential parts in the anamnesis of the patient with palpitations is this frog sign. Table 2 shows the questions to be asked by the attending physician to a patient with paroxysmal palpitations in order to come to a putative diagnosis of the cause.[4] A well-taken clinical history can immediately suggest a diagnosis.

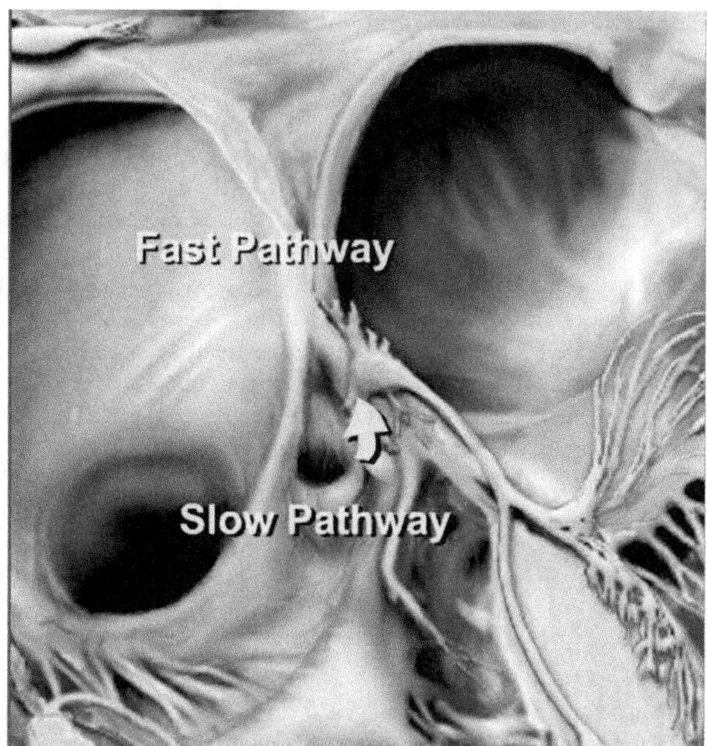

Figure 1. A schematic representation of the mechanisms of AVNRT. A slow (S) and a fast (F) AV nodal pathway are connected to each other at the level of the His bundle.

Diagnosis based on characteristics of palpitations	
Characteristics	Suspected arrhythmia
Rapid, regular, frog +	AV nodal tachycardia
Rapid, regular, frog -	CMT, AT, VT
Rapid irregular	Atrial fibrillation
Slow, regular, frog +	Ventricular premature
Slow, regular, frog -	Any extrasystoles

Table 2.

In terms of AVNT the anamnestic clues are clear (see table 2): if the patient suffers from fast, regular palpitations that are also felt in the neck, the diagnosis is almost certainly AVNT; if the patient is, in addition, a young female, the chances are close to 100% that AVNT is the cause of the palpitations and not anxiety disorders, hyperventilation or stress.

2   Is ECG documentation of an arrhythmia necessary in a patient with paroxysmal palpitations before undergoing definitive diagnosis and cure?

Many patients with paroxysmal, fast, regular palpitations do not suffer from sufficiently long episodes to enable recording of the arrhythmia on an ECG. In the majority of patients the episodes are also too scattered as to allow registration of the arrhythmia by means of 24-hour or even 7-day long-term ECG continuous recordings. Exercise tests do not trigger the arrhythmia in these individuals with, in general, an otherwise normal heart. The question arises then as to what is the fastest and most effective approach to diagnosis and treatment. The most common approach in clinical practice is to tell the patient to come to the emergency room for an ECG during the complaints. For the reasons previously explained, this approach has a very low chance of success. And, in the case that the arrhythmia is documented, what next? Obviously, to undergo a curative treatment the patient will require an electrophysiological study and catheter ablation. We have nowadays provided sufficient scientific evidence to state that if a paroxysmal supraventricular tachycardia is suspected based on the clinical history of the patient as delineated in table 2, the best approach is a direct electrophysiological investigation followed by catheter ablation. In patients with the Wolff-Parkinson-White syndrome, electrophysiologists no longer doubt that this is the fastest and most effective approach in addition to being the best approach from the prognostic point of view as demonstrated by the Pappone Group.[5] Similarly, in patients with paroxysmal palpitations without documented tachycardia if the electrophysiological study demonstrates a concealed accessory pathway, no electrophysiologist will hesitate to ablate that accessory pathway. But what should be done if during the electrophysiological study dual AV nodal pathways are documented in a patient with paroxysmal palpitations and no documented arrhythmia? For 3 years we have electrophysiologically studied on a prospective basis all individuals with paroxysmal palpitations without documented tachycardia in which a diagnosis of AVNT was suspected because of regular, fast palpitations with a positive "frog" sign.[6] In all these individuals demonstration of dual AV nodal pathways was considered sufficient evidence to explain the palpitations, and ablation of the slow AV nodal pathway was undertaken. Of the 135 patients studied, ablation of the slow pathway resulted in control of symptoms in 98% during a follow-up of a mean of 14 months. These results are identical to those that are obtained in patients with documented AVNT. As expected, 80% of the patients included in the study were female, and 40% of patients had received antiarrhythmic drugs empirically without any beneficial effect. These results clearly show that an electrophysiological approach to the patient with paroxysmal palpitations with a positive "frog" sign is the fastest way to effective cure of the symptoms. If dual AV nodal pathways are documented (with or without induction of AVNT during the electrophysiological study) ablation of the slow AV nodal pathway is justified.

3   Referring the patient with suspected or proven cardiac arrhythmia

Every physician should be aware of the diagnostic power of a well-taken clinical history. It is evident that a rapid referral of a patient for correct diagnosis and treatment is the best way to practice medicine irrespective of the medical problem. For the patient with documented or suspected cardiac arrhythmias this reasoning is particularly important. When a patient complains of symptoms that may suggest cardiac arrhythmias, the physician has to keep a quite open eye on the ultimate aim to be reached. Because cardiac arrhythmias have a wide range of clinical presentation and of prognostic consequences, it is the obligation of the doctor to try to assess them in a correct way. Some symptoms represent true medical emergencies, like syncope. A syncopal episode may be the first and last warning sign of a severe arrhythmia that may result in sudden cardiac death the next time. Unfortunately, many individuals who die suddenly never get the "benefit" of this warning syncope. They simply die suddenly as first manifestation of their disease.

Symptoms suggesting arrhythmias are shown in table 3. Any type of symptoms with a paroxysmal ("in crisis") character always has to include the possibility of a cardiac arrhythmia in the differential diagnosis.

Symptoms caused by cardiac arrhythmias
– None (asymptomatic)   – Palpitations (most frequent in SVT's)   – Dizziness   – Polyuria   – Syncope (most frequent in ventricular arrhythmias and severe bradyarrhythmias)   – Chest pain, fair, anxiety, dyspnea   – Sudden death

Table 3.

4   How to electrophysiologically approach documented or suspected AVNT

During the electrophysiological investigation of patients with paroxysmal palpitations with a positive frog sign, the demonstration of dual AV nodal pathways must be considered as sufficient evidence of the demonstration of an arrhythmia substrate. Figure 2 shows a classic example of a

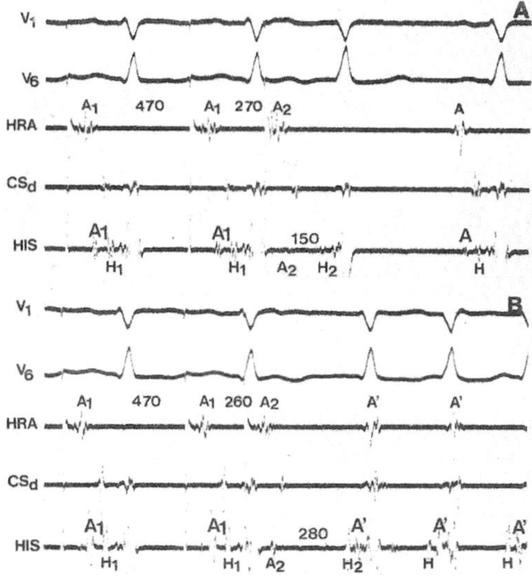

Figure 2. AV nodal conduction curves in a patient with AVNRT. See text for explanation.

jump in AV nodal anterograde conduction by more than 50 ms when the interval of the stimulated atrial premature beat is shortened from 270 (panel A) to 260 ms (panel B). Note how the A2H2 interval suddenly prolongs from 150 (panel A) to 280 ms (panel B). The jump is associated with an atrial echo (A') and initiation of AVNT. It is not always possible to initiate AVNT even in patients with documentation of the arrhythmia. Therefore, a jump in AV nodal conduction is sufficient proof for the demonstration of a potential arrhythmia substrate. As discussed previously, demonstration of this substrate is for us sufficient to indicate ablation of the slow AV nodal pathway in patients with paroxysmal fast and regular palpitations and a positive frog sign.

5   Curing AVNT: ablation strategy

The approach to the ablative cure of AVNT has changed over the years. Initially, ablation of the fast pathway was used, although nobody ever exactly described why. There were three major complications in this approach: *1)* complete AV block; *2)* first degree AV block; and *3)* inappropriate sinus tachycardia. These complications prompted the development of techniques for the ablation of the slow AV nodal pathway.[7] Ablation of the slow AV nodal pathway is associated with less chance of complete AV block, the PR interval does not prolong, and inappropriate sinus tachycardia does not occur after ablation in the area of the slow AV nodal pathway. Why the differences in the complications rates while using the same energy source (radiofrequency) and settings? It is clear that the differences can be only explained by the anatomic location of the fast and the slow AV nodal pathways and their proximity to other structures and the functional characteristics of the two pathways. The complexity of the AV node is so great that the surprise is not that AVNT exists, but on the contrary, why the majority of human beings and animals do not suffer from AVNT. Figure 3 shows the conduction of the cardiac

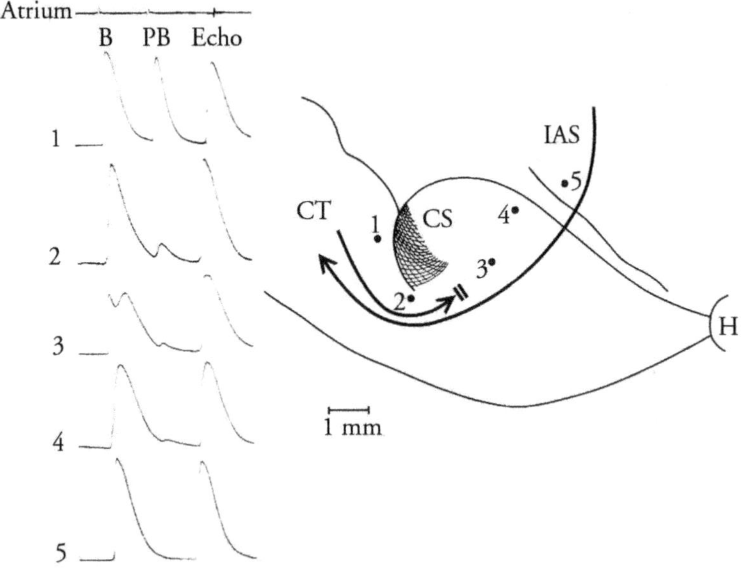

Figure 3. Electrophysiological recording during initiation of an AV nodal echo.

impulse during the initiation of an AV nodal echo.[8] Note how the input into the compact AV node coming from the crista terminalis (CT) blocks and the one coming from the interatrial septum (IAS) reenters. This is a block in conduction in the fast (1 to 2 to 3 cell recording) with retrograde conduction from the slow (5 to 4 to 3 to 2 to 1 cell recording). Further retrograde conduction into the CT results in the first atrial echo. Perpetuation of this activation results in AVNT (panel B). This schema taken from experiments from the rabbit heart illustrates that the two AV nodal pathways are anatomically distinct. The normal location of the two pathways in the human heart is that the fast pathway is close to the His bundle and superiorly located with respect to the compact AV node. The slow pathway is located inferiorly and far from the His bundle. Although variations and exceptions exist, these anatomical relations explain the differences in the incidence of complete AV block.

The prolongation of the PR interval (1st degree AV block) after ablation of the fast AV nodal pathway is explained by the electrophysiological properties of the fast and slow AV nodal pathway. Figure 4 illustrates a typical AV nodal conduction curve in a patient with dual AV nodal pathways and AVNT. The fast pathway conducts, as indicated by its name, fast, and the slow pathway, as also indicated by its name, slowly. Ablation of the fast pathway switches anterograde conduction over the AV node from the fast conducting to the slowly conducting pathway and the PR interval prolongs. That is, in itself, not a major problem, unless the PR interval prolongs so much that the P wave and the QRS complex come together during sinus rhythm. If that happens, the patient may again experience paroxysmal palpitations with the frog sign in spite of being cured of AVNT! The complaints are now not caused by AVNT, but by the prolongation of the PR interval that leads also to simultaneous contraction of atria and ventricles and to the frog sign.

Inappropriate sinus tachycardia following ablation of AVNT occurs almost exclusively after ablation of the fast AV nodal pathway.[9] It is suspected, but not proven, that ablation in the anatomic area of the fast pathway can cause destruction of some nerve terminals related to one or another reflex mechanism that leads to the acceleration of the sinus node rate.

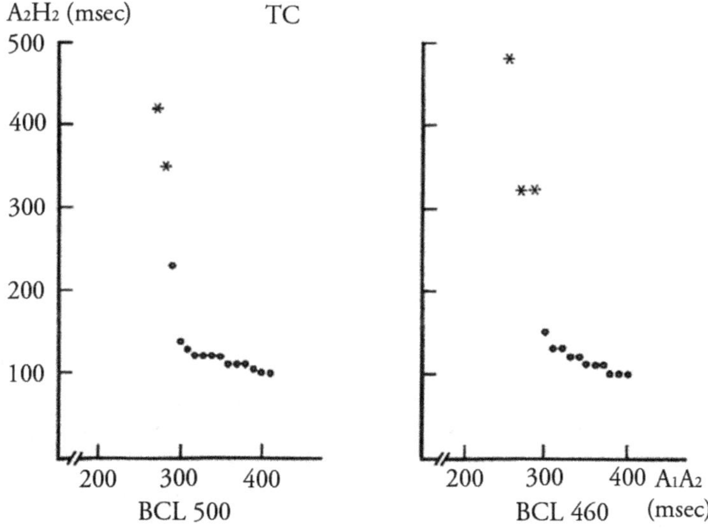

Figure 4. AV nodal conduction curves in a patient with dual AV nodal pathways and AVNT.

Because of these potential complications, clearly related to ablation of the fast AV nodal pathway, ablation of the AV nodal slow pathway is the treatment of choice. Figure 5 illustrates the three steps to place the ablation catheter in the adequate area while using fluoroscopy. First (step 1) the catheter is placed to record a His bundle potential. Second (step 2) the catheter is fully bent. A large ventricular potential will usually be recorded. Third (step 3) the catheter is pulled back until a small atrial electrogram is recorded together with a moderate size ventricular electrogram. Once in that position, radiofrequency or cryoenergy is applied to ablate the slow pathway. Observation of an accelerated junctional rhythm during radiofrequency ablation is a good predictor of success.

After ablation, programmed atrial stimulation is repeated to confirm conduction block over the slow AV nodal pathway. If no conduction can be shown during the same conditions as before the ablation, we consider that the substrate has been ablated and the procedure is stopped. With this approach a recurrence rate of less than 1% can be expected.

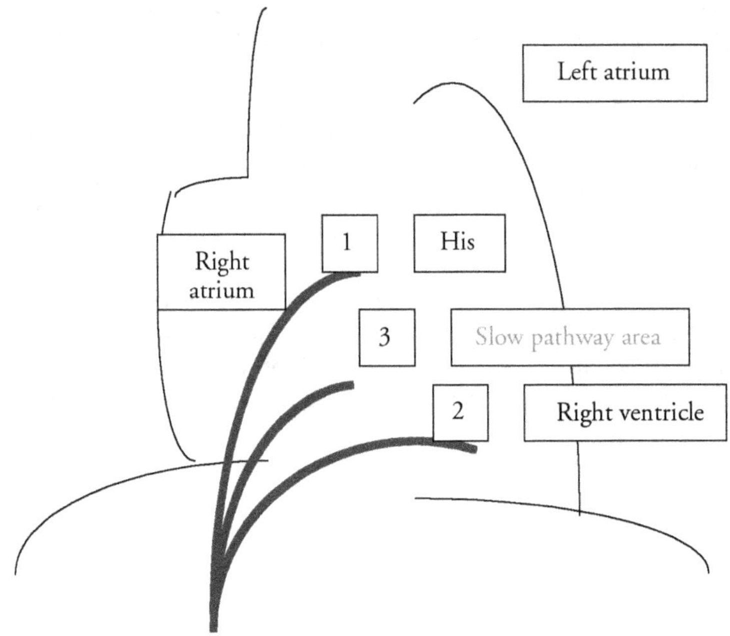

Figure 5. Steps in the ablation of AVNRT as seen fluoroscopically.

Conclusions

AV nodal reentrant tachycardia is a very common arrhythmia. Because it usually occurs in individuals with a normal heart, normal ECG, young age and female sex, the diagnosis is very frequently missed unless the patient is seen during the tachycardia. However, it is a relatively easy to diagnose arrhythmia if the physician asks the appropriate questions. Rapid, regular palpitations with a frog sign are pathognomonic of AV nodal reentrant tachycardia. Cure can be rapidly and effectively achieved by means of an electrophysiological investigation and ablation of the slow AV nodal pathway.

References

1. Kalbfleisch SJ, el-Atassi R, Calkins H, *et al.* Differentiation of paroxysmal narrow QRS complex tachycardias using the 12-lead electrocardiogram. J Am Coll Cardiol 1993; 21(1): 85-89.

2. Josephson ME, Wellens HJJ. Differential diagnosis of supraventricular tachycardia. Cardiol Clin 1990; 8: 411-442.

3. Gursoy S, Steurer G, Brugada J, *et al.* The hemodynamic mechanism of pounding in the neck in atrioventricular nodal reentrant tachycardia. N Eng J Med 1992; 327: 772-774.

4. Brugada P, Gursoy S, Brugada J, *et al.* Investigation of palpitations. The Lancet 1993; 341: 1254-1258.

5. Santinelli V, Radinovic A, Manguso F, *et al.* Asymptomatic ventricular preexcitation: A long-term followup study of 293 patients. Circ Arrhyth Electrophysiol 2009; 2: 102-107.

6. Muller-Burri SA, Personal communication.

7. Elvas L, Gursoy S, Brugada J, *et al.* Atrioventricular nodal reentrant tachycardia: A review. Can J Cardiol 1994; 10: 342-348.

8. Wellens HJJ, Lie KI, Janssen MJ. The conduction system of the heart. HE Stenfert Kroese BV. Leiden 1976: 296-315.

9. Skeberis V, Simonis F, Andries E, *et al.* Inappropriate sinus tachycardia following radiofrequency ablation of atrioventricular nodal reentrant tachycardia. Incidence and clinical significance. J Am Coll Cardiol 1993; 21: 314.

Chapter 11. Ablation of atrial tachycardias: a combination of ECG and EP may allow a simpler and faster approach

A.W. Teh, P.M. Kistler, C. Medi, K. Roberts-Thomson,
J.M. Kalman

Department of Cardiology
Royal Melbourne Hospital
Melbourne, Australia

Department of Medicine
University of Melbourne
Melbourne, Australia

Address for correspondence:
Dept. of Cardiology
Royal Melbourne Hospital
Prof. Jonathan M. Kalman
jon.kalman@mh.org.au

Introduction

Focal atrial tachycardia is an unusual form of supraventricular tachycardia but like other mechanisms of SVT is highly suited to curative catheter ablation. Over recent years with the widespread use of sophisticated mapping technology and a better understanding of anatomic distribution, reported success rates for atrial tachycardia ablation have been high. However, in an era of sophisticated 3D mapping solutions, it is important to remember that P-wave analysis and simple mapping techniques targeted to anatomic structures can rapidly and accurately localize many, if not most, atrial tachycardia foci.

1   P-wave morphology

Several algorithms for localizing atrial tachycardias based on P-wave morphology have been developed.[1-4] P-waves are generally described as isoelectric, positive, negative, or biphasic (positive-negative or negative-positive) and a full description will include the presence of notching. Analysis of the initial P-wave vector is paramount, and maneuvers such as carotid sinus massage, administration of intravenous adenosine or transient ventricular pacing will allow a clear demonstration of the "unencumbered" P-wave morphology by avoiding fusion of the P-wave and T-wave. Although atrial tachycardias may arise from anywhere within the atria, they tend to be distributed to typical anatomic locations (see figure 1). In the right atrium, these sites include the crista terminalis, tricuspid annulus, coronary sinus ostium, perinodal region, right atrial septum and right atrial appendage.[1] In the left atrium, sites of origin include the pulmonary veins, mitral annulus, CS body, left atrial septum and left atrial appendage.[1]

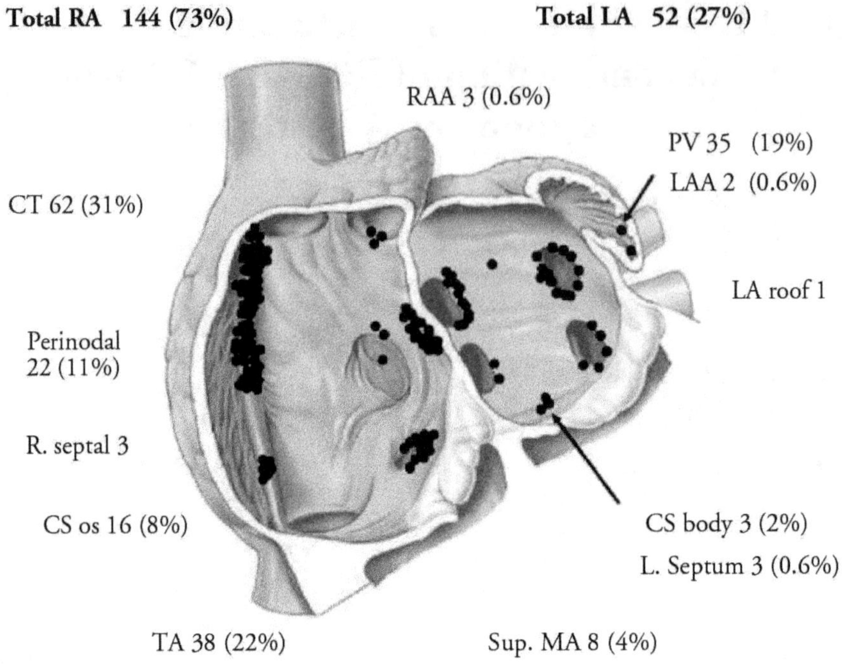

Figure 1. A schematic representation of the anatomic distribution of focal atrial tachycardias. The atrioventricular valvular annuli have been removed. Reprinted from Kistler, PM et al., P-wave morphology in focal atrial tachycardia: development of an algorithm to predict the anatomic site of origin. J Am Coll Cardiol, 2006; 48(5): 1010-7. With permission from Elsevier.
CS = coronary sinus; CT = crista terminalis; LA = left atrium; LAA = left atrial appendage; MA = mitral annulus; PV = pulmonary vein; RA = right atrium; RAA = right atrial appendage; TA = tricuspid annulus.

2   Right or left atrial site of origin

Differentiating the atrium of origin prior to ablation has important implications for planning whether left atrial access via trans-septal puncture is necessary. Tang *et al.* studied 31 consecutive patients undergoing catheter ablation for atrial tachycardia and found that a positive or biphasic P-wave in aVL predicted a right atrial focus with a sensitivity of 88%, specificity of 79%, positive predictive value of 83% and negative predictive value of 85%.[3] Three patients with right superior pulmonary vein foci had positive P-waves in aVL. However, in these patients the P-wave in V1 was biphasic during sinus rhythm and changed to positive during tachycardia in comparison with superior crista terminalis foci, where this change did not occur. They also noted that a positive P-wave in V1 predicted a left atrial focus with a sensitivity of 93%, specificity of 88%, positive predictive value of 87% and negative predictive value of 94%. An isoelectric or negative P-wave in lead I was 100% specific for a left atrial focus, but was only present in 50% of patients with left atrial foci.

Kistler *et al.* recently developed an algorithm to localize focal atrial tachycardia from any location (see figure 2).[1] This algorithm prospectively identified 93% of focal tachycardia anatomic origin correctly. In this algorithm, V1 was most useful differentiating right from left

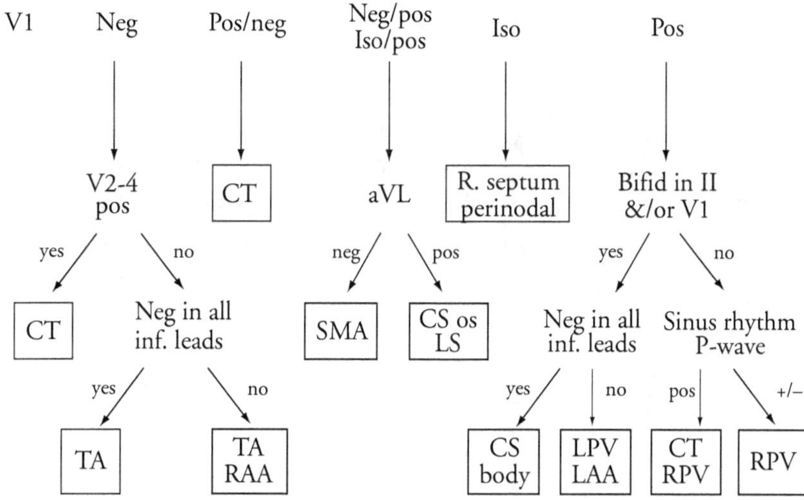

Figure 2. P-wave algorithm for localizing site of atrial tachycardia. Reprinted from Kistler, P.M. et al., P-wave morphology in focal atrial tachycardia: development of an algorithm to predict the anatomic site of origin. J Am Coll Cardiol 2006; 48(5): 1010-7. With permission from Elsevier.
CS = coronary sinus; CT = crista terminalis; ECG = electrocardiogram; LA = left atrium; LAA = left atrial appendage; LIPV = left inferior pulmonary vein; LSVP = left superior pulmonary vein; LS = left septum; MA = mitral annulus; SMA = superior mitral annulus; PWM = P-wave morphology; RA = right atrium; RAA = right atrial appendage; RFA = radiofrequency ablation; RIPV = right inferior pulmonary vein; RSPV = right superior pulmonary vein; SVC = superior vena cava; TA = tricuspid annulus.

atrial tachycardias. A negative or biphasic (positive-negative) V1 predicted a right atrial origin with 100% specificity, 100% positive predictive value, 69% sensitivity and 66% negative predictive value. Conversely, a positive or negative-positive biphasic P-wave in V1 had 100% sensitivity, 81% specificity, 76% positive predictive value and 100% negative predictive value for a left atrial origin. In this series, the P-wave morphology could not distinguish reliably between tachycardias located in close proximity to the septum (left versus right septal or perinodal).

3   Anatomic sites of origin

3.1   Crista terminalis

The crista terminalis (see figure 3) is the most common site for right atrial tachycardia accounting for two-thirds of right atrial foci in an early series.[5] The majority of these foci arose from the superior and mid crista terminalis[1] and therefore may have similar P-wave morphology (PWM) to sinus rhythm.[6] Tada and co-workers found that a negative P-wave in aVR predicted a cristal origin compared with anterior right atrial foci with a sensitivity of 100% and specificity of 93%.[2] Kistler *et al.* found that a positive-negative V1 P-wave (or positive V1 during tachycardia and sinus rhythm), positive lead I and II and negative aVR predicted a cristal origin with 93% sensitivity, 95% specificity, 84% positive predictive value and 98% negative predictive value.[1] Although there may be overlap between superior crista and right superior pul-

Right Atrial Foci

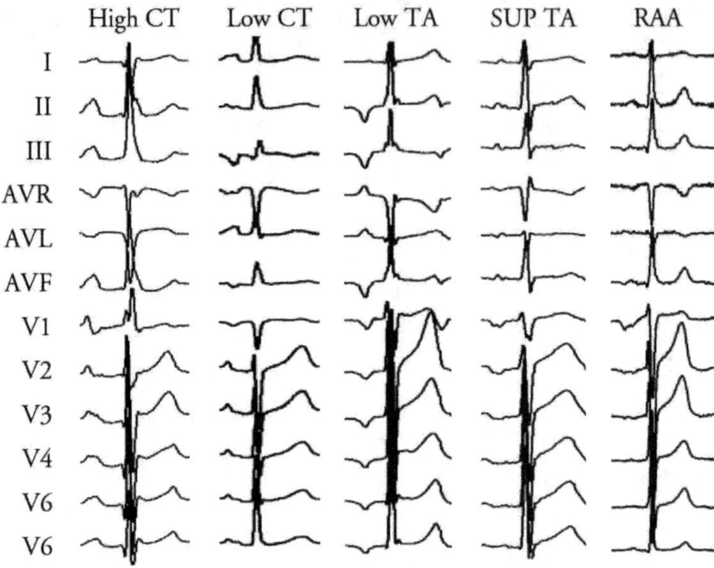

Figure 3. Representative examples of P-wave morphology for right atrial foci. Reprinted from
Teh, AW et al., Using the 12-lead ECG to localize the origin of ventricular and atrial tachycardias: part 1.
Focal atrial tachycardia. J Cardiovasc Electrophysiol 2009; 20: 706-709; quiz 705. With permission from
Blackwell-synergy.

monary vein P-wave morphology due to the anatomic proximity of the two sites, these may be distinguishable on the basis of changes to the P-wave in lead V1 during tachycardia compared with sinus rhythm.[1] In an RSPV AT, V1 will invariably be upright in V1 in tachycardia and biphasic (pos-neg) in SR. When a CT AT has an upright P-wave in V1 (approximately 10%) it is invariably also upright during SR.

3.2   *Tricuspid annulus and right atrial appendage*

A number of series have described origin of focal atrial tachycardias from anywhere around the circumference of the tricuspid annulus and this is the second most common site of origin for right atrial tachycardias. Obviously, the P-wave morphology can vary markedly according to where on the annulus the focus is located (see figure 2). Nevertheless, a common feature of tricuspid annular tachycardias is the presence of an inverted P-wave in V1 and V2 with late precordial transition to an upright appearance. In general, the polarity of leads II and III is deeply negative for an inferoanterior location, and low amplitude, positive, or biphasic for a superior location. Other P-wave characteristics were: positive in aVL and positive or isoelectric in lead I.

Recently, a number of series have described the origin of focal tachycardias from the right atrial appendage (see figure 2). The majority of these originates from the lateral base of the appendage but is also well described from an apical location. Due to their close anatomic proximity, these tachycardias are generally indistinguishable from superior tricuspid annular foci.[1]

In a recent series, V1 and V2 were negative in 10/10 patients (V1 notching was present in 6/10) with variable precordial transition to positive in V6. Inferior leads were characteristically low amplitude positive in 9/10 patients.[7]

3.3   Coronary sinus: ostium and mid-body

The coronary ostium (see figure 4) is also a well-recognized location of origin for focal atrial tachycardias.[8] The P-wave morphology is highly characteristic with deeply inverted (negative) P-waves in II, III and aVF. V1 is usually isoelectric-positive or negative-positive, with variable precordial transition. P-waves are invariably positive in aVL and aVR.

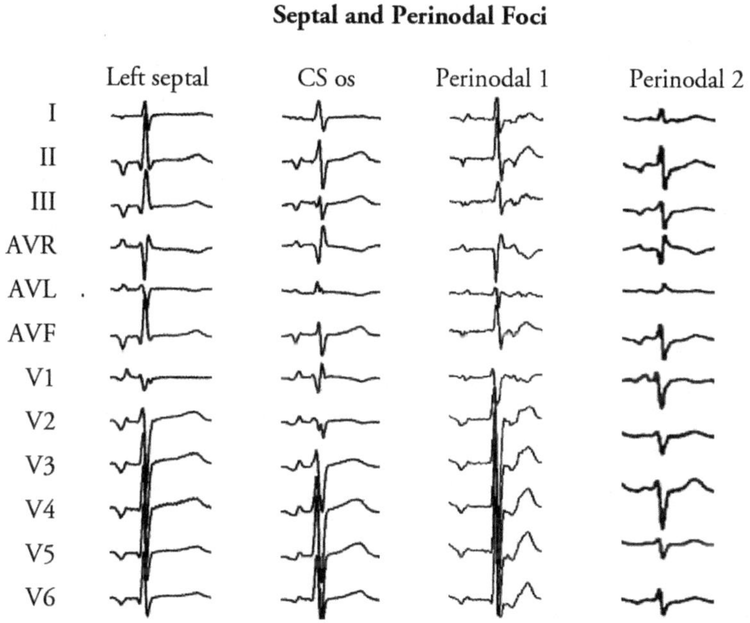

Septal and Perinodal Foci

Figure 4. Representative examples of P-wave morphology for septal and perinodal foci. Reprinted from Teh, AW et al., Using the 12-lead ECG to localize the origin of ventricular and atrial tachycardias: part 1. Focal atrial tachycardia. J Cardiovasc Electrophysiol 2009; 20: 706-709; quiz 705. With permission from Blackwell-synergy.

Recently focal AT has been described originating from 3-4 cm into the body of the coronary sinus. The distinguishing P-wave feature is that V1 is broad and upright as the site of origin is leftward and posterior compared with the CS ostium. The inferior leads are also deeply inverted and aVR is positive (see figure 3).

3.4   Perinodal region and interatrial septum

The P-wave morphology of perinodal and septal tachycardias (see figure 5) is variable and there is overlap between the left and right sides. For right perinodal and right septal foci, an

Left atrial foci

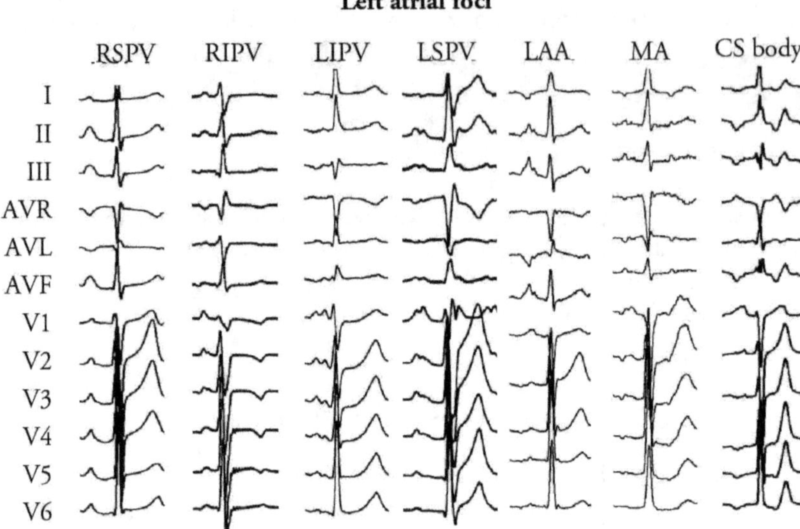

Figure 5. Representative examples of P-wave morphology for left atrial foci. Reprinted from Teh, AW et al., Using the 12-lead ECG to localize the origin of ventricular and atrial tachycardias: part 1. Focal atrial tachycardia. J Cardiovasc Electrophysiol 2009; 20: 706-709; quiz 705. With permission from Wiley-Blackwell.

isoelectric P-wave in V1 is helpful if present (specificity and PPV of 100%) but is only present in 50% of cases.[1] Alternately the P-wave in V1 has been reported to be low amplitude negative, positive-negative biphasic or in some instances negative-positive biphasic. Left septal and left perinodal foci may demonstrate either a positive P-wave in V1 or commonly a biphasic negative-positive appearance. Variable findings in limb leads have been reported. Some of the reported differences in P-wave morphology in this area may relate to how the septal region is defined. In some reports this has included the fossa ovalis region and the septum primum (infolding between superior caval vein and right superior pulmonary vein) and in others has referred to the region of Kochs triangle (so-called anterior, mid- or postero-septal areas).

3.5　*Pulmonary veins and left atrial appendage*

The pulmonary vein ostia are the most common site for focal tachycardias in the left atrium. Their posterior location within the left atrium is reflected by the universal finding of a positive P-wave in V1 and across the precordial leads (see figure 3).[1] Almost all foci are also negative in aVR and negative or isoelectric in aVL.[1] Compared with the right-sided veins, the left-sided veins have a broader notched P-wave in V1 and in the inferior leads.[1] Right-sided PV foci usually have a positive P-wave in lead I.[1] The superior pulmonary veins invariably have a positive P-wave in the inferior leads. The inferior veins may have inverted, low amplitude positive or isoelectric inferior P-waves. Due to the close proximity of the superior and inferior veins and marked anatomical variation, distinguishing superior from inferior foci may be difficult.

The left atrial appendage (LAA) is closely approximated with the left superior pulmonary vein and as such has a similar P-wave morphology (see figure 3).[6] In our experience, a P-wave morphology that suggests an LSPV focus (broad upright and notched in V1 and inferior leads) together with a deeply inverted P-wave in lead I will most usually indicate an LA appendage focus.[1] In one recent study, 7/7 patients had negative P-waves in I and aVL, along with positive P-waves in the inferior leads.[9] Another study observed that a negative P-wave in leads I and aVL predicted an LAA focus with a sensitivity and specificity of 92% and 97% respectively.[10]

3.6   Aortomitral continuity and non-coronary cusp AT

Although AT foci have been described from a range of mitral annular sites, several studies have reported that the majority cluster at the aortomitral continuity adjacent to the left fibrous trigone. Atrial tachycardias arising from this region characteristically have a biphasic negative-positive appearance in V1 and an isoelectric or negative P-wave in aVL (see figure 3) (sensitivity of 88%, specificity 99%, PPV 88%, and NPV 99%). Inferior leads were usually low amplitude or isoelectric.[1] Recently atrial tachycardia has been described originating from the non-coronary cusp of the aortic valve. Using an approach from within the aortic root these tachycardias could be mapped and successfully ablated. Due to the close anatomic proximity, the P-wave description is similar to that of those arising from the aortomitral continuity. The P-waves in leads V1 and V2 are also characteristically negative.[11] In this study, all nine patients had an upright P-wave in leads I and aVL and this may serve as a distinguishing feature from aortomitral AT. In most patients the inferior leads were biphasic negative-positive but of low amplitude.

3.7   Limitations of P-wave localization

While mapping may be targeted to an anatomic structure or structures of interest on the basis of P-wave morphology, it is important to remember that foci have been described form virtually any atrial location.

The spatial resolution of the P-wave has been estimated at 17 mm in a pace mapping study. This will limit the ability of the P-wave to distinguish between sites in close proximity.

Any analysis of P-wave morphology must be made on a P-wave which is not partially obscured by QRS or T-wave.

P-wave morphology has only proven useful for AT localization in patients without structural heart disease. In patients with prior surgery or extensive atrial ablation or in those with significant structural heart disease, activation patterns may alter significantly rendering P-wave morphology unhelpful. P-wave morphology is also of minor utility only in patients with macroreentrant AT.

4   Mapping and ablation

A variety of different and complementary approaches may be used for mapping and ablation of focal atrial tachycardia. However, a combination of P-wave analysis and targeted endocardial activation mapping will facilitate rapid localization of many atrial foci.

4.1 *Endocardial activation zapping*

Endocardial activation mapping is the most commonly used technique to identify the location of the AT focus. Mapping of focal AT as defined[12] will demonstrate atrial activation starting at a small area (focus) from which it spreads out centrifugally. It is very helpful to deploy standard mapping catheters which may give a rapid guide to the anatomic region of interest. Multipolar catheters will also give a rapid visual guide to when there is a change in tachycardia or in some cases when termination to a sinus tachycardia occurs. Most usually, catheters will be placed in the bundle of His area and the coronary sinus. Other catheters may be deployed to provide higher density mapping in the anatomic region of interest. These include multipolar catheters such as a crista terminalis catheter or a catheter deployed around the tricuspid annulus in the right atrium. In the left atrium, when a pulmonary vein tachycardia is suspected a lasso catheter may help to locate the focus or facilitate PV isolation. Most often, precise localization will be achieved with detailed mapping using the ablation catheter in the anatomic region of interest. Generally activation times of >20-30 ms before the P-wave are observed at successful sites but this is highly variable. When P-wave onset cannot be consistently observed, mapping can be performed to a stable intracardiac fiducial point with a known relationship to P-wave onset. Techniques to unmask the P-wave to facilitate fiducial marking include ventricular pacing to dissociate the "V" or adenosine bolus, provided that this does not terminate the tachycardia.

4.2 *Anatomic relationships and mapping atrial tachycardias*

The anatomic relationships described above under P-wave identification are also important during catheter mapping. As examples:

- Atrial tachycardias apparently originating from the superior crista terminalis or superior posterior right atrium should arouse suspicion of a possible right superior pulmonary vein tachycardia.
- Early activation at the coronary sinus ostium may suggest a CS os tachycardia but is also consistent with an origin from deeper into the CS, from the inferior tricuspid annulus or from the perinodal region.
- Tachycardias originating from the superior tricuspid annulus will have a very similar activation pattern to those from the base of the right atrial appendage. Those apparently from a left superior pulmonary vein will need to be distinguished from those arising within the left atrial appendage. Finally, early activation in the perinodal region may indicate a tachycardia originating from the tricuspid annulus in that region or alternately the left atrial septum or aortic root. Knowledge of these critical anatomic relationships and of the likely sites of AT origin will greatly facilitate mapping.

4.3 *Right versus left atrium: endocardial mapping*

In addition to information from the P-wave morphology, the endocardial activation pattern can provide early clues to the need to perform transeptal puncture to map the left atrium. Clearly, when CS activation is distal to proximal in sequence this immediately denotes a left atrial site of origin. However, a proximal to distal sequence is also compatible with a left atrial origin, particularly for sites at the septum, aortomitral continuity or right-sided pulmonary veins. Generally, for tachycardias originating at these sites, there will be a large region with similar activation timing on the right side of the septum and in the perinodal region. Further, this is usually less than 15 msec pre-P-wave.

When earliest right-sided activation suggests a "perinodal" site of origin, it is important to map adjacent structures. In the right atrium, these will include the perinodal tricuspid annulus and adjacent RA septum. However, when earliest RA activity is perinodal, it is important to map the left side of the septum and also consider aortic root mapping for a coronary cusp origin.

4.4   3D mapping

In recent years the use of 3D mapping systems during mapping and ablation of atrial tachycardias has become virtually universal. This technology registers the mapping information and provides a far greater anatomic resolution than can be achieved with biplane fluoroscopy alone. A number of studies have demonstrated the ability of electroanatomic mapping to provide a high resolution map in the region of earliest activation and precisely locate the focus in relation to endocardial geometry (see figure 6).[13-17] The ability to import an MRI or CT scan has further enhanced our appreciation of anatomic relationships and individual anatomic variations and as a result has further facilitated zapping.[18,19] In recent years it has become our approach to routinely supplement multipolar mapping with the use of a 3D mapping system.

The main limitation of a sequential mapping approach is the requirement for regular ectopics or sustained tachycardia. Hoffmann *et al.*[14] found that in 12% of patients, electroanatomic maps were unable to be constructed due to non-sustained or non-inducible tachycardia.

The non-contact mapping system (EnSite balloon) allows reconstruction of chamber geometry and simultaneous recording of >3,300 virtual unipolar electrograms enabling entire activation from a single beat. In theory therefore, this system might be helpful in cases of atrial tachycardia where ectopic activity is infrequent or sporadic.[20-22] In practice, the uncertainty that infrequent ectopics reflect the clinical arrhythmia (or are simply catheter induced) and the uncertainty of the endpoint are some of the reasons why many electrophysiologists still prefer detailed mapping of an active focus.

4.5   Paced endocardial activation sequence mapping

Paced activation sequence mapping has been used to complement activation mapping. The ablation catheter is maneuvered to a position where the paced activation sequence reproduces the spontaneous endocardial sequence. Tracy *et al.*[23] matched the paced endocardial map to the spontaneous map for right atrial tachycardias. Using this technique combined with activation mapping they reported a success rate of 80%. Paced activation sequence mapping may be helpful when the tachycardia is non-sustained or difficult to induce. Using a standarized set of right atrial catheters, Deen *et al.*[24] demonstrated a characteristic right atrial activation map created by pacing each pulmonary vein corresponded closely with the map from the same pulmonary vein during rapid atrial tachycardia and initiation of focal AF. The pulmonary vein of origin could be distinguished on the basis of this characteristic pattern.

Ultimately, however, this technique can only give an approximate idea as to the region of interest but may be helpful when activity from a tachycardia focus is infrequent.

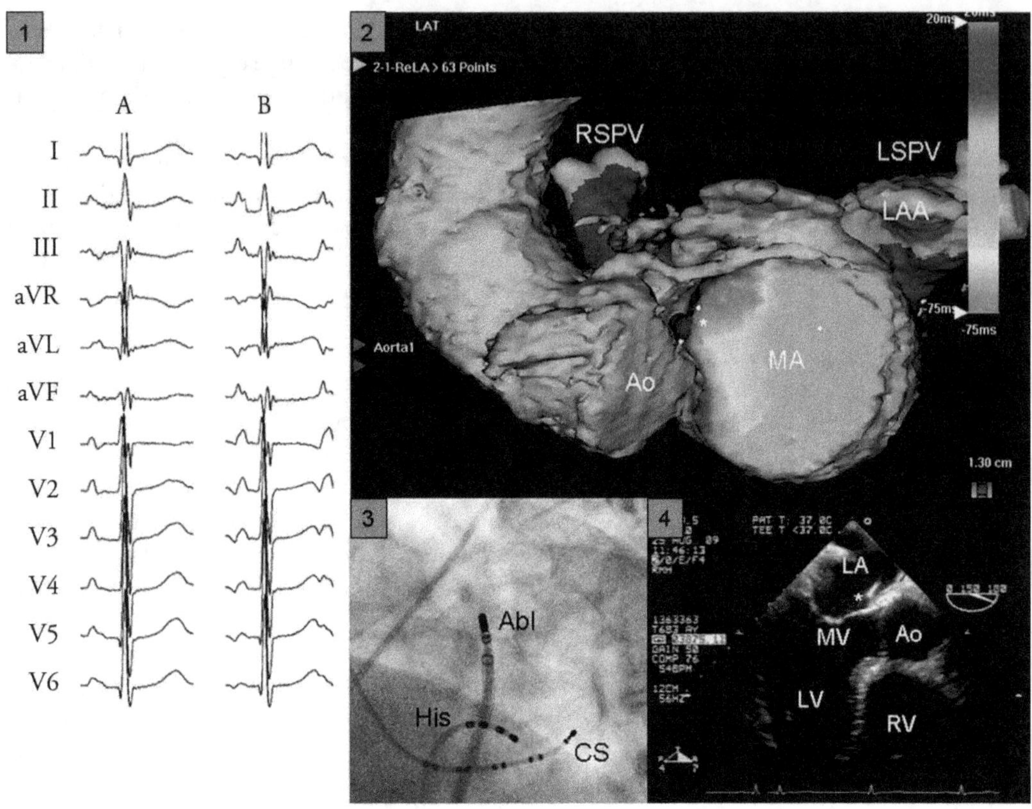

Figure 6. Representative case of focal atrial tachycardia from aortomitral continuity.
Reprinted from Teh AW et al., A case of focal atrial tachycardia from the aortomitral continuity.
J Cardiovasc Electrophysiol 2009: 1-2. With permission from Wiley-Blackwell.
Panel 1. 12-lead ECG demonstrating P-wave morphology in sinus rhythm "A" and tachycardia "B".
Panel 2. Color-coded activation map in left lateral projection from CARTO 3D mapping system
(red = early, purple = late). Note centrifugal spread from successful ablation site (red dot, *).
Ao = aorta; RSPV = right superior pulmonary vein. LSPV = left superior pulmonary vein;
MA = mitral annulus; LAA = left atrial appendage.
Panel 3. fluoroscopic image in left-anterior-oblique projection showing position of ablation catheter
(Abl) at successful site.
His = His-bundle electrogram catheter. CS = coronary sinus catheter.
Panel 4. transesophageal echocardiogram showing ablation catheter tip (*) in contact with aortomitral
continuity at successful ablation site.
LA = left atrium; MV = mitral valve; LV = left ventricle; RV = right ventricle; Ao = aorta.

4.6   Entrainment

Recently, Mohamed *et al.* described an approach to tachycardia mapping which involves atrial overdrive pacing.[25] Although many focal atrial tachycardias cannot be entrained, they
demonstrated that the site at which the PPI-TCL is closest to zero is the likely site of tachycardia origin.

4.7   *Characteristics of the ablation signal*

Several criteria have been proposed to identify the signal at the AT focus. Fractionated electrograms are frequently found at the successful ablation site,[5, 20, 26-28] however not all studies have reported this.[29-31] In patients with AT located mainly on the crista terminalis, Kalman *et al.*[5] observed fractionated signals at the site of successful ablation. In studies by both Lesh *et al.*[26] and Wang *et al.*,[28] a fractionated ablation signal was seen in a variety of right and left atrial sites. Fractionated electrograms may reflect localized abnormalities in atrial conduction, with poor cell to cell coupling causing slowed conduction from a poorly coupled automatic focus or small reentrant circuit.

Unipolar recordings have also been used to successfully identify the site of tachycardia origin.[30,32] The presence of a pure negative deflection (QS-pattern) with a rapid initial slope theoretically localizes the site of origin of the AT. Tang *et al.*[3] analyzed the unipolar electrogram at both the successful and unsuccessful ablation sites of focal AT. All the successful sites were characterized by the presence of the QS-morphology. An RS-pattern was observed at unsuccessful sites. Poty *et al.*[30] reported an acute success rate of 86% using unipolar recordings to identify the target site for ablation.

4.8   *Focal ablation*

Radiofrequency ablation has become the treatment of choice in symptomatic patients with atrial tachycardia. AT ablation series have reported success rates between 69 and 100%.[5,14,16,17,20, 22, 23, 26, 28-31, 33-38] Recurrence rates are generally low, varying between 0 and 33%. In an analysis of 16 studies by Chen *et al.*[39] the recurrence rate was 7%. In that study, the authors analyzed predictors of success of radiofrequency ablation. A right atrial location was the only independent predictor of successful radiofrequency ablation. In contrast, Anguera *et al.*[36] noted that patients who were male, had multiple foci, and had repetitive forms of AT, had lower acute success rates. Similarly, older patients, patients with other cardiac diseases and those with multiple foci had a higher risk of recurrence.[39]

Conclusion

The majority of focal atrial tachycardias originate from defined anatomic structures or sites within the atria. In patients without structural heart disease (or prior surgery or extensive ablation) these sites have a characteristic P-wave appearance which can facilitate targeted mapping. However, sites in close anatomic proximity will have overlap in P-wave appearance and detailed mapping will be required. Endocardial activation mapping targeted to anatomic structures and facilitated by multipolar catheters can rapidly and simply identify critical regions of anatomic interest. 3D mapping systems with imported CT or MRI enhance mapping resolution and provide a precise appreciation of individualized anatomy. Radiofrequency ablation is the treatment of first choice for patients with symptomatic atrial tachycardia and success rates are high.

References

1. Kistler PM, Roberts-Thomson KC, Haqqani HM, *et al.* P-wave morphology in focal atrial tachycardia: development of an algorithm to predict the anatomic site of origin. J Am Coll Cardiol 2006; 48:1010-7.

2. Tada H, Nogami A, Naito S, *et al.* Simple electrocardiographic criteria for identifying the site of origin of focal right atrial tachycardia. Pacing Clin Electrophysiol 1998; 21: 2431-9.

3. Tang CW, Scheinman MM, Van Hare GF, *et al.* Use of P-wave configuration during atrial tachycardia to predict site of origin. J Am Coll Cardiol 1995; 26: 1315-24.

4. Teh AW, Kistler PM, Kalman JM. Using the 12-lead ECG to localize the origin of ventricular and atrial tachycardias: part 1. Focal atrial tachycardia. J Cardiovasc Electrophysiol 2009; 20: 706-9; quiz 705.

5. Kalman JM, Olgin JE, Karch MR, *et al.* "Cristal tachycardias": origin of right atrial tachycardias from the crista terminalis identified by intracardiac echocardiography. J Am Coll Cardiol 1998; 31: 451-9.

6. Roberts-Thomson KC, Kistler PM, *et al.* Focal atrial tachycardia II: management. Pacing Clin Electrophysiol 2006; 29: 769-78.

7. Roberts-Thomson KC, Kistler PM, Haqqani HM, *et al.* Focal atrial tachycardias arising from the right atrial appendage: electrocardiographic and electrophysiologic characteristics and radiofrequency ablation. J Cardiovasc Electrophysiol 2007; 18: 367-72.

8. Kistler PM, Fynn SP, Haqqani H, *et al.* Focal atrial tachycardia from the ostium of the coronary sinus: electrocardiographic and electrophysiological characterization and radiofrequency ablation. J Am Coll Cardiol 2005; 45: 1488-93.

9. Wang YL, Li XB, Quan X, *et al.* Focal atrial tachycardia originating from the left atrial appendage: electrocardiographic and electrophysiologic characterization and long-term outcomes of radiofrequency ablation. J Cardiovasc Electrophysiol 2007; 18: 459-64.

10. Yamada T, Murakami Y, Yoshida Y, *et al.* Electrophysiologic and electrocardiographic characteristics and radiofrequency catheter ablation of focal atrial tachycardia originating from the left atrial appendage. Heart Rhythm 2007; 4: 1284-91.

11. Ouyang F, Ma J, Ho SY, *et al.* Focal atrial tachycardia originating from the non-coronary aortic sinus: electrophysiological characteristics and catheter ablation. J Am Coll Cardiol 2006; 48: 122-31.

12. Saoudi N, Cosio F, Waldo A, *et al.* Classification of atrial flutter and regular atrial tachycardia according to electrophysiologic mechanism and anatomic bases: a statement from a joint expert group from the Working Group of Arrhythmias of the European Society of Cardiology and the North American Society of Pacing and Electrophysiology. J Cardiovasc Electrophysiol 2001; 12: 852-66.

13. Hoffmann E, Nimmermann P, Reithmann C, *et al.* New mapping technology for atrial tachycardias. J Interv Card Electrophysiol 2000; 4 Suppl 1: 117-20.

14. Hoffmann E, Reithmann C, Nimmermann P, *et al.* Clinical experience with electroanatomic mapping of ectopic atrial tachycardia. Pacing Clin Electrophysiol 2002; 25: 49-56.

15. Marchlinski F, Callans D, Gottlieb C, *et al.* Magnetic electroanatomical mapping for ablation of focal atrial tachycardias. Pacing Clin Electrophysiol 1998; 21: 1621-35.

16. Natale A, Breeding L, Tomassoni G, *et al.* Ablation of right and left ectopic atrial tachycardias using a three-dimensional nonfluoroscopic mapping system. Am J Cardiol 1998; 82: 989-92.

17. Weiss C, Willems S, Rueppel R, *et al.* Electroanatomical Mapping (CARTO) of ectopic atrial tachycardia: impact of bipolar and unipolar local electrogram annotation for localization the focal origin. J Interv Card Electrophysiol 2001; 5: 101-7.

18. Rosso R, Morton JB, Aggarwal A, *et al.* Image Integration to Guide Ablation of Incessant Left Atrial Appendage Tachycardia. Heart Rhythm 2009. doi: 10.1016/j.hrthm.2009.11.033

19. Teh AW, Lee G, Kalman JM: A case of focal atrial tachycardia from the aortomitral continuity. J of Cardiovasc Electrophysiol 2009: 1-2. doi: 10.1111/ j.1540-8167. 2009. 01675.x

20. Higa S, Tai CT, Lin YJ, *et al.* Focal atrial tachycardia: new insight from noncontact mapping and catheter ablation. Circulation 2004; 109: 84-91.

21. Higa S, Tai CT, Lin YJ, *et al.* Mechanism of adenosine-induced termination of focal atrial tachycardia. J Cardiovasc Electrophysiol 2004; 15: 1387-93.

22. Schmitt H, Weber S, Schwab JO, *et al.* Diagnosis and ablation of focal right atrial tachycardia using a new high-resolution, non-contact mapping system. Am J Cardiol 2001; 87: 1017-21; A1015.

23. Tracy CM, Swartz JF, Fletcher RD, *et al.* Radiofrequency catheter ablation of ectopic atrial tachycardia using paced activation sequence mapping. J Am Coll Cardiol 1993; 21: 910-17.

24. Deen VR, Morton JB, Vohra JK, *et al.* Pulmonary vein paced activation sequence mapping: comparison with activation sequences during onset of focal atrial fibrillation. J Cardiovasc Electrophysiol 2002; 13: 101-7.

25. Mohamed U, Skanes AC, Gula LJ, *et al.* A novel pacing maneuver to localize focal atrial tachycardia. J Cardiovasc Electrophysiol 2007; 18: 1-6.

26. Lesh MD, Van Hare GF, Epstein LM, *et al.* Radiofrequency catheter ablation of atrial arrhythmias. Results and mechanisms. Circulation 1994; 89: 1074-89.

27. Iesaka Y, Takahashi A, Goya M, *et al.* Adenosine-sensitive atrial reentrant tachycardia originating from the atrioventricular nodal transitional area. J Cardiovasc Electrophysiol 1997; 8: 854-64.

28. Wang L, Weerasooriya HR, Davis MJ: Radiofrequency catheter ablation of atrial tachycardia. Aust N Z J Med 1995; 25: 127-32.

29. Kay GN, Chong F, Epstein AE, *et al.* Radiofrequency ablation for treatment of primary atrial tachycardias. J Am Coll Cardiol 1993; 21: 901-9.

30. Poty H, Saoudi N, Nair M, *et al.* Radiofrequency catheter ablation of atrial flutter. Further insights into the various types of isthmus block: application to ablation during sinus rhythm. Circulation 1996; 94: 3204-13.

31. Walsh EP, Saul JP, Hulse JE, *et al.* Transcatheter ablation of ectopic atrial tachycardia in young patients using radiofrequency current. Circulation 1992; 86: 1138-46.

32. Tang K, Ma J, Zhang S, *et al.* Unipolar electrogram in identification of successful targets for radiofrequency catheter ablation of focal atrial tachycardia. Chin Med J (Engl) 2003; 116: 1455-8.

33. Chen SA, Chiang CE, Yang CJ, *et al.* Sustained atrial tachycardia in adult patients. Electrophysiological characteristics, pharmacological response, possible mechanisms, and effects of radiofrequency ablation. Circulation 1994; 90: 1262-78.

34. Kammeraad JA, Balaji S, Oliver RP, Chugh SS, *et al.* Nonautomatic focal atrial tachycardia: characterization and ablation of a poorly understood arrhythmia in 38 patients. Pacing Clin Electrophysiol 2003; 26: 736-42.

35. Pappone C, Stabile G, De Simone A, *et al.* Role of catheter-induced mechanical trauma in localization of target sites of radiofrequency ablation in automatic atrial tachycardia. J Am Coll Cardiol 1996; 27: 1090-7.

36. Anguera I, Brugada J, Roba M, *et al.* Outcomes after radiofrequency catheter ablation of atrial tachycardia. Am J Cardiol 2001; 87: 886-90.

37. Chen SA, Chiang CE, Yang CJ, *et al.* Radiofrequency catheter ablation of sustained intra-atrial reentrant tachycardia in adult patients. Identification of electrophysiological characteristics and endocardial mapping techniques. Circulation 1993; 88: 578-87.

38. Goldberger J, Kall J, Ehlert F, *et al.* Effectiveness of radiofrequency catheter ablation for treatment of atrial tachycardia. Am J Cardiol 1993; 72: 787-93.

39. Chen SA, Tai CT, Chiang CE, *et al.* Focal atrial tachycardia: reanalysis of the clinical and electrophysiologic characteristics and prediction of successful radiofrequency ablation. J Cardiovasc Electrophysiol 1998; 9: 355-65.

Chapter 12. Ablation of accessory pathways: a simplified approach

L. MONT, J. BRUGADA

Arrhythmia Section
Thorax Institute
Hospital Clínic Universitari
de Barcelona
Barcelona, Spain

Address for correspondence:
Thorax Institute
Hospital Clínic Universitari
de Barcelona
Dr. Lluís Mont
Dr. Josep Brugada
LMONT@clinic.ub.es
jbrugada@clinic.ub.es

Introduction

About 20 years ago, the treatment of arrhythmias took a huge step forward with the introduction of radiofrequency catheter ablation. Ablation of the accessory pathways (AP) became the treatment of choice due to its nearly 95% efficacy[1-3] and low risk for complications[4]. However, once the initial methodology became established, little has changed in terms of technical approaches. In many laboratories, the process is still complex, requiring multiple catheters, pacing maneuvers, and long procedures. On the other hand, following the initial descriptions of single catheter ablation by Kuck,[5] others have simplified the procedures, achieving results equal to complex procedures, with less time, less radiation and probably lower risk.[6,7] Whether these simplified approaches represent a real advantage and can be generalized is still under debate.[8] This chapter describes the simplified approach and discusses some advantages.

AP ablation implies, first, a correct diagnosis and, second, a detailed localization of the AP insertion at the AV groove, by measuring the shortest AV or VA activation time. Diagnosis is the first step. Whereas in overt pre-excitation the diagnosis is obvious, and easily achieved by pattern recognition of the delta wave, concealed APs often require some extra time and a differential diagnosis. Correct diagnosis requires careful analysis of the 12-lead ECG in sinus rhythm and during tachycardia.

1   Electrocardiographic recognition

The usefulness of the surface ECG in establishing the initial diagnosis and designing the ablation strategy has probably been underestimated. A good initial diagnosis based on the ECG may spare some work and help in planning the procedure.

2 Overt preexcitation

The presence of preexcitation on the surface ECG quite accurately defines the AP location. Several algorithms have been defined,[9,10] but generally for locating the pathway, determining right or left and then anterior, inferior and lateral (see figures 1, 2 and 3), three simple points may be useful to remember:

- Delta and QRS positive in V1 establishes the diagnosis of left-sided AP; negative delta and QRS in lead V1 define a right-sided pathway location.
- Negative delta and QRS in inferior leads (II, III and aVF) suggest an inferior location (also called posterior, due to the surgical exposure).
- Positive delta and QRS in II, III, and aVF suggest a superior location (also called anterior, due to the surgical exposure).

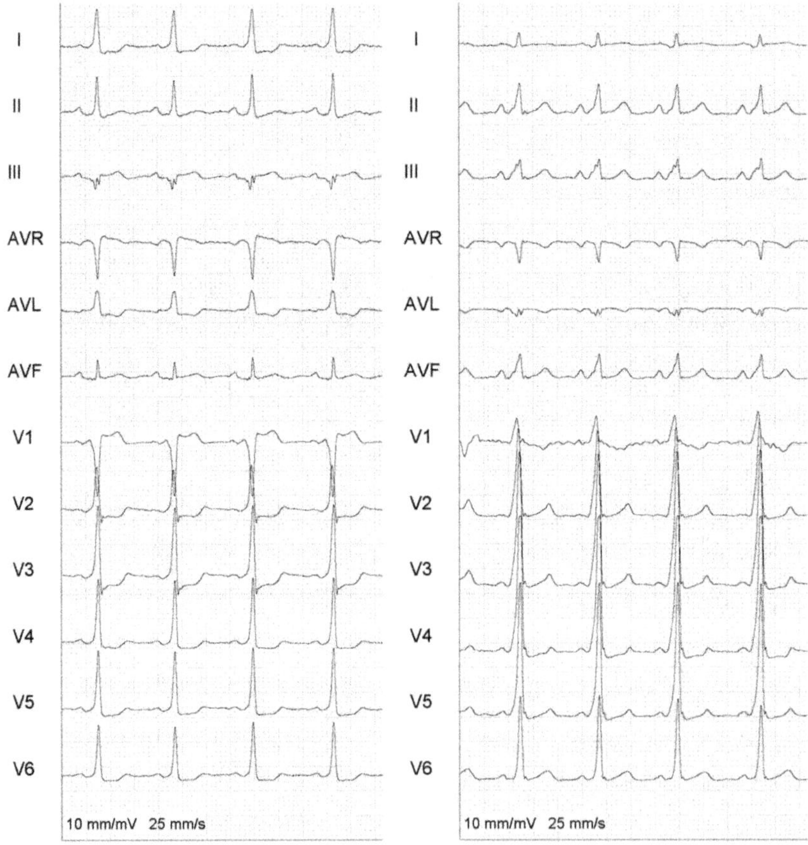

Figure 1. Left panel depicts a 12-lead ECG of a patient with Wolff-Parkinson-White syndrome. Negative delta wave and QRS in lead V1 define the presence of a right-sided accessory pathway. Right panel shows ECG of a patient with a left-sided accessory pathways it is suggested by the positive delta wave and QRS in lead V1.

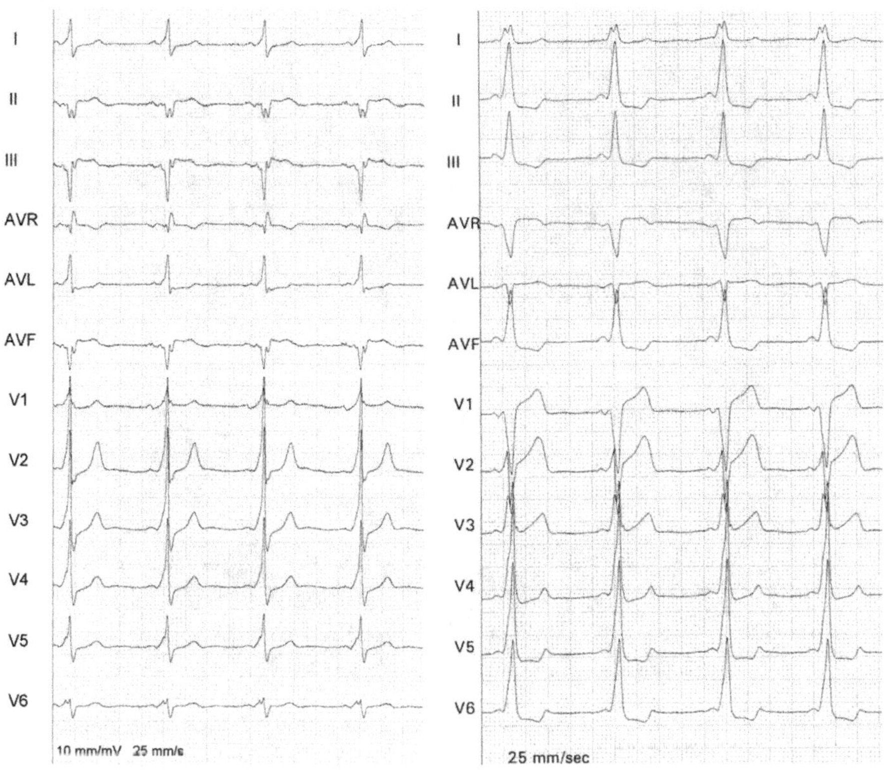

Figure 2. Polarity of the delta wave and the QRS in inferior leads (II, III, avF) suggest the location of the accessory pathway. Negative polarity suggests an inferior (posterior) localisation (right panel). Positive polarity suggested a superior (anterior) localization (left panel).

3   Concealed accessory pathways

Careful analysis of the surface ECG during tachycardia will usually suggest a clear diagnosis (AV reentrant tachycardia versus atrial tachycardia or intranodal reentry), depending on the location of the P-wave and the polarity. In atrioventricular reentry, the P-wave is usually located about 120-140 ms after the onset of the QRS (see figure 4). In intranodal tachycardia, the P-wave is within or usually fused at the terminal portion of the QRS; it is small, symmetrical and negative in inferior leads, in agreement with its midseptal origin (see figure 5). Finally, atrial tachycardia is usually recognized because the RP is longer than the PR, or is changing due to the PR interval (PR changes precede RP changes). Valsalva maneuver or adenosine are often helpful in establishing the diagnosis of atrial tachycardia, by dissociating or changing the AV ratio, and may also make pacing maneuvers unnecessary. On the other hand, a craneo-caudal and right-to-left axis of the P-wave exclude an accessory AP, since the P-wave from the AP originates at the AV groove and excites the atrium from the AV groove to the posterior part (the AV groove is anterior and inferior in relation to the atrium) (see figure 6). The morphology of the retrograde P-wave may also localize the AP. There are two main steps in determining the polarity:

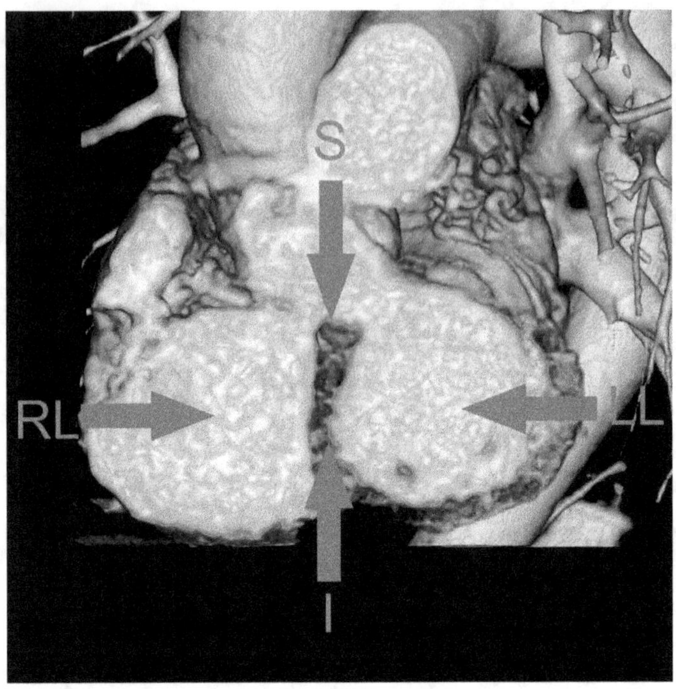

Figure 3. Coronal views at the level of the interauricular septum obtained by a computed tomography. The arrow shows the direction of the ventricular activation of an accessory pathway. According to two main axis (right-left and inferior-superior).

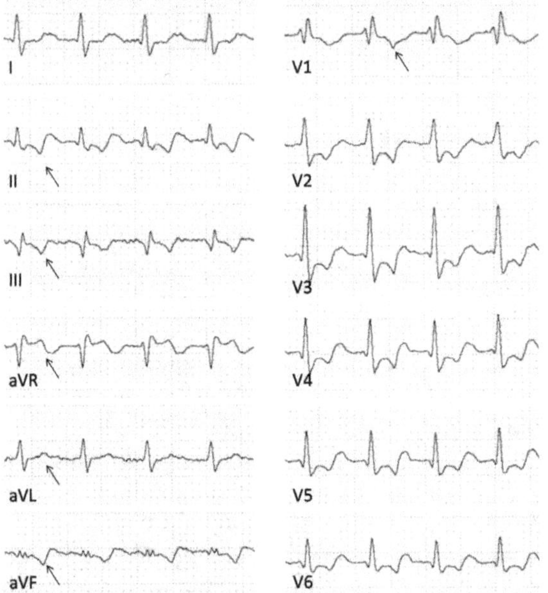

Figure 4. 12-lead ECG showing a narrow QRS tachycardia with a retrograde P-wave, negative in the inferior leads and in lead V1, suggestive of a right inferior pathway.

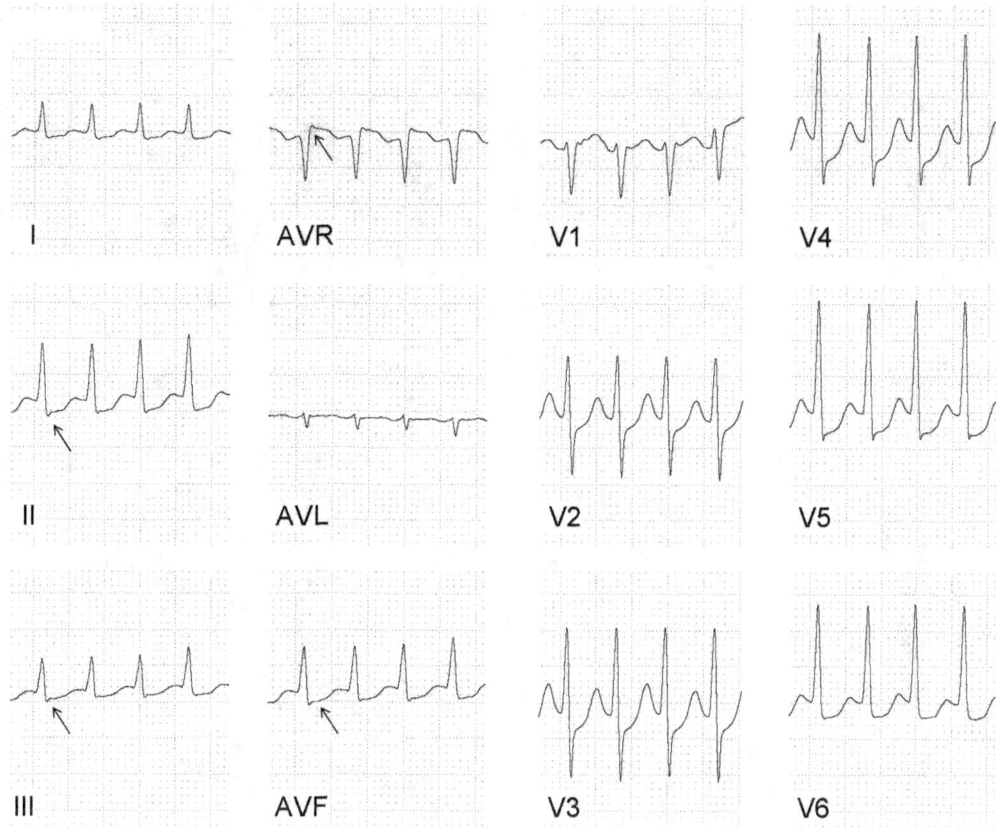

Figure 5. 12-lead ECG showing a narrow QRS tachycardia, with a small S-wave at the terminal part of the QRS at the inferior leads, suggestive of a retrograde P-wave fused with the QRS due to AV nodal reentry.

- A positive P-wave in lead V1 and negative in aVL and lead I suggest a left-sided pathway, whereas the opposite is found in a right-sided AP.
- A negative P-wave in inferior leads identifies an inferior (posterior) pathway.

4　Procedure details

As a general rule, it is useful to adapt the procedure to an individual patient, using the minimum number of punctures and catheters. The standard approach involves usually two catheters. A quadripolar catheter, initially positioned at the lateral right atrium, is used to pace and record. The ablation catheter is advanced through the right femoral vein into the right side of the heart, unless the preexcitation clearly shows a left-sided AP. X-ray exposure can be minimized by using PA projection and avoiding non-essential multiple projections (RAO, LAO). This approach is particularly important in children (see chapter 14).

The simplified approach implies a dynamic technique, rather than the traditional static technique. In the traditional approach, several catheters are left in place (coronary sinus, right

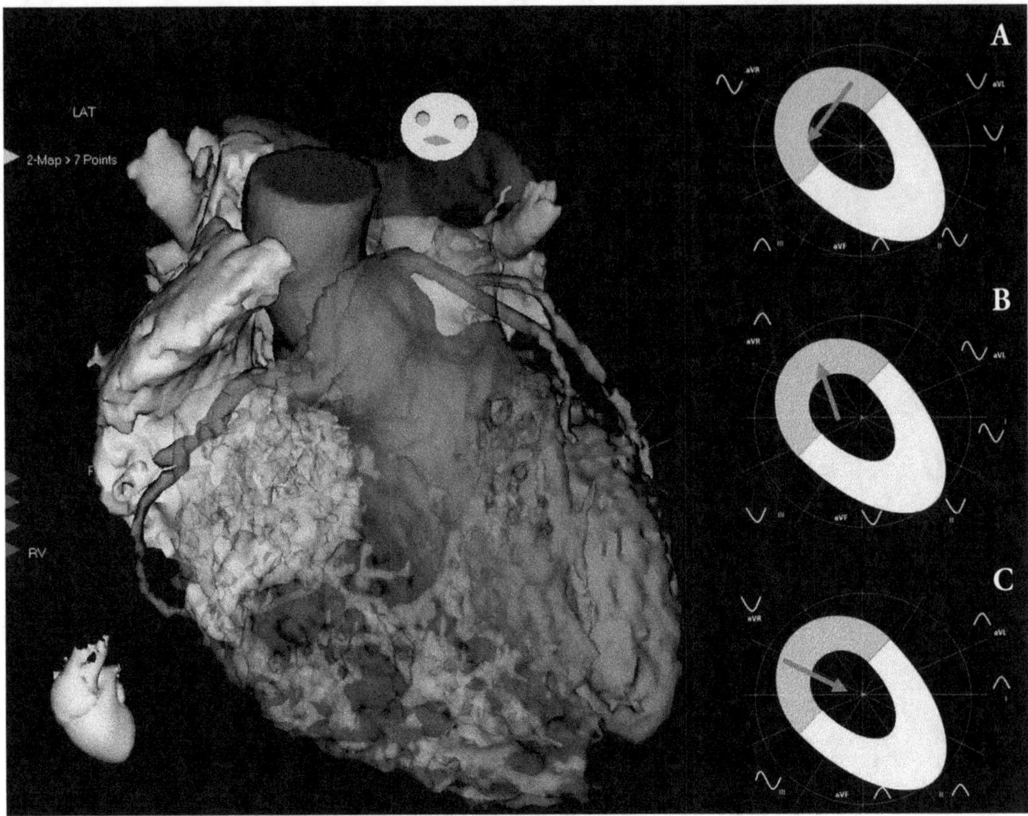

Figure 6. The left panel shows a coronal view of the heart depicting the right and anterior position of the right atrium (yellow) in relation to the left atrium (orange) located posteriorly. The right ventricle (green transparent) is also anterior in relation to the left ventricle. The right panel depicts three examples of the polarity of the P-wave, depending on the origin of the atrial activation. Panel A. Left to right activation. Panel B. Caudocraneal, activation. Panel C. Craneocaudal activation.

atrium, His, right ventricle, mapping catheter) and the activation is studied by looking at multiple simultaneous recordings. In the simplified technique, the mapping-ablation catheter is moved; the mapping is dynamic, positioning the catheter in several places to find the earliest activation, usually by using the recording system's trigger mode. The screen is refreshed every beat with static QRS position, allowing fast and careful measurements of AV and VA intervals, using a 300 mm/s screen speed.

5   Strategy in overt preexcitation

In overt preexcitation, no systematic pacing maneuvers to determine the refractory period of the AP are performed. This shortens and simplifies the procedure. Pacing is only performed to uncover preexcitation if needed. At the same time, tachycardia or atrial fibrillation are not intentionally induced. Therefore, the AP insertion is directly mapped.

- In *left-sided accessory pathways,* the ablation catheter is advanced through the right femoral artery and retrogradely positioned at the AV ring (see figure 7A), through the aortic valve. The mitral ring is mapped in detail, if possible in sinus rhythm, looking for the earliest V in the local electrogram, taking the onset of the delta wave on the surface ECG as a reference. A negative delta to V electrogram interval is required, because it shows that the ventricular activation begins at the tip of the catheter and starts earlier than at the surface ECG. The analysis of the morphology of the electrogram also helps, by showing the tiny presumed AP potential fused with the ventricular potential, or a fractionated signal in between AV electrograms (see figure 8). A "clean" atrial and ventricular potential, without activity in between, is rarely the insertion point.[11]
- The AV groove is mapped without any catheter in the coronary sinus, following the technique initially described by Kuck *et al.*[5] The recording system's trigger mode at 300 mm/s allows very accurate mapping; measures are made every beat by placing a caliper at the beginning of the delta wave. Very subtle changes in the electrogram precocity and morphology are rapidly recognized.
- Usually, the mapping is performed from the ventricular aspect of the mitral valve, because it allows greater stability. Sometimes the power of the application cannot go over 5-10 W, because the catheter is exerting great pressure and there is no cooling effect under the mitral valve. Therefore, the tip temperature rises to the preset limit of 55 ºC at a very low power. If this occurs, application at the atrial aspect may solve the problem; alternatively, the use of an irrigated tip cathether will allow higher power. If the catheter cannot be appropriately positioned, mapping can be performed from the atrial aspect of the valve. However, this may produce atrial premature beats and pain during RF ablation, which

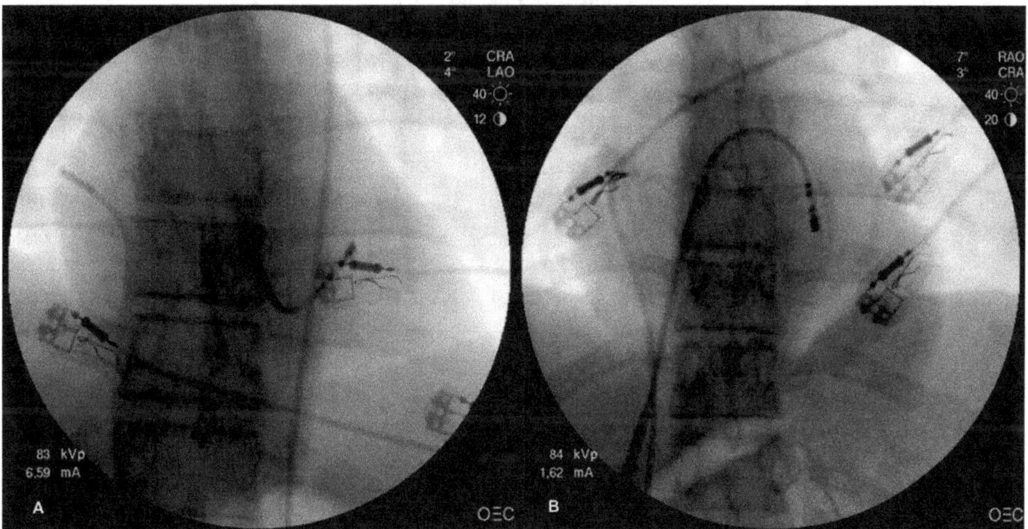

Figure 7. The left panel (image A) shows the position of the ablation catheter in anteroposterior projection. The catheter is positioned retrogradedly, through the aortic valve, at the ventricular aspect of the mitral valve. Right panel (image B) depicts the ablation catheter located at the mitral AV ring, through a transeptal approach.

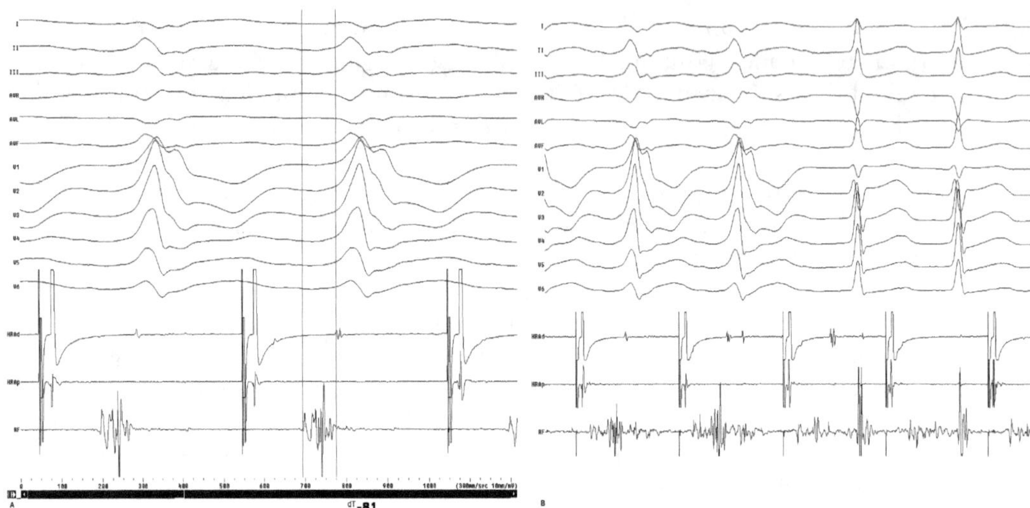

Figure 8. Left panel depicts the local electrogram recorded at the ventricular insertion of the accessory pathway. The electrogram shows the atrial and ventricular component, with an intermediate signal, suggestive of an accessory pathway potential. The right panel shows the interruption of the conduction through the accessory pathway during RF application.

can add some difficulty and increase the risk of tamponade if the catheter exerts intense pressure against the thin atrial wall, particularly during tachycardia and isoprenaline infusion. Alternatively, a transeptal approach may provide access in difficult cases (see figure 7B).

- The *right-sided accessory pathways* may pose diverse difficulties, depending on the location of the pathways.
- The *inferior pathways (posteroseptal)* may be located at the pyramidal space and can be difficult to ablate, probably because of an epicardial position in relation to the mouth of the coronary sinus. Some of them may require application within the ostium of the coronary sinus (CS). Others may have the atrial entrance located to the right and the exit to the left, with an oblique course. In any case, irrigated tip catheters are often needed to achieve complete ablation. The presence of CS diverticula has been associated with the presence of AP in that region.
- The *right free-wall pathways* create a problem of stability. Coming from the inferior vena cava, it is usually difficult to stabilize the catheter at the lateral tricuspid ring. The use of long sheaths, whether steerable or not, may be of help. Irrigated catheters have also improved the success rate in these locations.
- The *mid-septal pathways* usually are in close proximity to the AV node, and imply some risk for AV block. It is always important to stop the application as soon as a nodal rhythm is triggered.
- The *anteroseptal or superior pathways* are usually located at the superior part of the tricuspid ring. In close proximity to the His bundle, therefore, they pose a risk of complete AV block. A jugular vein approach has been advocated to reach that region, entering the

atrium from the superior vena cava. In that way, the tip of the catheter remains more stable, theoretically allowing a safer ablation.[12] However, the standard approach at Hospital Clínic in Barcelona is usually femoral. The most useful strategy to prevent complete AV block is to monitor nodal rhythm and tritrate the power, starting from 30 W. Sometimes, however, a delayed AV block can be seen after a few hours or days. Therefore, it is wise to carefully discuss the risk/benefit with the patient, particularly in young individuals. The use of cryoablation also has been proposed as a safer approach.[13]

6   Strategy in concealed accessory pathways

The traditional approach starts by positioning several catheters, including a catheter in the coronary sinus. Alternatively, in the 2-catheter strategy a quadripolar diagnostic catheter and the ablation catheter are advanced through the right femoral vein. The tachycardia is induced with atrial or ventricular extrastimulus, using isoprenaline if needed. The next step is to exclude common intranodal reentry, which is easily done by mapping the activation. If the retrograde P-wave is hidden within the QRS, or negative and fused with the QRS, the diagnosis of intranodal tachycardia is highly probable. The earliest retrograde atrial activation is observed at the His position, almost with the QRS electrogram; an eccentric retrograde activation excludes intranodal tachycardia. Therefore, the dynamic mapping, using the right atrial catheter as a reference, allows the localization of the earliest activation.

A fixed AV interval in some atrial tachycardias may pose some diagnostic difficulties. The first, and easy, maneuver is to perform a carotid sinus massage and determine whether an AV change precedes the VA change. On the other hand, careful mapping of earliest activation using the right atrial catheter as a reference allows localization of the onset of the atrial activation. Usually, this maneuver is also diagnostic because the earliest activation in the AP takes place at the AV groove (see chapter 11).

Once the onset of the activation is localized in the right atrium or in the left atrium (by mapping the CS if needed), the femoral artery is punctured when the AP is located in the left AV ring.

Mapping strategy will depend on the individual characteristics of the patient:

- *Mapping with ventricular pacing or in tachycardia.* As a general rule, we prefer to map during tachycardia. This avoids the confusing factor of retrograde nodal conduction. However, some patients are highly susceptible to atrial fibrillation. To avoid the need for repeated cardioversions in these patients, it is wise to map during ventricular pacing, always being aware of the possibility of nodal retrograde conduction that may fuse with VA conduction in the AP.
- *RF ablation during tachycardia or in sinus rhythm.* Applying energy during tachycardia documents the interruption of the tachycardia, which blocks retrograde conduction in the AP. Sometimes, however, when sinus rhythm resumes there is a jump in the cardiac movement that dislodges the ablation catheter. In these patients, once the proper position has been established by ventricular pacing, application of RF during sinus rhythm may be a good option.
- *Influence of pathway localization.* Special considerations regarding the localization of the pathway are described in the section on ablation of overt APs.

7　Confirmation of ablation

The quadripolar catheter is advanced into the ventricle to confirm VA dissociation or nodal conduction and thereby confirm the success of the ablation. The ablation catheter is used to record atrial activation.

If ventricular pacing detects VA dissociation, no further maneuvers are needed. However, atrial extrastimulus is recommended to exclude uncommon but possible associations (e.g., intranodal tachycardia, or atrial tachycardias).

If VA conduction still exists, activation mapping of the retrograde conduction will show whether activation is eccentric or occurring normally through the AV node. Finally, decremental VA conduction using ventricular extrastimuli will further confirm the successful ablation of the AP. In the past, a 30-minute waiting period, and further pacing maneuvers, was recommended before retrieving the catheters. However, we have reduced this time to 15 minutes of pacing maneuvers, without encountering a higher rate of recurrences.

Special techniques are recommended for challenging cases:

- *Transeptal approach in left-sided pathways.* In our experience, this approach is seldom needed. However, it is a helpful alternative when the retrograde approach is not successful. Doing the transeptal approach during the same procedure poses an additional risk because the patient receives heparin after the femoral artery puncture. Therefore, we prefer to reschedule the ablation. Mapping from the transeptal approach may be more appropriate in left anterior and free-wall pathways than in inferior (posteroseptal) pathways.
- *Epicardial approach.* In some patients, particularly in pathways arising from the pyramidal space but also in left-sided pathways, an epicardial approach may be successful. An epicardial approach should probably be attempted only in centers with previous experience in epicardial ablation, due to the risk of tamponade, or coronary artery lesion.[14]
- *Robotic navigation.* Some authors have suggested that robotic navigation may facilitate the access to difficult locations and can ensure good contact, particularly when the catheter is in an unstable position. However, no comparative studies are available. Further studies and technical developments will eventually determine whether robotic navigation is a useful tool to improve success.

8　Complications

The use of a simplified approach may decrease the risk of complications. In a recent randomized study, a simplified approach showed a lower percentage of vascular complications and a non-significant difference in major complications.[15] This may be due to fewer punctures, particularly avoiding the subclavian punctures systematically used in many laboratories, to place the CS catheter. Despite the potential decrease in the risk for hematomas and vascular complications, such as fistulae and pseudo-aneurysms, the use of a more dynamic approach also implies the need to carefully move and reposition the catheters. This in turn increases the risks associated with the manipulation of the catheters.

Other complications, such as tamponade, stroke, aortic retrograde dissection, coronary occlusion, valvular entrapment of the catheters, or valvular rupture, are extremely uncommon. Most of these are related to left heart catheterization. Therefore, experience in left heart catheterization should be mandatory before an operator attempts ablation of left-sided APs.

9   Decreasing radiation

The use of a simplified technique may decrease x-ray exposure, although the only comparative study to date failed to find significant differences.[15] The mean radiation time for RF ablation of an AP using the simplified approach in our laboratory is 17±11 min. The reported times do reflect the fact that our center is a teaching hospital and include the learning process of graduate fellows in electrophysiology.

10   Limitations of the simplified approach

If the simplified approach has significant advantages over the traditional multicatheter approach, why has it not been widely adopted? The easy answer is that teaching centers apply the orthodox approach and the new electrophysiologist simply has not been taught the simplified method. But there are other considerations. Using multiple simultaneous recordings and structured diagnostic maneuvers leaves little room for improvisation and therefore supports consistency. The traditional approach allows a picture of the whole activation, within a single beat, once all the catheters are in place. The simplified approach is less structured and therefore requires decision making on how to proceed. These decisions require experience with traditional ablation. Furthermore, the traditional use of multiple catheters produces anatomic references that are visible on the screen. Using only two catheters, the anatomy has to be visualized, which requires that the individual operator have the ability to imagine a 3-dimensional structure. Therefore, it could be argued that the simplified approach requires longer training and relies more on an individual's skills and abilities.

Conclusions

The use by an experienced operator of a simplified approach, with just two catheters, in AP ablations may shorten the duration, resulting in a more cost-effective procedure and potentially fewer complications without compromising success.

References

1. Kuck KH, Schluter M, Geiger M, *et al.* Radiofrequency current catheter ablation of accessory atrioventricular pathways. Lancet 1991; 337(8757): 1557-61.

2. Jackman WM, Wang XZ, Friday KJ *et al.* Catheter ablation of accessory atrioventricular pathways (Wolff-Parkinson-White syndrome) by radiofrequency current. N Engl J Med 1991; 324(23): 1605-11.

3. Calkins H, Sousa J, el-Atassi R *et al.* Diagnosis and cure of the Wolff-Parkinson-White syndrome or paroxysmal supraventricular tachycardias during a single electrophysiologic test. N Engl J Med 1991; 324(23): 1612-8.

4. Hindricks G. The Multicentre European Radiofrequency Survey (MERFS): complications of radiofrequency catheter ablation of arrhythmias. The Multicentre European Radiofrequency Survey (MERFS) investigators of the Working Group on Arrhythmias of the European Society of Cardiology. Eur Heart *J* 1993; 14(12): 1644-53.

5. Kuck KH, Schluter M. Single-catheter approach to radiofrequency current ablation of left-sided accessory pathways in patients with Wolff-Parkinson-White syndrome. Circulation 1991; 84(6): 2366-75.

6. Brugada J, Matas M, Mont L, *et al.* One thousand consecutive radiofrequency ablation procedures. Indications, results, and complications. Rev Esp Cardiol 1996 November; 49(11): 810-4 (in spanish).

7. Brugada J, Garcia-Bolao I, Figueiredo M, *et al.* Radiofrequency ablation of concealed left free-wall accessory pathways without coronary sinus catheterization: results in 100 consecutive patients. J Cardiovasc Electrophysiol 1997; 8(3): 249-53.

8. Mont L, Brugada J. Electrophysiology: it is time to simplify! Europace 2009; 11(8): 985-6.

9. Boersma L, Garcia-Moran E, Mont L, *et al.* Accessory pathway localization by QRS polarity in children with Wolff-Parkinson-White syndrome. J Cardiovasc Electrophysiol 2002; 13(12): 1222-6.

10. Basiouny T, de CC, Fareh S *et al.* Accuracy and limitations of published algorithms using the twelve-lead electrocardiogram to localize overt atrioventricular accessory pathways. J Cardiovasc Electrophysiol 1999; 10(10): 1340-9.

11. Cappato R, Schluter M, Mont L, *et al.* Anatomic, electrical, and mechanical factors affecting bipolar endocardial electrograms. Impact on catheter ablation of manifest left free-wall accessory pathways. Circulation 1994; 90(2): 884-94.

12. Schluter M, Kuck KH. Catheter ablation from right atrium of anteroseptal accessory pathways using radiofrequency current. J Am Coll Cardiol 1992; 19(3): 663-70.

13. Atienza F, Arenal A, Torrecilla EG *et al.* Acute and long-term outcome of transvenous cryoablation of midseptal and parahissian accessory pathways in patients at high risk of atrioventricular block during radiofrequency ablation. Am J Cardiol 2004; 93(10): 1302-5.

14. Valderrabano M, Cesario DA, Ji S *et al.* Percutaneous epicardial mapping during ablation of difficult accessory pathways as an alternative to cardiac surgery. Heart Rhythm 2004; 1(3): 311-6.

15. Liew R, Baker V, Richmond L, *et al.* A randomized-controlled trial comparing conventional with minimal catheter approaches for the mapping and ablation of regular supraventricular tachycardias. Europace 2009; 11(8): 1057-64.

Chapter 13. Diagnosis and therapy of complex accessory pathways (Mahaim fibers, Coumel tachycardia, uncommon locations)

K.R. Julian Chun, F. Ouyang, B. Schmidt, K. Heinz Kuck

II. Medizinische Abteilung
Asklepios Klinik St. Georg
Hamburg, Germany

Address for correspondence:
II. Medizinische Abteilung
Asklepios Klinik St. Georg
Prof. Dr. Karl-Heinz Kuck
k.kuck@asklepios.com

Introduction

Catheter ablation has become the curative therapy of choice for patients with atrioventricular reentrant tachycardias (AVRT). This chapter will focus on rare but important subforms of AVRT with anterograde slow decremental conduction properties, retrograde decremental conduction properties and accessory pathways (APs) associated with uncommon anatomic locations.

1 Accessory pathways with slow anterograde decremental conduction properties ("Mahaim fibers")

Preexcitation syndromes were traditionally classified on the basis of their anatomical location and course and named according to the original investigator. This resulted in the terminology of Mahaim, James and Kent fibers. However, with growing anatomic evidence and increasing electrophysiological understanding this description was found to be inadequate. For APs with anterograde slow decremental conduction properties the description of "Mahaim fibers" however remained despite the introduction of a novel terminology. Originally, Mahaim *et al.* described APs connecting the AV node and the distal right bundle branch or adjacent ventricular myocardium[1,2] which exhibited slow anterograde decremental conduction properties. Ablation of the AV node was considered to be the logical therapy for these tachycardias. This concept was challenged by the observation that "Mahaim preexcitation" was not abolished after AV node ablation but after AP ablation at the lateral RA annulus.[3,4] These observations were in agreement with the concept of a distinct AP with AV node-like conduction properties. This was supported by Tchou *et al.*, 1988,[5] who demonstrated that ventricular activation was preceded during tachycardia by an atrial extrastimulus during AV node refractoriness. It is now believed that most nodoventricular and nodofascicular "Mahaim tachycardias" can be contributed to atriofascicular APs which account for approximately 80% of Mahaim fibers. They mostly have an anatomically long course with insertion into the distal right bundle near the right ventricular apex, often with arborisation.[6] Atrioventricular decremental APs with a short course and ventricular insertion near the AV annulus account for approximately 20% of Mahaim fibers.[6] Overall, the prevalence of Mahaim fibers is low and comprises approximately 2-3% of all overt APs.[7] Interestingly, in 40% of patients with Mahaim fibers additional APs or dual AV nodal pathways are present[8,9] which has been commonly observed in Ebstein's anomaly.[10] We will refer to the term Mahaim fiber as a synonym for slow anterograde (unidirectional) conducting decremental APs and focus on the most common form: the atriofascicular AP.

1.1 Surface ECG features and localization

In sinus rhythm there is no or only discrete preexcitation.[11,12] It has been suggested that an rS pattern in lead III without Q wave in lead I may indicate the presence of a Mahaim fiber.[13] Preexcited QRS complexes and/or Mahaim tachycardias display a left bundle branch block morphology with a leftward axis (see figure 1). Mahaim fibers are typically located along the tricuspid annulus[14] (see figure 2).

1.2 Intracardiac ECGs and diagnosis

The clinical arrhythmia is characterized by a regular wide QRS complex tachycardia with left axis and left bundle branch block morphology. This reentrant tachycardia uses the Mahaim fiber as the anterograde limb and the right or left bundle, His and AV node as the retrograde limb of the

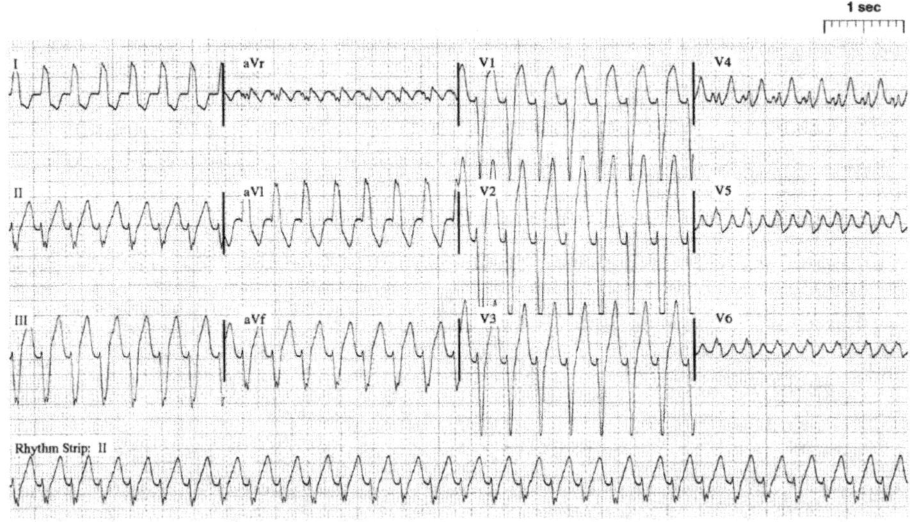

Figure 1. 12-lead ECG of Mahaim tachycardia with left bundle branch block morphology and left axis.

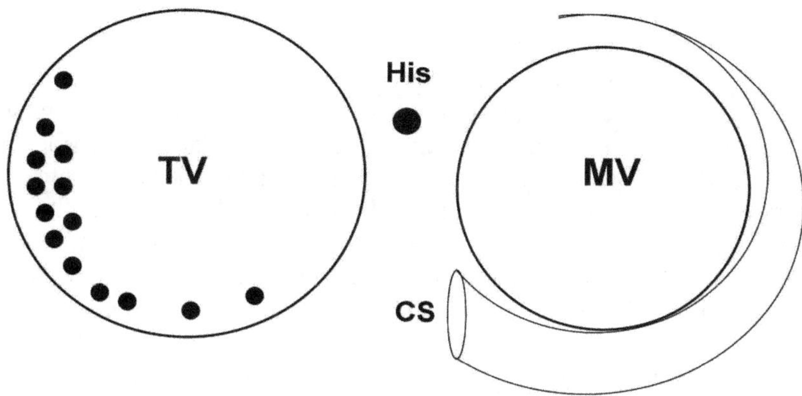

Figure 2. Schematic view of typical Mahaim atriofascicular fiber locations along the tricuspid annulus. CS = coronary sinus; MV = mitral valve; TV = tricuspid valve.

circuit (see figure 3). Definite diagnosis of such a Mahaim tachycardia requires intracardiac ECG recordings and can be established based on subsequent electrophysiological characteristics:

- *Rate-dependent anterograde conduction time.* During programmed atrial stimulation there is progressive AH interval prolongation combined with decreasing HV interval resulting in a greater preexcitation. At maximal preexcitation the His bundle deflection can be inscribed after the right bundle potential [5] due to distal to proximal His activation (figure 3)

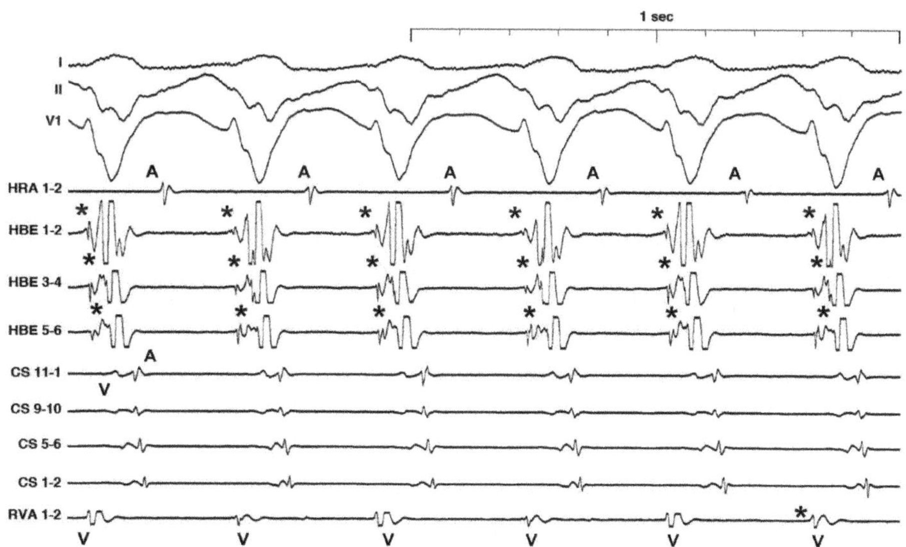

Figure 3. Lead I, II, V1 and intracardiac recordings of a Mahaim tachycardia; activation of the RV via the atriofascicular fiber (anterograde limb) and via the right bundle branch distal to proximal His activation (*) representing the retrograde limb of the tachycardia circuit.
HRA = high right atrium; HBE = His bundle; CS = coronary sinus; RVA = right ventricular apex.

and there is a constant QRS to His bundle relationship without changes during shortening the atrial pacing cycle length.

- *Ventricular preceding by an atrial stimulus when the AV node is refractory.* Delivery of a late atrial stimulus near the atrial insertion at the time of AV nodal refractoriness results in advancing the next ventricular activation (figure 4). This stimulation maneuver helps to distinguish the presence of an atriofascicular versus a nodofascicular/ nodoventricular AP and AV nodal reentry tachycardia with an atriofascicular AP as a bystander.
- *Long cycle length pacing from the right atrium (RA) but not left atrium (LA) generally leads to pronounced preexcitation.* The atrial insertion of the atriofascicular fiber is typically located along the RA free wall near the tricuspid annulus.[14,15] Thus RA pacing at longer cycle length is associated with preexcitation whereas stimulation from the LA (coronary sinus catheter) is not. In the presence of such an atriofascicular fiber, ventricular activation from the RA can bypass the tricuspid annulus and preexcite the ventricles independent of the AV node.

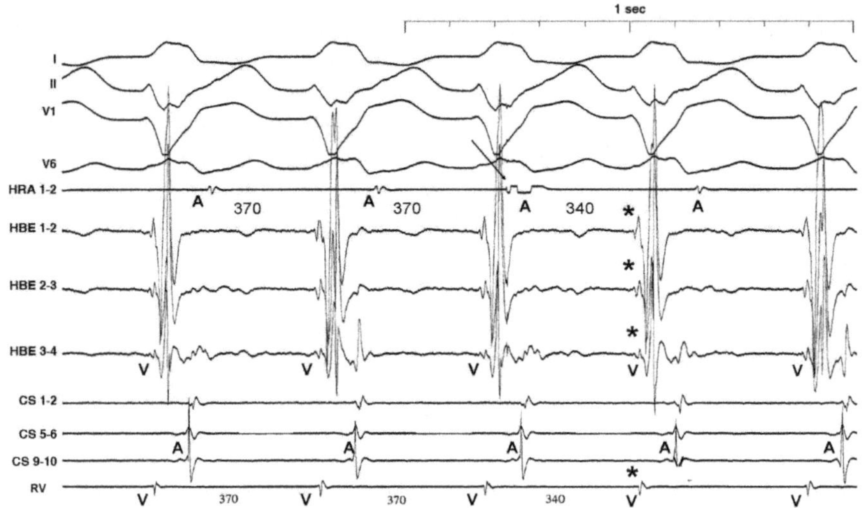

Figure 4. Lead I, II, V1 and intracardiac recordings of a Mahaim tachycardia (cycle length 370 ms). An atrial extrastimulus (arrow) precedes ventricular activation (*) demonstrating atrial participation of tachycardia.
A = atrium; HRA = high right atrium,; HBE = His bundle; CS = coronary sinus;
RVA = right ventricular apex; V = ventricle.

1.3   Techniques for mapping and ablation

Although there is evidence of retrograde penetration into the Mahaim fiber during ventricular pacing, there is no evidence of retrograde atriofascicular fiber conduction into the atria. Therefore, mapping of the atrial insertion during ventricular stimulation is not possible due to unique unidirectional anterograde AP conduction. Presence of eccentric atrial activation during tachycardia or ventricular stimulation indicates the presence of an additional rapidly conducting AP tract. In principle, both the atrial or ventricular atriofascicular fiber insertion site can be targeted.

1.3.1   Atrial insertion

Searching for the so-called "M potential" is critical for successful ablation. Identification of this local AP potential should be the preferred mapping strategy to guide ablation. The local M potential resembles a "His potential" and may display a high frequency potential with low or high amplitudes widely separated from the atrial and ventricular activation (see figure 5). The ablation catheter should be moved cautiously along the tricuspid annulus to avoid mechanical bumps of "Mahaim fiber tissue" which can cause transient AP conduction abolition indicating a subendocardial AP location. This susceptibility to mechanical trauma may also be utilized to guide successful catheter ablation.[14] The use of a long sheath to facilitate catheter stability should be considered when mapping and ablating Mahaim "atriofascicular fibers" typically located at the right free wall.[14] An alternative mapping strategy aims to identify the shortest stimulus to QRS interval of fully preexcited beats during atrial pacing along the tricuspid annulus.[16]

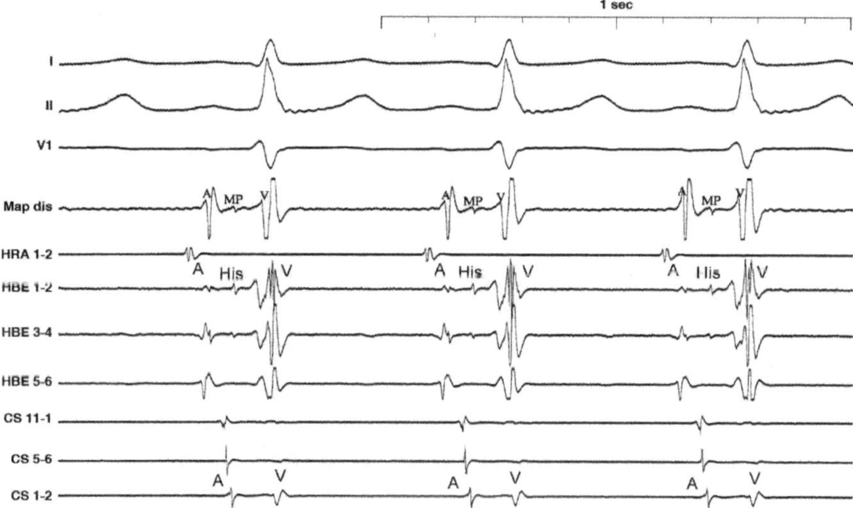

Figure 5. Lead I, II, V1 and intracardiac recordings in sinus rhythm. Local map catheter in an anterolateral tricuspid annulus position. Identification of the "M potential" suggesting a successful ablation site. A = atrium; HRA = high right atrium; HBE = His bundle; CS = Coronary sinus; MP = Mahaim potential; RVA = right ventricular apex; V = ventricle.

1.3.2   Ventricular insertion

Strategies to identify the ventricular insertion aim to identify the earliest ventricular activation of fully preexcited beats or to obtain a perfect 12-lead ECG pace map. However, AP arborisation at the level of ventricular insertion may complicate mapping and successful ablation.

2   Permanent junctional reciprocating tachycardia (PJRT, Coumel tachycardia)

The permanent junctional reciprocating tachycardia (PJRT) was originally described by Coumel *et al.* in 1967.[17] This rare supraventricular tachycardia predominantly occurs in children but may persist into adulthood.[18] This tachycardia is often resistant to medical treatment and may cause tachycardia-induced cardiomyopathy.[19] Recent studies have indicated the presence of an AP with slow decremental retrograde conduction properties as the underlying substrate for orthodromic circus movement tachycardia.[20,21] However, the term PJRT may be misleading since an AP and not the AV node represents the retrograde tachycardia limb.

2.1 Surface ECG features and localization

Patients typically present with an incessant narrow QRS complex tachycardia ranging from 120-250 beats/minute. The characteristic ECG features are a long RP tachycardia consistent with slow retrograde conduction and inverted P-waves in leads II, III and aVF (figure 6). Negative P-waves in inferior leads indicate an AP insertion near the coronary sinus (CS) ostium but AP insertion may also occur along the right or left free wall.[22] The QRS complex is normal during sinus rhythm due to unidirectional retrograde AP conduction properties in patients with preserved AV node conduction.[19]

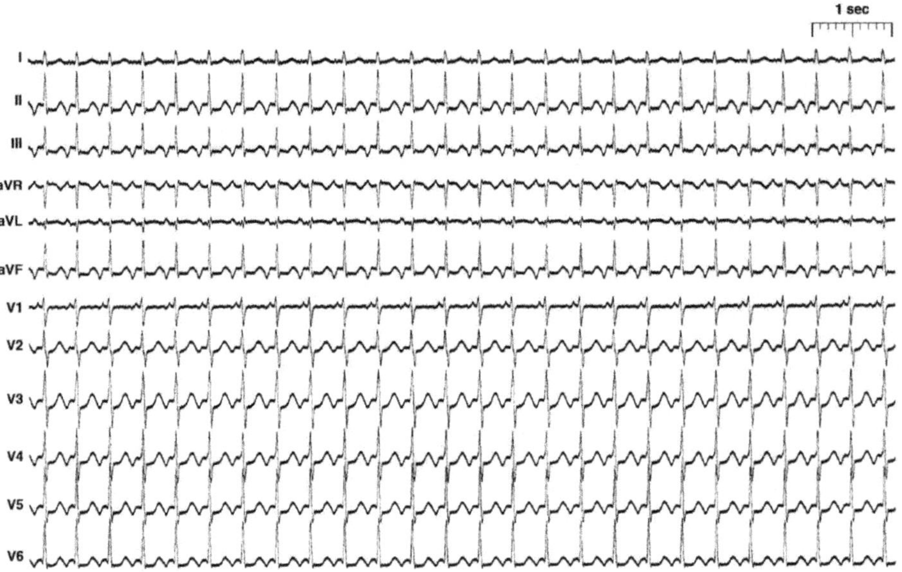

Figure 6. 12-lead ECG of a permanent junctional reciprocating tachycardia (PJRT).
Please note long RP tachycardia with inverted P-waves in inferior lead (II, III, aVF).

2.2 Intracardiac ECGs and diagnosis

Since the AP is anatomically separated from the AV node/His-Purkinje system, a ventricular extrastimulus delivered when the His bundle is refractory can reset the next atrial activation without changing the atrial activation sequence (see figure 7). This response cannot occur during uncommon fast-slow AV nodal reentrant tachycardia or atrial tachycardia and

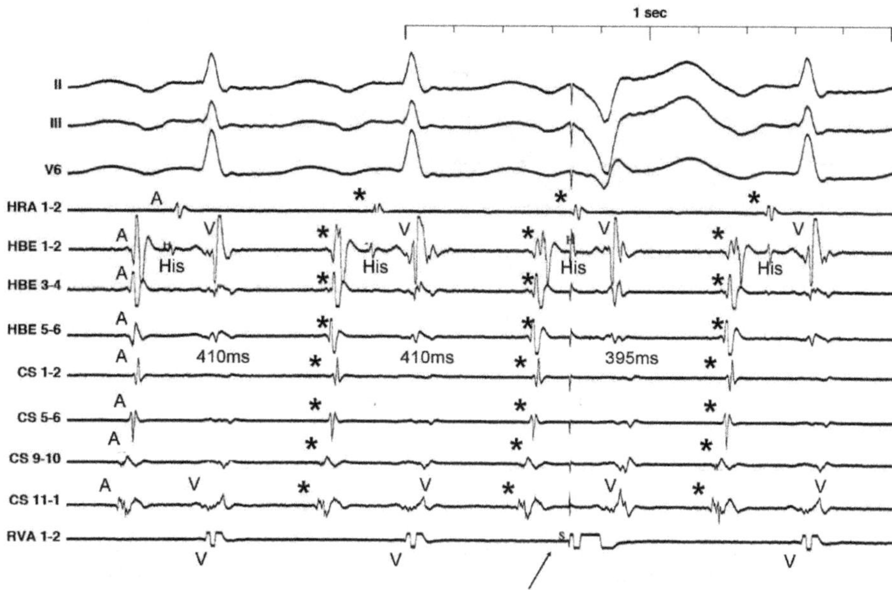

Figure 7. Lead II, III, V6 and intracardiac recordings during PJRT. Delivery of ventricular extrastimulus (arrow) precedes atrial activation without changing the atrial activation sequence (*).
A- = atrium; HRA = high right atrium; HBE = His bundle; CS = coronary sinus;
RVA = right ventricular apex; V = ventricle.

is useful for differentiation among long RP supraventricular tachycardias.[23] Because the AP conducts decrementally during PJRT, the atrial activation and tachycardia cycle reset response to the ventricular extrastimulus may actually either preexcite or delay atrial activation.[24] Tachycardia termination occurring spontaneously or following vagal maneuvers frequently results from block in the AP; the ECG and intracardiac recordings show the last tachycardia event as a QRS complex and ventricular electrogram without a subsequent P-wave and atrial activation.

2.3   Techniques for mapping and ablation

Identification of the ablation target site is guided by the earliest retrograde atrial activation either during tachycardia or pacing. The presence of a discrete AP potential may indicate a successful ablation site (see figure 8). Successful ablation sites are typically found using a right-sided approach in the region of the CS ostium, but some variability of AP locations has been reported requiring a left-sided approach.[18,25]

3   Accessory pathways arising from uncommon locations

Usually, APs directly connect the atria and ventricle bypassing the AV node and are typically located along the AV groove as discussed in Chapter 12. Following characterization of anatom-

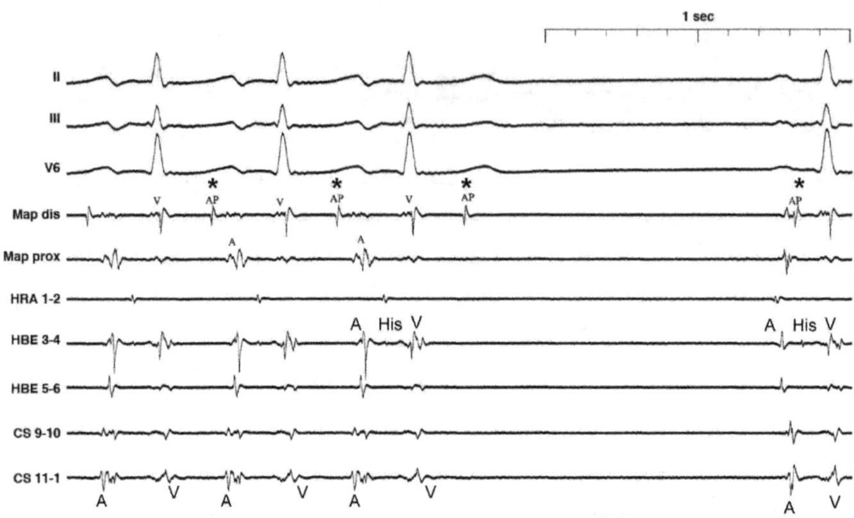

Figure 8. Lead II, III, V6 and intracardiac recordings during PJRT. Identification of local AP potential (*) (Map). Radiofrequency current application terminates tachycardia blocking the retrograde conduction in the AP without subsequent atrial activation. Please note preserved anterograde AP penetration in sinus rhythm (*).
A = atrium; AP = accessory pathway potential; HRA = high right atrium; HBE = His bundle; CS = coronary sinus; RVA = right ventricular apex; V = ventricle.

ical and electrophysiological properties, catheter ablation of APs is commonly highly successful.[26,27] However, atypical anatomic AP connections may be present and account for ablation failures requiring special mapping and ablation techniques.

3.1 Sub/epicardial atrioventricular accessory pathways

Inferoparaseptal (posteroseptal) APs are frequently located to the region of the proximal CS and linked to CS anatomy variations such as a middle cardiac vein, ventricular branches or a diverticulum with a subepicardial AP location. Mapping and subsequent ablation should be guided by direct angiography to visualize the patient's individual CS anatomy.[28] Recently, this facilitated successful identification and ablation of an inferoparaseptal (posteroseptal) AP related to the presence of two uncommon CS diverticula in one of our patients (see figure 9). A superior access from the jugular vein can be considered for mapping and ablation at a diverticulum. In a small group of patients a large AP potential can be detected within the distal CS indicating a left epicardial AP location. Successful catheter ablation abolishing AP conduction can be performed from within the CS,[29] which requires irrigated tip ablation in the majority of cases due to high impedance. In rare cases AP connections between the right or left atrial appendage (RAA or LAA) and the ventricle have been described.[30-32] LAA to ventricular connections should be mapped for within the CS or its branches, whereas mapping and ablation for the ventricular insertion from the RAA is often futile and can be attempted from within the RAA. However, it may become necessary to obtain an epicardial access to ablate the AP.[33,34]

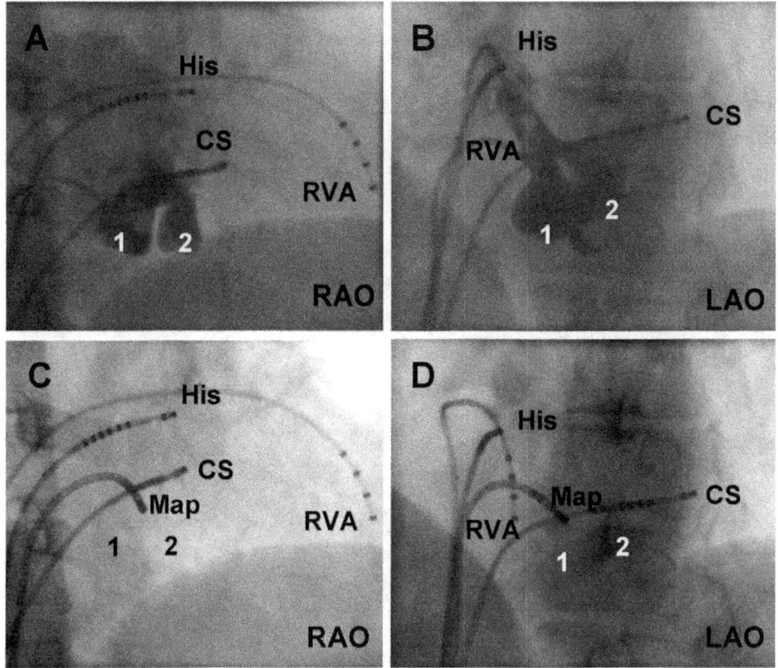

Figure 9. A and B. RAO and LAO projections of CS angiography relvealing the presence of two uncommon CS diverticula (1; 2).
C and D. RAO and LAO projections demonstrating the local map position at the successful ablation site (neck of diverticulum 1) of an inferoparaseptal (posteroseptal) AP.
CS = coronary sinus; His = His bundle; LAO = left anterior oblique; RAO = right anterior oblique;
RVA = right ventricular apex.

3.2 Aortoventricular accessory pathways

Atrial and ventricular tachycardias can originate from the aortic root due to the presence of cardiac muscle fibers.[35,36] An uncommon AP origin from the aortic root should be considered in patients with earliest superoparaseptal (anteroseptal) activation. We recently encountered one patient from a referring center after a previous futile ablation of a superoparaseptal (anteroseptal) AP with incessant AVRT and tachycardia-induced cardiomyopathy. Careful mapping revealed earliest endocardial activation along the His region which prompted additional mapping in the aortic root and revealed such an uncommon AP in the aortic root (non-coronary cusp) (see figure 10). To facilitate catheter orientation within the aortic root angiography in standard angulations should be performed (see figure 10). Conventional radiofrequency current ablation resulted in tachycardia termination but only transient AP block. Permanent AP block required use of irrigated radiofrequency current energy which strongly suggests that the AP was located deeply in the epicardial region of the non-coronary cusp. Subsequently, a normal heart rate was established and left ventricular ejection fraction normalized after ablation.[37]

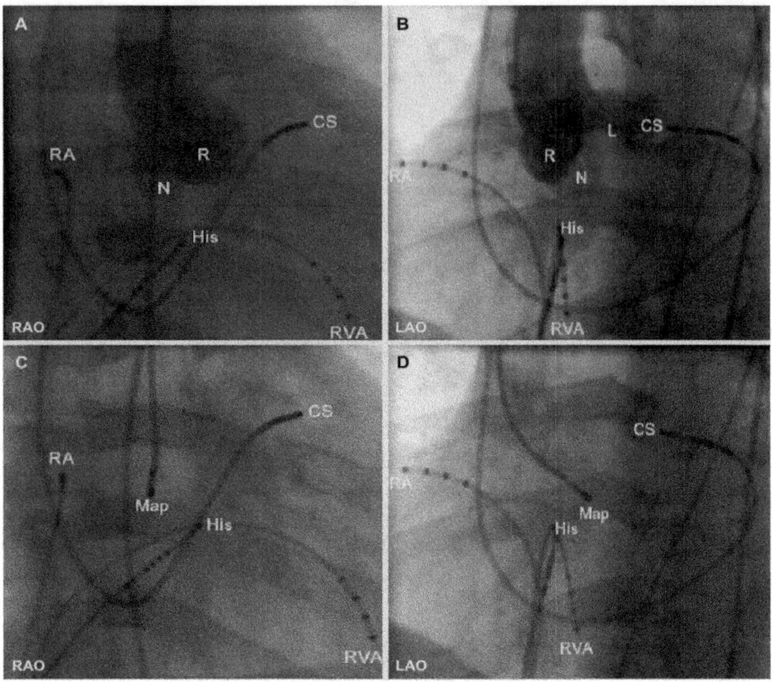

Figure 10. A and B. RAO and LAO projections of aortic root angiography.
C and D. RAO and LAO projections of Map catheter position at the successful ablation
site of an anteroseptal AP from the non-coronary cusp.
CS = coronary sinus; His = His bundle; LAO = left anterior oblique; RA = right atrium;
RAO = right anterior oblique; RVA = right ventricular apex; N = non-coronary cusp;
L = left coronary cusp; R = right coronary cusp.

Conclusion

Catheter ablation of simple accessory pathways has been established as the preferred curative treatment option for atrioventricular reentry tachycardias. Detailed understanding of cardiac anatomy and electrophysiology is essential to guide ablation of complex accessory pathways and can be associated with high success rates.

References

1. Mahaim I, Benatt A. Nouvelles recherches sur les connexions superieures de la branches gauche du faisceau de His-Tawara avec cloison interventriculaire. Cardiologia, 1938; 1(61).

2. Mahaim I, Winston MR. Recherches d'anatomique comparée et de pathologie experimentale sur les connexions hautes du faisceau de His-Tawara. Cardiologica 1941; 5(189).

3. Bhandari A, Morady F, Shen EN, *et al.* Catheter-induced His bundle ablation in a patient with reentrant tachycardia associated with a nodoventricular tract. J Am Coll Cardiol 1984; 4(3): 611-6.

4. Klein GJ, Guiraudon GM, Kerr CR, *et al.* "Nodoventricular" accessory pathway: evidence for a distinct accessory atrioventricular pathway with atrioventricular node-like properties. J Am Coll Cardiol 1988; 11(5): 1035-40.

5. Tchou P, Lehmann MH, Jazayeri M, *et al.* Atriofascicular connection or a nodoventricular Mahaim fiber? Electro-

physiologic elucidation of the pathway and associated reentrant circuit. Circulation 1988; 77(4): 837-48.

6. Haissaguerre M, Cauchemez B, Marcus F, *et al.* Characteristics of the ventricular insertion sites of accessory pathways with anterograde decremental conduction properties. Circulation 1995; 91(4): 1077-85.

7. Miller JM, Olgin JE. Catheter ablation of free-wall accessory pathways and "Mahaim" fibers. In: Zipes DP, Haissaguerre M, eds. Catheter ablation of Cardiac Arrhythmias, 2nd ed Armonk, NX 2002: 277.

8. Gallagher JJ, Smith WM, Kasell JH, *et al.* Role of Mahaim fibers in cardiac arrhythmias in man. Circulation 1981; 64(1): 176-89.

9. Sung RJ, Styperek JL. Electrophysiologic identification of dual atrioventricular nodal pathway conduction in patients with reciprocating tachycardia using anomalous bypass tracts. Circulation 1979; 60(7): 1464-76.

10. Cappato R, Schluter M, Weiss C, *et al.* Radiofrequency current catheter ablation of accessory atrioventricular pathways in Ebstein's anomaly. Circulation 1996; 94(3): 376-83.

11. Bardy GH, Fedor JM, German LD, *et al.* Surface electrocardiographic clues suggesting presence of a nodofascicular Mahaim fiber. J Am Coll Cardiol 1984; 3(5): 1161-8.

12. McClelland JH, Wang X, Beckman KJ, *et al.* Radiofrequency catheter ablation of right atriofascicular (Mahaim) accessory pathways guided by accessory pathway activation potentials. Circulation 1994; 89(6): 2655-66.

13. Sternick EB, Timmermans C, Sosa E, *et al.* The electrocardiogram during sinus rhythm and tachycardia in patients with Mahaim fibers: the importance of an "rS" pattern in lead III. J Am Coll Cardiol 2004; 44(8): 1626-35.

14. Cappato R, Schluter M, Weiss C, *et al.* Catheter-induced mechanical conduction block of right-sided accessory fibers with Mahaim-type preexcitation to guide radiofrequency ablation. Circulation 1994; 90(1): 282-90.

15. Bohora S, Dora SK, Namboodiri N, *et al.* Electrophysiology study and radiofrequency catheter ablation of atriofascicular tracts with decremental properties (Mahaim fibre) at the tricuspid annulus. Europace 2008; 10(12): 1428-33.

16. Klein LS, Hackett FK, Zipes DP, *et al.* Radiofrequency catheter ablation of Mahaim fibers at the tricuspid annulus. Circulation 1993; 87(3): 738-47.

17. Coumel P, Gourgon R, Fabiato A, *et al.* Studies of assisted circulation. I. Methods of repetitive provoked extrasystole and slowing of effective heart rate. Arch Mal Coeur Vaiss 1967; 60(1): 67-88.

18. Dorostkar PC, Silka MJ, Morady F, *et al.* Clinical course of persistent junctional reciprocating tachycardia. J Am Coll Cardiol 1999; 33(2): 366-75.

19. Critelli G, Gallagher JJ, Monda V, *et al.* Anatomic and electrophysiologic substrate of the permanent form of junctional reciprocating tachycardia. J Am Coll Cardiol 1984; 4(3): 601-10.

20. Farre J, Ross D, Wiener I, *et al.* Reciprocal tachycardias using accessory pathways with long conduction times. Am J Cardiol 1979; 44(6): 1099-109.

21. Lerman BB, Greenberg M, Overholt ED, *et al.* Differential electrophysiologic properties of decremental retrograde pathways in long RP' tachycardia. Circulation 1987; 76(1): 21-31.

22. Ticho BS, Saul JP, Hulse JE, *et al.* Variable location of accessory pathways associated with the permanent form of junctional reciprocating tachycardia and confirmation with radiofrequency ablation. Am J Cardiol 1992; 70(20): 1559-64.

23. Brugada P, Farre J, Green M, *et al.* Observations in patients with supraventricular tachycardia having a P-R interval shorter than the R-P interval: differentiation between atrial tachycardia and reciprocating atrioventricular tachycardia using an accessory pathway with long conduction times. Am Heart J 1984; 107(3): 556-70.

24. Cain ME, Luke RA, Lindsay BD. Diagnosis and localization of accessory pathways. Pacing Clin Electrophysiol 1992; 15(5): 801-24.

25. Meiltz A, Weber R, Halimi F, *et al.* Permanent form of junctional reciprocating tachycardia in adults: peculiar features and results of radiofrequency catheter ablation. Europace 2006; 8(1): 21-8.

26. Jackman WM, Wang XZ, Friday KJ, *et al.* Catheter ablation of accessory atrioventricular pathways (Wolff-Parkinson-White syndrome) by radiofrequency current. N Engl J Med 1991; 324(23): 1605-11.

27. Kuck KH, Schluter M, Geiger M, *et al.* Radiofrequency current catheter ablation of accessory atrioventricular pathways. Lancet 1991; 337(8757): 1557-61.

28. Tebbenjohanns J, Pfeiffer D, Schumacher B, *et al.* Direct angiography of the coronary sinus: impact on left posteroseptal accessory pathway ablation. Pacing Clin Electrophysiol 1996; 19(7): 1075-81.

29. Haissaguerre M, Gaita F, Fischer B, *et al.* Radiofrequency catheter ablation of left lateral accessory pathways via the coronary sinus. Circulation 1992; 86(5): 1464-8.

30. Soejima K, Mitamura H, Miyazaki T, *et al.* Catheter ablation of accessory atrioventricular connection between right atrial appendage to right ventricle: a case report. J Cardiovasc Electrophysiol 1998; 9(5): 523-8.

31. Lam C, Schweikert R, Kanagaratnam L, *et al.* Radiofrequency ablation of a right atrial appendage-ventricular accessory pathway by transcutaneous epicardial instrumentation. J Cardiovasc Electrophysiol 2000; 11(10): 1170-3.

32. Servatius H, Rostock T, Hoffmann BA, *et al.* Catheter ablation of an atrioventricular bypass tract connecting a funnel-shaped bilobular left atrial appendage with the ventricular free wall. Heart Rhythm 2009; 6(7): 1075-6.

33. Schweikert RA, Saliba WI, Tomassoni G, *et al.* Percutaneous pericardial instrumentation for endo-epicardial mapping of previously failed ablations. Circulation 2003; 108(11): 1329-35.

34. Valderrabano M, Cesario DA, Ji S, *et al.* Percutaneous epicardial mapping during ablation of difficult accessory pathways as an alternative to cardiac surgery. Heart Rhythm 2004; 1(3): 311-6.

35. Ouyang F, Ma J, Ho SY, *et al.* Focal atrial tachycardia originating from the non-coronary aortic sinus: electrophysiological characteristics and catheter ablation. J Am Coll Cardiol 2006; 48(1): 122-31.

36. Ouyang F, Fotuhi P, Ho SY, *et al.* Repetitive monomorphic ventricular tachycardia originating from the aortic sinus cusp: electrocardiographic characterization for guiding catheter ablation. J Am Coll Cardiol 2002; 39(3): 500-8.

37. Huang H, Wang X, Ouyang F, *et al.* Catheter ablation of anteroseptal accessory pathway in the non-coronary aortic sinus. Europace 2006; 8(12): 1041-4.

Chapter 14. Radiofrequency ablation in infants and children: the simpler, the better

G. SARQUELLA-BRUGADA[1], J. BRUGADA[1,2]

[1] Arrhythmia Unit, Cardiology Section
Sant Joan de Déu Hospital
Barcelona, Spain

[2] Cardiology Service
Hospital Clínic de Barcelona
Barcelona, Spain

Address for correspondence:
Cardiology Service
Hospital Clínic de Barcelona
Dr. J. Brugada
jbrugada@clinic.ub.es

Introduction

It took twenty years from first intracavitary electrocardiographic registries[1] to first description of pediatric cardiac ablations.[2] In 2009, twenty years later, ablation procedures have become extensible to pediatric population, to the point of being considered first-line treatment in some centers.[3-6] In others, ablation is still considered a risky and long procedure, advocating for an intense pharmacological treatment, not free from side effects, in order to control some arrhythmias. Personal and center experience might account for these differences in management among the centers.

Several issues increase the complexity on pediatric procedures: small body surface, radiation exposure potential effects,[7-10] vascular access limitations and concomitant congenital heart disease.[11, 12]

Control with medical therapy alone is possible, but treatment failures are not rare, and drug side effects are not negligible. In experienced hands, radiofrequency catheter ablation (RFA) is a safe and effective treatment option for children with refractory arrhythmias, to the point of being considered a first-line therapy for some of the arrhythmias, such as supraventricular tachycardias. Success rates for RFA are high, over 90% in most of the series, with low complications rates associated with the procedure.[3, 4]

In most centers, several catheters (3 to 5) are used for mapping the arrhythmia mechanism. This takes long procedure and radiation times, and compromises vascular access (often three catheters inserted in femoral approach, plus a fourth from jugular vein). Hence, general anesthesia is often needed even for older patients.[3, 4]

Probably the use of complex studies, requiring many vascular accesses, long procedure times and complex room settings, by some of the groups performing them, has created the view in some pediatric cardiologists that this is a very risky procedure.

We present our approach, which is based on a very simplified technique that allows short procedural times, short radiation times, fewer anaesthesia demands, and fewer complications.

1   Arrhythmias in children

Supraventricular tachycardia (SVT) constitute the most common tachyarrhythmia in the pediatric population, affecting 1 in 250 to 1,000 paediatric patients with structurally normal hearts.[13] The prevalence of the different mechanisms of the SVT has been shown to vary among different age groups.

- *Atrioventricular reentrant tachycardia (AVRT) using an accessory pathway* often presents in the first year of life, with two other peaks of presentation at 10 years and 15 years of age.[14] In Wolff-Parkinson-White syndrome (WPW) diagnosed in infancy, a decrease in the recurrence has been shown in the first years of life, with an increase of episodes at the end of the first decade. Around 90% of infants diagnosed with WPW have remission of tachycardia episodes by the age of 18 months with recurrence of tachycardia later in life,[15-19] up to 70% in late follow-up. A main concern is the reported risk of sudden death in patients with WPW, estimated to be 0.1 to 0.6 % per patient-year of follow-up.[20,21] As the risk of probability of life-threatening arrhythmias is considered higher with respect to the risk related to ablation,[22] some groups consider RFA for asymptomatic WPW patients after a certain age or above a certain body weight. A particular form of AVRT is "persistent junctional reciprocating tachycardia" (PJRT) described by Coumel *et al.* in 1976,[23] PJRT diagnosed, mostly in infants, and often in heart failure phase due to tachycardiomyopathy, difficult to control with drugs.
- *Atrioventricular nodal reentry tachycardia* (AVNRT*)* is uncommon in infancy,[24] with increasing incidence beyond the age of 5 years.[25]
- *Automatic atrial tachycardia* has a constant prevalence throughout infancy, childhood and adolescence, occurring in 10 to 12 % of pediatric patients with SVT.[25] When sinus rhythm is achieved with medication, around 50% will have spontaneous resolution of tachycardia.[26-29] When refractory to medication, multiple foci may be implicated, and can lead to tachycardiomyopathy. Ablation is indicated at this point.
- *Atrial flutter in normal hearts* is seen at the early neonatal period, but low recurrence rates later in life.[30]
- *Junctional ectopic tachycardia or "automatic Junctional tachycardia"* is a rare disorder, most commonly seen in infants, and difficult to manage with drugs,[31] with high mortality rates beyond the series.[32]
- *Ventricular tachycardia* (VT) is an uncommon entity in childhood (0.8 per 1,000 children in school-based heart screening),[33] with a tendency to recur in the absence of an identifiable predisposing cause, mostly in adolescence.[34] When VT associates cardiomyopathy or genetic disorders (long QT syndrome, Brugada syndrome or catecholaminergic, dilated or hypertrophic cardiomyopathy or arrhythmogenic right ventricle dysplasia) the tendency is to progress and worsen.

1.1   Patients and methods

We describe our experience, collected from patients under 18 years of age, referred to our Arrhythmia Unit during the last fifteen years.

Indications for RFA were incessant tachycardia refractory to double drug therapy, recurrent paroxysmal tachycardia refractory to single drug therapy or patient-family decision (for asymptomatic WPW over 35 kg).

1.2　Procedure

1.2.1　Anesthesia

RFA can be stressful, uncomfortable and painful. Hence, anesthesiologist collaboration is crucial. Our simplified RFA protocol (see below) allows short procedural times, and anesthesia is adapted to the procedure. Therefore, adolescents are softly sedated with midazolam and local anesthesia; infants procedures are performed under deep sedation (midazolam with phentanyl) with propophol continuous infusion to achieve spontaneous ventilation or, eventually, assistance with laryngeal mask; finally, RFA in neonates and toddlers are performed under balanced general anesthesia.

1.2.2　Energy sources

Radiofrequency ablation has been used in ALL patients. No other sources of energy have been necessary so far. Our usual setting is 20 to 40 W application under temperature control for 5-60 sec. depending on the location of the target, age and weight of the patient and immediate result during application.

1.2.3　Approach

Close and detailed examination of the surface 12-lead ECG is essential for choosing the appropriate approach for each procedure. Several algorithms have been proposed for accessory pathway localization.[35] Once the target (accessory pathway, atrial focus or circuit, AV nodal pathway or ventricular circuit) is presumably located, vascular access is taken based on the following:

- For left sided accessory pathways, retrograde approach from the femoral artery is the standard, except for those patients having a persistent foramen ovale, in which femoral vein is chosen. Transeptal puncture approach has only been used in two patients with left-sided atrial tachycardias and no patent foramen ovale.
- For right sided accessory pathways, femoral vein approach is used.

Only in three cases other than femoral approaches were used: one severely compromised newborn in which femoral access was not achieved, and subclavian vein in one and internal jugular vein in the other were used to perform the RFA. In a third case, internal jugular vein access was needed to ensure catheter stability in an anteroseptal accessory pathway ablation.

1.2.4　Simplified catheter technique

We perform RFA in patients trying to use the so-called "single catheter technique", consisting of the introduction of a single catheter for stimulation, registration and ablation. To perform the single catheter RFA safely, an EP system with beat-by-beat trigger capability is mandatory.

In our series, 80% of small patients (less than 15 kg) could be ablated using this technique. In the rest, only two catheters were needed. We have never used more than two catheters simultaneously (see figures 1 and 2).

Simplified catheter technique is indicated in the following situations:

- *Pre-excitation* on the ECG: location of the accessory pathway is achieved with the same single 5F ablation catheter, trying to find the area where atrial and ventricular activation is the closest. RFA is performed in this area. When applied on the right place, early disappearance

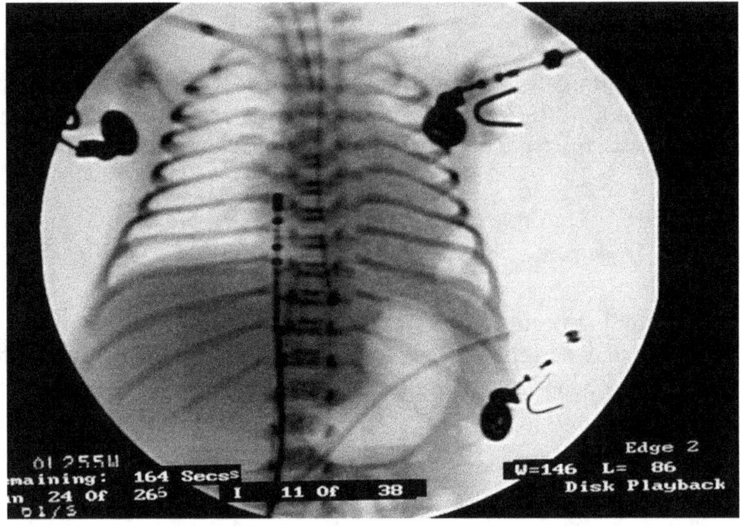

Figure 1. Single catheter technique in a newborn.

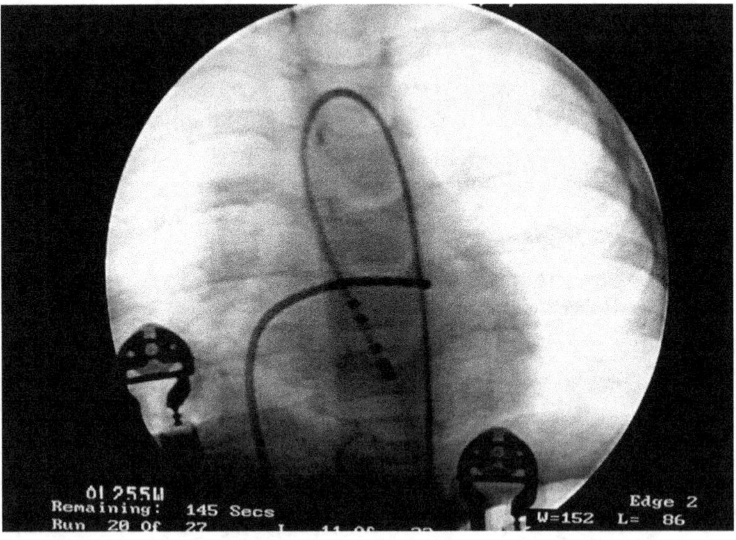

Figure 2. Two-catheter technique for left-sided accesory pathways.

of the delta wave is observed, and then energy is maintained for 30 to 60 seconds, carefully looking for AV prolongation. If after around 5 seconds of application, no effect is observed on AP conduction, energy delivery is stopped and the procedure is restarted looking for a better location. Following a successful ablation, electrophysiological testing using atrial and ventricular pacing is performed to ensure that AP conduction does not resume. Atrial pacing is performed using single and double extrastimulus until refractoriness and rapid atrial pacing until 1 to 1 conduction to the ventricle is lost. Ventricular pacing is performed using single and double extrastimulus and rapid pacing to ensure: *1)* that no tachycardia is induced; *2)* that VA conduction, if present, is not done using the AP; and *3)* that no AV conduction over the AP is observed after the ventricular pause that usually follows ventricular premature beats. Again, beat to beat trigger is mandatory to be able to observe VA conduction on the surface ECG since a single catheter is used. The most reliable situation is, of course, observation of VA dissociation, but also careful analysis allows for observation of progressive VA prolongation while extrastimuli coupling intervals are shortened. Normally a 5 to 10-minute observation in the EP lab is sufficient to confirm success.

- *Supraventricular tachycardia without pre-excitation* on the ECG: by inducing the tachycardia, electrophysiological properties arise with the diagnostic (simultaneous activation of the ventricles and atria for intranodal reentry tachycardia versus non-simultaneous activation suggesting a concealed accessory pathway).
  - For *intranodal reentry tachycardia* (AVNRT), a second catheter is always inserted and positioned in the RA to be able to monitor carefully the VA conduction during RF application. Careful anatomic localization of the His bundle activation and the coronary sinus (CS) entrance will reflect the area to ablate. The ablation catheter is positioned in the area immediately superior to the CS entrance where atrial and ventricular signals are obtained (approximately 1 to 10 ratio). In this area RF current is applied, trying to obtain a slow AV nodal rhythm, and as already stated, VA conduction during this AV nodal rhythm is carefully followed on the screen. In case of any minor increase in the VA time, or occurrence of very fast AV nodal rhythm, RF energy delivery is immediately stopped and the ablation catheter withdrawn 1 to 2 centimeters to avoid any residual effect. This is the most critical point to avoid inadvertent AV block during ablation. Our feeling is that 1 or 2 additional seconds of RF delivery can result in complete AV block. Immediate reaction requires full concentration on the screen in a beat to beat basis to ensure any minor change in VA is immediately detected. After a successful application, programmed electrical stimulation is repeated during basal conditions and during isoproterenol infusion using doses that increase heart rate by 25%. Non inducibility of AV nodal reentrant tachycardia is the endpoint of the procedure. Single AV nodal reentrant beats are accepted. In case the application does not result in AV nodal rhythm, the catheter is gently moved upwards and application restarted until the desired effect during application (occurrence of slow AV nodal rhythm) is obtained.
  - For *concealed accessory pathways*, location of the pathway can be achieved during tachycardia. Gross location of the shortest VA interval is performed in the right (anterior, inferior, septal or lateral) and if no short VA is observed, the catheter is positioned in the CS entrance. In case this location shows the shortest VA interval, the same catheter is positioned inside the CS to map the left side of the heart. Depending on whether the VA interval gets even shorter when inside the CS, then a left-sided approach will be used. If the short VA interval is located in the right side, then a fine mapping is per-

formed, looking for the shortest one during tachycardia. In this position, RF energy is delivered, and if in the right position tachycardia will terminate due to VA block. The position of the catheter is maintained and application pursued until 30 to 60 seconds as already explained. If tachycardia does not terminate after around 5 seconds of application, energy delivery is stopped and a new position is looked for. In the case that tachycardia cannot be maintained, a second catheter might be necessary to stimulate the ventricle in order to map VA conduction during pacing and to ensure correct location and effectiveness of the ablation. During ventricular pacing the VA conduction is mapped first locating the atrial activity at the AV node level and then looking for a shorter VA interval. If the shortest one is at the AV node level, suggesting either VA nodal conduction or simultaneous VA nodal and VA AP conduction, the mapping is performed during fast atrial pacing or even during a single or a double extrastimulus looking for a change in the activation pattern that suggests VA conduction over the AP and not over the AV node. Again, beat to beat trigger mode at fast screen speed (250 to 500 mm/sec) is mandatory to ensure proper analysis of the VA conduction. Once the ablation has been performed, success is verified by trying to induce tachycardia or VA conduction over the AP by atrial and ventricular pacing. As in the previous case of ventricular preexcitation, the most reliable situation is of course observation of VA dissociation, but also careful analysis allows for observation of progressive VA prolongation while extrastimuli coupling intervals are shortened.

– For *atrial tachycardias*, again a single catheter approach is usually used. The tachycardia is induced during atrial pacing and a beat to beat trigger is used taking as reference the beginning of the P wave. The catheter is moved around the atria trying to identify the earliest atrial deflection. Once this earliest site is located, RF energy is delivered until tachycardia terminates and it is continued for 30 to 60 seconds, or for a maximum of 5 to 10 seconds if ineffective. In that case, the mapping is restarted and identification of a new "better" location is tried. Verification of non-inducibility after a successful ablation is performed using programmed electrical stimulation during basal conditions and after isoproterenol infusion.

1.3 Follow-up

After the procedure, patients remain hospitalized for one night. Twelve-lead surface ECG is performed before discharge. Daily aspirin is recommended for 4 weeks for all patients. One month after the procedure, another ECG is performed. If normal, general pediatric cardiologist is in charge of the follow-up.

1.4 Results

In the last 15 years we have performed 936 ablations in patients under 18 years. There is a slight male predominance (55.4%), with a mean age of 12.03 ± 4.2 years, and mean weight 38.8 ± 19.8 kg.

Overall, this technique can be performed in a short time, with no differences between small children (less than 15 kg) and larger ones: procedure mean time is 51 ± 26 min *versus* 49 ± 33 min; radiation mean time 10 ± 7 min *versus* 11 ± 11 min, respectively.

In our series, final diagnostics were as shown in table 1. Mainly, the most frequent diagnostic in small children is tachycardia by concealed accessory pathway (32.3%), followed by Coumel type tachycardia (22.0%) and WPW (20.5%). In older patients, most common, by far, is WPW (51.7%), followed by tachycardia by concealed accessory pathway (20.4%) and AVNRT (16.5%).

Acute success or efficacy (no anterograde and/or retrograde conduction on ablated accessory pathway and no inducible tachycardia, with or without isoproterenol infusion) is 95% in small patients and 96% older ones (see table 2.)

Recurrence, considered as the electrophysiological demonstration of conduction on a previously ablated accessory pathway is 9% and 5% in both groups, probably associated to the fact that low temperature and short application time is preferred in order to avoid complications. Almost 90% of these patients are definitely cured with a second RFA. Only 2% need a third procedure. Overall efficacy is 98% in both groups. Right-sided accessory pathways are responsible for 87% of recurrence in WPW, probably due to instability of the catheter during ablation (see table 3).

Complications are rare in our series. We have had four complications among the 936 ablations performed (0.42%). These are a severe mitral regurgitation, requiring surgical mitral valve plasty, and an acute cardiac tamponade, solved by immediate drainage, both in patients weighing less than 5 kg. Another patient, with a septal accessory pathway developed a complete heart block, well tolerated to date, but probably requiring a pacemaker in the near future. Finally, a 10-year-old boy had femoral vein obstruction, requiring catheter repermeabilization of the vessel.

Diagnostic	Weight < 15 kg	Weight > 15 kg	Total
Atrial tachycardia	7 (10.3%)	44 (5.1%)	51
Atrial flutter	4 (5.9%)	5 (0.06%)	9
Atrial fibrillation	0	1 (0.01%)	1
AVNRT	2 (2.9%)	144 (16.5%)	146
WPW	14 (20.5%)	450 (51.6%)	464
AVRT by concealed accessory pathway	22 (32.3%)	178 (20.4%)	200
Coumel type tachycardia	15 (22%)	22 (2.5%)	37
AVRT by Mahaim accessory pathway	0	8 (0.09%)	8
Ventricular tachycardia	3 (4.4%)	16 (1.8%)	19
Junctional ectopic tachycardia	1 (1.5%)	0	1
Total	**68**	**868**	**936**

Table 1. Diagnostics by weight (less than 15 kg, and more than 15 kg).
WPW = Wolf-Parkinson-White syndrome; AVRT = atrioventricular reentry tachycardia;
AVNRT = atrioventricular nodal reentry.

	Efficacy	**Recurrence**
WPW	448 (96.5%) Non-efficacy: 67% septal	33 (7.11%) 87% right-sided
AVRT by concealed accessory pathway	192 (96%)	19 (9,5%) 37% right sided 37% perihissian
AVNRT	144 (98.7%)	1 (0.6%)
Coumel type tachycardia	37 (100%)	4 (10.8%)
Ventricular tachycardia	17 (89.4%)	2 (10.5%)
Atrial tachycardia	47 (92.2%)	5 (9.8%)

Table 2. Efficacy and recurrence rates by diagnostic. Note that 67% of inefficacy in WPW is in septal accessory pathways, and 87% of recurrence are in right-sided accessory pathways.
WPW = Wolf-Parkinson-White syndrome; AVRT = atrioventricular reentry tachycardia;
AVNRT = atrioventricular nodal reentry tachycardia.

Accessory pathway localization	**WPW**	**AVRT concealed accessory pathway**
Left lateral	35.3%	44.3%
Left septal	6.0%	6.3%
Right lateral	22.2%	5.7%
Right septal	3.4%	14.6%
Right anterior	12.0%	10.1%
Perihissian	13.5%	12.7%
Multiples	7.6%	6.3%

Table 3. Localization of accessory pathways.
WPW = Wolf-Parkinson-White syndrome; AVRT = artioventricualr reentry tachycardia.

Conclusions

Radiofrequency ablation using a simplified catheter technique can be performed successfully and safely in children, even in infants. This technique allows short procedural and radiation exposure times, and low complications.

References

1. Scherlag BJ, Lau SH, Helfant RH, *et al.* Catheter technique for recording his bundle activity in man. Circulation 1969; 39: 13-18.

2. Bromberg BI, Dick M, 2nd, Scott WA, *et al.* Transcatheter electrical ablation of accessory pathways in children. Pacing Clin Electrophysiol 1989; 12: 1787-1796.

3. Kugler JD, Danford DA, Deal BJ, *et al.* Radiofrequency catheter ablation for tachyarrhythmias in children and adolescents. The pediatric electrophysiology society. N Engl J Med 1994; 330: 1481-1487.

4. Kugler JD, Danford DA, Houston K, *et al.* Radiofrequency catheter ablation for paroxysmal supraventricular tachycardia in children and adolescents without structural heart disease. Pediatric EP society, radiofrequency catheter ablation registry. Am J Cardiol 1997; 80: 1438-1443.

5. Kugler JD, Danford DA, Houston KA, *et al.* Pediatric radiofrequency catheter ablation registry success, fluoroscopy time, and complication rate for supraventricular tachycardia: Comparison of early and recent eras. J Cardiovasc Electrophysiol 2002; 13: 336-341.

6. Kantoch MJ. Supraventricular tachycardia in children. Indian J Pediatr 2005; 72: 609-619.

7. Wigle DT, Arbuckle TE, Walker M, *et al.* Environmental hazards: Evidence for effects on child health. J Toxicol Environ Health B Crit Rev 2007; 10: 3-39.

8. Perisinakis K, Damilakis J, Theocharopoulos N, *et al.* Accurate assessment of patient effective radiation dose and associated detriment risk from radiofrequency catheter ablation procedures. Circulation 2001; 104: 58-62.

9. Kovoor P, Ricciardello M, Collins L, *et al.* Risk to patients from radiation associated with radiofrequency ablation for supraventricular tachycardia. Circulation 1998; 98: 1534-1540

10. Cohen M. Are we doing enough to minimize fluoroscopic radiation exposure in children? Pediatr Radiol 2007; 37: 1020-1024

11. Chetaille P, Walsh EP, Triedman JK. Outcomes of radiofrequency catheter ablation of atrioventricular reciprocating tachycardia in patients with congenital heart disease. Heart Rhythm 2004; 1: 168-173.

12. Hebe J, Hansen P, Ouyang F, *et al.* Radiofrequency catheter ablation of tachycardia in patients with congenital heart disease. Pediatr Cardiol 2000; 21: 557-575.

13. Etheridge SP, Judd VE. Supraventricular tachycardia in infancy: Evaluation, management, and follow-up. Arch Pediatr Adolesc Med 1999; 153: 267-271.

14. Perry JC, Garson A, Jr. Supraventricular tachycardia due to Wolff-Parkinson-White syndrome in children: Early disappearance and late recurrence. J Am Coll Cardiol 1990; 16: 1215-1220.

15. Lundberg A. Paroxysmal atrial tachycardia in infancy: Long-term follow-up study of 49 subjects. Pediatrics 1982; 70: 638-642.

16. Nadas AS, Daeschner CW, Roth A, *et al.* Paroxysmal tachycardia in infants and children; study of 41 cases. Pediatrics 1952; 9: 167-181.

17. Mantakas ME, McCue CM, Miller WW. Natural history of Wolff-parkinson-white syndrome discovered in infancy. Am J Cardiol 1978; 41: 1097-1103.

18. Flensted-Jensen E. Wolff-Parkinson-White syndrome. A long-term follow-up of 47 cases. Acta Med Scand 1969; 186: 65-74.

19. Deal BJ, Keane JF, Gillette PC, *et al.* Wolff-Parkinson-White syndrome and supraventricular tachycardia during infancy: Management and follow-up. J Am Coll Cardiol 1985; 5: 130-135.

20. Munger TM, Packer DL, Hammill SC, *et al.* A population study of the natural history of Wolff-Parkinson-White syndrome in Olmsted County, Minnesota, 1953-1989. Circulation 1993; 87: 866-873.

21. Bromberg BI, Lindsay BD, Cain ME, *et al.* Impact of clinical history and electrophysiologic characterization of accessory pathways on management strategies to reduce sudden death among children with Wolff-Parkinson-White syndrome. J Am Coll Cardiol 1996; 27: 690-695.

22. Pappone C, Manguso F, Santinelli R, *et al.* Radiofrequency ablation in children with asymptomatic Wolff-Parkinson-White syndrome. N Engl J Med 2004; 351: 1197-1205.

23. Coumel P, Attuel P, Motte G, Slama R, Bouvrain Y. [paroxysmal junctional tachycardia. Determination of the inferior point of junction of the reentry circuit. Dissociation of the intra-nodal reciprocal rhythms] Arch Mal Coeur Vaiss. 1975; 68: 1255-1268 (in french).

24. Crosson JE, Hesslein PS, Thilenius OG, *et al.* Av node reentry tachycardia in infants. Pacing Clin Electrophysiol 1995; 18: 2144-2149.

25. Ko JK, Deal BJ, Strasburger JF, *et al.* Supraventricular tachycardia mechanisms and their age distribution in pediatric patients. Am J Cardiol 1992; 69: 1028-1032.

26. Koike K, Hesslein PS, Finlay CD, *et al.* Atrial automatic tachycardia in children. Am J Cardiol 1988; 61: 1127-1130.

27. Mehta AV, Sanchez GR, Sacks EJ, *et al.* Ectopic automatic atrial tachycardia in children: Clinical characteristics, management and follow-up. J Am Coll Cardiol 1988; 11: 379-385.

28. Naheed ZJ, Strasburger JF, Benson DW, *et al.* Natural history and management strategies of automatic atrial tachycardia in children. Am J Cardiol 1995; 75: 405-407.

29. Klersy C, Chimienti M, Marangoni E, *et al.* Factors that predict spontaneous remission of ectopic atrial tachycardia. Eur Heart J 1993; 14: 1654-1656.

30. Mendelsohn A, Dick M, 2nd, Serwer GA. Natural history of isolated atrial flutter in infancy. J Pediatr 1991; 119: 386-391.

31. Collins KK, Van Hare GF, Kertesz NJ, *et al.* Pediatric nonpost-operative junctional ectopic tachycardia medical management and interventional therapies. J Am Coll Cardiol 2009; 53: 690-697.

32. Villain E, Vetter VL, Garcia JM, *et al.* Evolving concepts in the management of congenital junctional ectopic tachycardia. A multicenter study. Circulation 1990; 81: 1544-1549.

33. Iwamoto M, Niimura I, Shibata T, *et al.* Long-term course and clinical characteristics of ventricular tachycardia detected in children by school-based heart disease screening. Circ J 2005; 69: 273-276.

34. Tsuji A, Nagashima M, Hasegawa S, *et al.* Long-term follow-up of idiopathic ventricular arrhythmias in otherwise normal children. Jpn Circ J 1995; 59: 654-662.

35. Boersma L, Garcia-Moran E, Mont L, *et al.* Accessory pathway localization by QRS polarity in children with Wolff-Parkinson-White syndrome. J Cardiovasc Electrophysiol 2002; 13: 1222-1226.

Chapter 15. Long QT syndrome and catecholaminergic VT. A wise and sensitive approach to the patient and family

M. CERRONE,[1] S. YAGHOUBIAN,[1] S. G. PRIORI[1-3]

[1] Cardiovascular Genetics Program
Leon H. Charney Division of Cardiology
New York University School of Medicine
New York, USA

[2] Molecular Cardiology Laboratories
Fondazione S. Maugeri IRCCS
Pavia, Italy

[3] Department of Cardiology
Universita' degli Studi di Pavia
Pavia, Italy

Address for correspondence:
Molecular Cardiology Laboratories
Fondazione S. Maugeri IRCCS
Dr. Silvia G. Priori
silvia.priori@fsm.it

Introduction

The term "inherited arrhythmogenic disease" refers to a genetic cardiac disorder characterized by altered cardiac excitability often in the absence of structural cardiac involvement. The groundbreaking discoveries starting from the 1990s until the beginning of the current decade gathered the fundamental knowledge on the major genes causing these conditions. Stems of such knowledge are the availability of genetic diagnosis, genotype-phenotype correlation and genotype-based risk stratification schemes that are currently used in clinical practice. Among genetic arrhythmias, the long QT syndrome (LQTS) and the catecholaminergic polymorphic ventricular tachycardia (CPVT) are two conditions in which data derived from experimental research achieved a major contribution that penetrates current clinical practice. In this chapter we will review the clinical and genetic features of these diseases, with emphasis on translational science and new frontiers in patients' counseling.

1   The long QT syndrome

1.1   *Clinical presentation*

The LQTS is an inherited arrhythmogenic disease in the structurally normal heart characterized by prolonged QT interval and T-wave anomalies. The estimated prevalence is between 1:7,000 and 1:3,000 but this value may be affected by its incomplete prevalence and/or misdiagnosis.[1]

Symptoms are syncope and cardiac arrest typically occurring in situations of increased adrenergic tone. However, in 10-15% of patients, cardiac events occur at rest.[2] Syncope is often triggered by the onset of rapid polymorphic ventricular tachycardia (VT) (torsades de pointes) (see figure 1) that can degenerate into ventricular fibrillation (VF) and cause sudden death. Both the risk and the triggers for events are modulated by the genotype.[2,3] The mean age of onset of symptoms is 12 years, and earlier onset is usually associated with a more severe form of the disease.[4]

Generally, the first and most effective therapeutic approach for all forms is beta-blockers at a high dosage. In the presence of recurrences in therapy or in high-risk patients the implant of an ICD should be considered.[4]

Several non-cardiac medications have an effect on the duration of the repolarisation phase, by blocking one of the ionic channels involved in LQTS; therefore, all patients, independently of their specific genotype, should avoid all these agents.

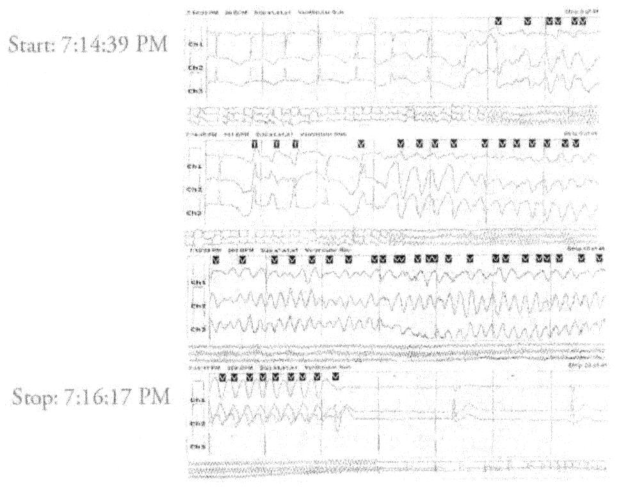

Figure 1. ECG Holter recording of torsade de pointes in a LQTS patient showing QTc >500 msec.

1.2   The ECG in LQTS

The diagnosis of LQTS is based on the evaluation of the ECG and on the measurement of the QT interval. Corrected QT interval (QTc) values >440 msec (in males) and >460 msec (in females after puberty) are considered abnormal. Albeit QTc assessment is the most important step for diagnosis of LQTS, ST-T wave abnormalities are often evident and can support the clinical diagnosis.[5,6] The evaluation of QT interval in the context of the diagnostic approach is not always straightforward. A careful selection of representative traces and several measurements at different values of heart rate should be performed and one should always select traces in which RR intervals are constant for at least 10-20 beats to avoid under- or overestimation. The evidence that in most affected individuals QTc interval fails to shorten when heart rate increases, leading to further QTc prolongation during tachycardia, emphasizes the need for a complete set of ECG recordings, including stress test and ECG Holter.

It is also evident that a "gray area" exists where QT values of normally and LQTS subjects overlap. The disease has incomplete penetrance and 10-35% of gene-carriers present a normal QTc interval.[1] However, their identification is important from a clinical standpoint, since at least 10% of them, if left without therapy, experience symptoms before age 40.[3] Accordingly, genetic screening becomes instrumental to integrate clinical evaluation for diagnostic purposes.

In the absence of genetic information, QT interval duration is the most important predictor of cardiac events[3]. This feature has been reproducibly confirmed in several cohorts.[3,7] The evidence of QTc interval >500 ms is associated with a fivefold increased risk of events. Additional risk factors are female sex[3] and the occurrence of a first event in early childhood[4] (see figure 2).

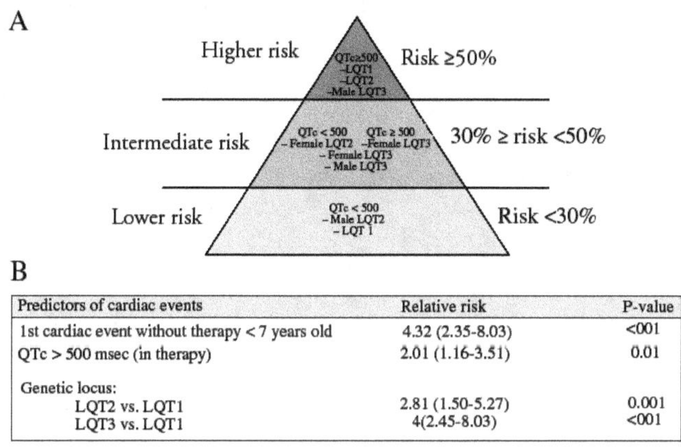

B

Predictors of cardiac events	Relative risk	P-value
1st cardiac event without therapy < 7 years old	4.32 (2.35-8.03)	<001
QTc > 500 msec (in therapy)	2.01 (1.16-3.51)	0.01
Genetic locus:		
LQT2 vs. LQT1	2.81 (1.50-5.27)	0.001
LQT3 vs. LQT1	4(2.45-8.03)	<001

Figure 2A. Risk factors for cardiac events in LQTS.
Figure 2B. Risk indicators of failure of beta-blocker therapy according to genotype in LQTS
(from references 3 and 4).

1.3   Genetic bases

Two patterns of inheritance are known for LQTS. The autosomal dominant variant is caused by mutations on at least 12 different genes (see table 1). The rare autosomal recessive form (Jervell-Lange Nielsen syndrome) presents with neurosensorial deafness associated with the cardiac phenotype (see table 1).

The list of LQTS-related genes is constantly expanding and it has now reached a count of 12[8,9] (see table 1). Despite this remarkable heterogeneity, the three forms (LQT1, LQT2, LQT3) reported in the early studies are still dominating the picture and account for more than 90% of affected patients with an identified mutation.[1,10] Even if mutations on the remaining variants account for only a minority of cases, they had the value of drawing attention to the concept that non-ion channel encoding genes may be associated with the disease. Yet, the concept that LQTS should be considered a channelopathy and that LQTS-related genes ultimately affect ionic currents, either directly (ion channel mutations) or indirectly (chaperones and other modulators), still holds true.

Locus name	Chromosomal locus	Inheritance	Gene symbol	Protein	Mutation effect	Phenotype
LQT1	11p15.5	AD	KCNQ1	IKs potassium channel alpha subunit (KvLQT1)	Loss of function	Long QT
LQT2	7q35-q36	AD	KCNH2	IKr potassium channel alpha subunit (HERG)	Loss of function	Long QT
LQT3	3p21	AD	SCN5A	Cardiac sodium channel alpha subunit (Nav 1.5)	Gain of function	Long QT
LQT4	4q25-q27	AD	ANK2	Ankyrin B, anchoring protein	Loss of function	Long QT, atrial fibrillation
LQT5	21q22.1-q22.2	AD	KCNE1	IKs potassium channel beta subunit (MinK)	Loss of function	Long QT
LQT6	21q22.1-q22.2	AD	KCNE2	IK potassium channel beta subunit (MiRP)	Loss of function	Long QT
AND/LQT7	17q23.1-q24.2	AD	KCNJ2	IK1 potassium channel (Kir2.1)	Loss of function	Long QT, potassium sensitive periodic paralysis, dysmorphic features
TS/LQT8	12p13.3	AD	CACNA1c	Voltage-gated calcium channel, CaV1.2	Gain of function	Long QT, syndactyly, septal defect, patent foramen ovale, mental retardation
LQT9	3p24	AD	Cav3	Caveolin	Gain of function (sodium current)	Long QT
LQT10	11q23.3	AD	SCNb4	Cardiac sodium channel beta subunit (SCN4B)	Gain of function (sodium current)	Long QT
LQT11	7q21-q22	AD	AKAP9	A-kinase-anchoring protein (yotiao)	Reduced IKs due to loss of cAMP sesitivity	Long QT
LQT12	20q11.2	AD	SNTA1	Alpha1-syntrophin	S-nitrosylation of SCN5A causing increased sodium current	Long QT
JLNS1	11p15.5	AR	KCNQ1	IKs potassium channel alpha subunit (KvLQT1)	Loss of function	Long QT, deafness
JLNS2	21q22.1-q22.2	AR	KCNE1	IKs potassium channel beta subunit (MinK)	Loss of function	Long QT, deafness

Table 1. Genetic loci and genes causing long QT syndrome.

The final common consequence of LQTS gene mutations is the disruption of one or more ion currents that generate the cardiac action potential. As a general concept, mutations affecting potassium channels cause a loss of function in the protein that ultimately prolongs the re-polarisation phase of the cardiac action potential, i.e., the QT interval. Mutations affecting the sodium channel or its modulators determine a gain of function, resulting in an excess of sodium entering the cell (see table 1).

Table 1 shows the list of all genes so far associated with the LQTS phenotype, highlighting which proteins and ionic currents are affected and if extracardiac phenotype is present.

The immediate consequence of the identification of the genetic substrate underlying LQTS is the availability of well-characterized genotype-based management for the most frequent forms, while much more blurred is the use of genetic information for the management of the "rare" LQTS variants due to the lack of large study cohorts.

1.4 Genotype-phenotype correlations

In LQTS genotype-phenotype correlation studies have been able to have a major impact and to influence the management of the patients. Gene-specific differences have been described in terms of morphology of the ST-T wave complex,[5,6] triggers[2] and risk for cardiac events.[3,4]

Moss *et al.*[5] and Zhang *et al.*[6] reported how the morphology of the T-wave could differ among LQT1, LQT2 and LQT3 patients and described up to ten distinguished ST-T-wave patterns associated with these LQTS variants. Even if overlap exists and the repolarisation pattern cannot be taken as a substitute for genotyping, it may however play a role to suggest from which variant the screening could be started.

In terms of triggers for cardiac events, LQT1 patients tend to have symptoms during physical activity, especially swimming; auditory stimuli and arousal are specific triggers for LQT2; LQT3 patients experience the majority of cardiac events at rest.[2]

Most importantly, genotype plays a relevant role in determining the risk of events and the response to beta-blocker therapy. Data from our LQTS registry have consistently shown that LQT2 and LQT3 patients have worse long-term prognosis than LQT1 patients. Therefore genotype has entered the risk stratification scheme as independent predictor of events, together with the "traditional" risk factors of QT duration and gender[3] (see figure 2).

LQTS genotype not only influences prognosis but also response to therapy. While beta-blockers are highly effective in LQT1, significantly higher recurrences of fatal arrhythmias are observed among LQT2 and LQT3.[4] Therefore, prophylactic ICD implant may be considered in these LQTS variants when associated with QTc >500ms and early onset of cardiac events (see figure 2).

1.5 Role of genetic test in the clinical management of LQTS patients

Genetic screening is an important diagnostic tool in all inherited arrhythmias. A positive genetic test confirms the diagnosis, allows identification of affected family members and potential silent carriers and could be used in reproductive counseling and prenatal screening.

Additionally, in the specific case of LQTS a positive genetic test (at least for LQT1, LQT2 or LQT3) bears the value of directing clinical management and risk stratification of the patients.

Until few years ago, genetic screening was only performed by few research laboratories. Recently, the availability of commercial tests has increased its accessibility to the medical community. The lack of rules and guidelines for the coverage of the costs of commercial genetic tests has limited the possibility of concretely incorporating it in the clinical practice in several instances. In an attempt to address this issue, our group has recently performed a cost-effectiveness analysis.[11] It emerged that the use of commercial screening in inherited arrhythmias could be reasonable and cost-effective depending on the disease and the clinical presentation. In the case of LQTS, in the presence of "definite" phenotype it reaches a yield of 64% and an average acceptable cost of $8,418 US per positive test. The presence/absence of symptoms is an additional determinant of cost-effectiveness in LQTS ($2,500 US per year of life saved)[11] (see figure 3).

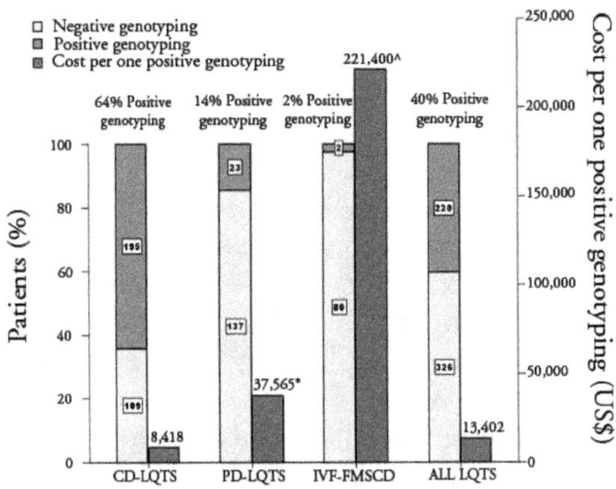

Figure 3. Cost-effectiveness analysis of genetic test in LQTS (from reference 11).
CD = conclusive diagnosis; PD = possible diagnosis; IVF-FMSCD = idiopathic ventricular fibrillation or family history for sudden cardiac death.

2   Catecholaminergic polymorphic ventricular tachycardia

2.1   *Clinical features and therapy*

CPVT is an inherited arrhythmia in the absence of structural cardiac anomalies, characterized by adrenergically mediated syncope or cardiac arrest often leading to sudden cardiac death.[12-15] Baseline ECG is unremarkable with the exception of sinus bradycardia and, occasionally, prominent U-wave.

Often cases of CPVT are misdiagnosed as "LQTS with normal QT interval", due to the association of adrenergic-induced arrhythmias and structurally normal heart. However, differential diagnosis is important in the clinical management because, as opposed to LQTS, CPVT is highly malignant. Available data show that 75-80% of patients experience at least one life-threatening event when younger than 40 years of age when left untreated.[15,16]

The original description of the disease includes a peculiar arrhythmia, the bidirectional VT, characterized by a beat-to-beat 180∞ rotation of the QRS axis (see figure 4). However, patients

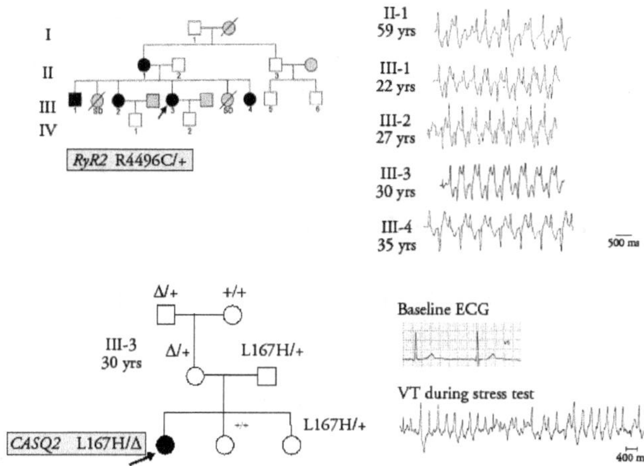

Figure 4. Upper panel: pedigree of a family affected by CPVT carrier of a heterozygous mutation on the RyR2 gene; on the right: exercise-induced bidirectional VT in all mutation carriers; lower panel: pedigree of the only family so far reported in which two CASQ2 mutations inherited in double heterozygosis caused CPVT phenotype; right lower panel: baseline ECG and exercise-induced-polymorphic VT in the proband (from references 13 and 21).

may fail to show bidirectional VT and present instead with polymorphic VT[14] (see figure 4) or idiopathic VF in the case sudden death is the first manifestation of the disease.[14,16] As compared to other inherited arrhythmias, CPVT has higher number of sporadic cases. This can be the consequence of higher mortality at young age that limits the transmission of the disease to the offspring.

The development of arrhythmias during graded exercise is highly reproducible. Isolated ventricular extrasystoles arise at a heart rate of 110-120 bpm, followed by runs of non-sustained VT. If the patients continue to exercise, the VT progressively becomes sustained. Supraventricular arrhythmias preceding the onset of VT are also common.[15] Therefore, exercise stress test represents the most important diagnostic test. ECG Holter monitoring is useful in patients who are more susceptible to emotional stressors and in children, in which it may be difficult to obtain a maximal exercise test.

Beta-blockers are the mainstay of treatment in CPVT[12,14] and the dose should be always titrated with exercise stress testing. Unfortunately a remarkable incidence of recurrences (up to 30%) of cardiac event despite beta-blockers has been reported.[15,16] Thus the implant of ICD remains indicated when sustained VT develops despite maximally tolerated beta-blocker dosage; 42% of patients implanted with an ICD received an appropriate shock at follow-up.[16] Recently a favorable long-term outcome in three patients who underwent left cardiac sympathetic denervation was reported.[17] Even if the surgery alone cannot guarantee a complete protection from sudden death it may be considered an option to prevent the occurrence of arrhythmic storms in patients who already have an ICD.

The discovery of the genetic and arrhythmogenic mechanisms of CPVT opened new possibilities in terms of therapeutic options. Calcium antagonists have been proposed since the earlier descriptions of CPVT. Data on a small cohort of patients suggested that verapamil could be considered an adjunctive treatment in non-responders, but are not yet a possible alternative to beta-blockers.[18]

Preliminary data in two CPVT patients, corroborated by results in animal models, suggested that flecainide might be effective.[19] Even if so far these should only be considered initial reports, they are opening new paths to be explored in the attempt to find novel antiarrhythmic strategies.

2.2   *Genetic bases and arrhythmogenic mechanisms*

Two genetic variants of CPVT have been identified. The autosomal dominant variant is due to mutations in the RyR2 gene, encoding for the cardiac ryanodine receptor[13] (see figure 4). The RyR2 is an intracellular Ca^{2+} release channel spanning the membrane of the sarcoplasmic reticulum and it is required for excitation-contraction coupling. Mutations in this gene account for 55-60% of clinically affected patients.[11]

The autosomal recessive variant is due to mutations of the calsequestrin 2 gene (*CASQ2*)[20] (see figure 4). Calsequestrin is a Ca^{2+} buffering protein. It binds Ca^{2+} ions to control the free Ca^{2+} concentration in the sarcoplasmic reticulum and it is also thought to directly modulate the RyR2 open probability.

At present, CASQ2 mutations account for 3-5% of all genotyped patients.[16] Aside from causing autosomal recessive CPVT, cases of double heterozygosity in non-consanguineous families have been reported[21] (see figure 4).

Several in vitro and in vivo studies helped clarify the mechanisms of arrhythmias in this disease. Overall, the common effect of both RyR2 and CASQ2 mutations is considered to lead to intracellular Ca^{2+} overload and the release of catecholamines during stress could then contribute to accentuating the imbalance in Ca^{2+} homeostasis caused by the genetic mutations.

Bidirectional VT has been described not only in CPVT patients, but also in cases of digitalis intoxication. Arrhythmias in digitalis toxicity are linked to intracellular Ca^{2+} overload that generate DADs-induced triggered activity. These observations suggested that arrhythmias in the setting of CPVT could be induced by the same mechanism. Experimental evidence obtained from animal models confirmed that indeed arrhythmias in CPVT are caused by abnormal propensity to DADs and triggered activity, increased by adrenergic stimulation.[22-24] This mechanism has also been supported by clinical evidence. Paavola *et al.*[25] showed the occurrence of DADs during monophasic action potential recordings in RyR2-CPVT patients.

2.3   *The role of genetic test in the clinical management of CPVT*

Genetic test in the setting of CPVT has a considerable positive yield (up to 70% of individuals with a clear phenotype result to be carriers of a mutation on the RyR2 or CASQ2 gene[11,16]). However, genetic analysis is complicated by the fact that RyR2 is one of the largest genes in the human genome, impacting turnaround time and accessibility. As with other inherited arrhythmias, CPVT involves a high degree of genetic heterogeneity with over 70 mutations reported so far; most of them are "private" mutations isolated to one or few families. Mutation scanning of the open reading frame regions of the gene is the most frequently used approach for mutation detection. Data from different groups showed that most of the CPVT-RYR2 mutations cluster in specific regions of the protein: the *N*-terminal domain (amino acids 77-466), the FKBP12.6 binding domain (amino acids 2246-2534) and the transmembrane/C-terminal domains from amino acid 3.778.[14,15,26] Based on this observation, some laboratories have limited the screening only to these selected regions[26] (61 exons out of the 105 total) and commercial companies have followed on these steps. At variance, preliminary observations from our CPVT cohort (personal communication, Priori SG) show that 12% of RYR2 probands have mutations outside of these clusters. Therefore, targeted exon analysis is likely to have lower detection sensitivity and carry implications in defining a partial test as "negative".

Performance analysis of CPVT genetic screening showed that the cost for one positive test was $9,170 US and it was reduced to $5,263 US in the presence of a clear clinical diagnosis, in which the yield of genetic testing reached 62%[11] (see figure 5).

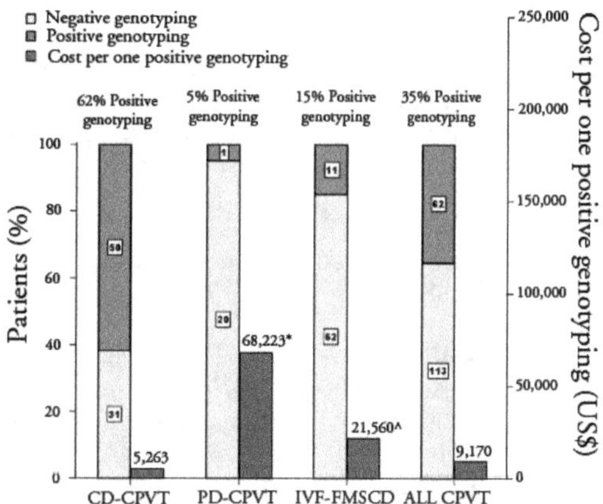

Figure 5. Cost-effectiveness analysis of genetic test in CPVT (from reference 11).
CD = conclusive diagnosis; PD = possible diagnosis; IVF-FMSCD = idiopathic ventricular fibrillation or family history for sudden cardiac death.

Conclusions

Recently, a remarkable body of knowledge derived from basic science allowed clinicians to achieve a better understanding of the substrate of some inherited arrhythmias. Most importantly, epidemiological evidence supports the idea that knowing the type of DNA abnormality is not only a diagnostic tool but it bears prognostic and therapeutic implications. However, the increasing availability of genetic screening has also highlighted the limitations and the complexity of handling genetic information. The detection of a mutation alone is not only a diagnostic tool anymore. Careful phenotyping, the availability of epidemiological data on relatively large series of affected patients and the study of the functional effects of a specific mutation are all factors that contribute to delivering a correct message to the families. All these needs are creating a new area of expertise, cardiovascular genetics, which is able to manage affected patients through the integration of clinical cardiology and insights derived from basic science.

References

1. Napolitano C, Priori SG, Schwartz PJ, *et al.* Genetic testing in the long QT syndrome: development and validation of an efficient approach to genotyping in clinical practice. JAMA 2005; 294(23): 2975-80.

2. Schwartz PJ, Priori SG, Spazzolini C, *et al.* Genotype-phenotype correlation in the long-QT syndrome: gene-specific triggers for life-threatening arrhythmias. Circulation 2001; 103(1): 89-95.

3. Priori SG, Schwartz PJ, Napolitano C, *et al.* Risk stratification in the long-QT syndrome. N Engl J Med 2003; 348(19): 1866-74.

4. Priori SG, Napolitano C, Schwartz PJ, *et al.* Association of long QT syndrome loci and cardiac events among patients treated with beta-blockers. JAMA 2004; 292(11): 1341-4.

5. AJ, Zareba W, Benhorin J, *et al.* ECG T-wave patterns in genetically distinct forms of the hereditary long QT syndrome. Circulation 1995; 92(10): 2929-34.

6. Zhang L, Timothy KW, Vincent GM, *et al.* Spectrum of ST-T-wave patterns and repolarization parameters in congenital long-QT syndrome: ECG findings identify genotypes. Circulation 2000; 102(23): 2849-55.

7. Hobbs JB, Peterson DR, Moss AJ, *et al.* Risk of aborted cardiac arrest or sudden cardiac death during adolescence in the long-QT syndrome. JAMA 2006; 296(10): 1249-54.

8. Lehnart SE, Ackerman MJ, Benson DW, Jr., *et al.* Inherited arrhythmias: a National Heart, Lung, and Blood Institute and Office of Rare Diseases workshop consensus report about the diagnosis, phenotyping, molecular mechanisms, and therapeutic approaches for primary cardiomyopathies of gene mutations affecting ion channel function. Circulation 2007; 116(20): 2325-45.

9. Ueda K, Valdivia C, Medeiros-Domingo A, *et al.* Syntrophin mutation associated with long QT syndrome through activation of the nNOS-SCN5A macromolecular complex. PNAS 2008; 105(27): 9355-60.

10. Splawski I, Shen J, Timothy KW, *et al.* Spectrum of mutations in long-QT syndrome genes. KVLQT1, HERG, SCN5A, KCNE1, and KCNE2. Circulation 2000; 102(10): 1178-85.

11. Rong B, Napolitano C, Bloise R, Monteforte N, Priori S. Yield of genetic screening in inherited cardiac channelopathies: how to prioritize access to genetic testing. Circ Arrhythmia Electrophysiol 2009; 2: 6-15.

12. Leenhardt A, Lucet V, Denjoy I, Grau F, Ngoc DD, Coumel P. Catecholaminergic polymorphic ventricular tachycardia in children. A 7-year follow-up of 21 patients. Circulation 1995; 91(5): 1512-9.

13. Priori SG, Napolitano C, Tiso N, *et al.* Mutations in the cardiac ryanodine receptor gene (hRyR2) underlie catecholaminergic polymorphic ventricular tachycardia. Circulation 2001; 103(2): 196-200.

14. Priori SG, Napolitano C, Memmi M, *et al.* Clinical and molecular characterization of patients with catecholaminergic polymorphic ventricular tachycardia. Circulation 2002; 106(1): 69-74.

15. Hayashi M, Denjoy I, Extramiana F, *et al.* Incidence and risk factors of arrhythmic events in catecholaminergic polymorphic ventricular tachycardia. Circulation 2009; 119(18): 2426-34.

16. Cerrone M, Colombi B, Bloise R, *et al.* Clinical and molecular characterization of a large cohort of patients affected with catecholaminergic polymorphic ventricular tachycardia. Circulation 2004; 110(Suppl): 552.

17. Wilde AA, Bhuiyan ZA, Crotti L, *et al.* Left cardiac sympathetic denervation for catecholaminergic polymorphic ventricular tachycardia. N Engl J Med 2008; 358(19): 2024-9.

18. Rosso R, Kalman JM, Rogowski O, *et al.* Calcium channel blockers and beta-blockers versus beta-blockers alone for preventing exercise-induced arrhythmias in catecholaminergic polymorphic ventricular tachycardia. Heart Rhythm 2007; 4(9): 1149-54.

19. Watanabe H, Chopra N, Laver D, *et al.* Flecainide prevents catecholaminergic polymorphic ventricular tachycardia in mice and humans. Nature Medi 2009;15(4): 380-3.

20. Lahat H, Pras E, Olender T, *et al.* A missense mutation in a highly conserved region of CASQ2 is associated with autosomal recessive catecholamine-induced polymorphic ventricular tachycardia in Bedouin families from Israel. Am J of Hum Genetics 2001; 69(6): 1378-84.

21. di Barletta MR, Viatchenko-Karpinski S, Nori A, *et al.* Clinical phenotype and functional characterization of CASQ2 mutations associated with catecholaminergic polymorphic ventricular tachycardia. Circulation 2006; 114(10): 1012-9.

22. Cerrone M, Noujaim SF, Tolkacheva EG, *et al.* Arrhythmogenic mechanisms in a mouse model of catecholaminergic polymorphic ventricular tachycardia. Circ Res 2007; 101(10): 1039-48.

23. Liu N, Colombi B, Memmi M, *et al.* Arrhythmogenesis in catecholaminergic polymorphic ventricular tachycardia: insights from a RyR2 R4496C knock-in mouse model. Circ Res 2006; 99(3): 292-8.

24. Knollmann BC, Chopra N, Hlaing T, *et al.* Casq2 deletion causes sarcoplasmic reticulum volume increase, premature Ca2+ release, and catecholaminergic polymorphic ventricular tachycardia. J Clin Invest 2006; 116(9): 2510-20.

25. Paavola J, Viitasalo M, Laitinen-Forsblom PJ, *et al.* Mutant ryanodine receptors in catecholaminergic polymorphic ventricular tachycardia generate delayed after depolarizations due to increased propensity to Ca2+ waves. Eur Heart J 2007; 28(9): 1135-42.

26. Medeiros-Domingo A, Bhuiyan ZA, Tester DJ, *et al.* The RYR2-encoded ryanodine receptor/calcium release channel in patients diagnosed previously with either catecholaminergic polymorphic ventricular tachycardia or genotype negative, exercise-induced long QT syndrome: a comprehensive open reading frame mutational analysis. J Am Coll Cardiol 2009; 54(22): 2065-74.

Chapter 16. Risk stratification in hypertrophic cardiomyopathy: who should receive an ICD?

M. Calcagnino, W. J. McKenna

Institute of Cardiovascular Science
and The Heart Hospital
University College London Partners
London, UK

Address for correspondence:
The Heart Hospital
Dr. William J. McKenna
william.mckenna@uclh.nhs.uk

Introduction

Hypertrophic cardiomyopathy (HCM) is an inherited heart muscle disorder which is phenotypically heterogeneous with clinical presentation from infancy to the later decades. HCM is defined clinically by the presence of left ventricular hypertrophy (LVH), typically asymmetric in distribution, in the absence of a detectable cause.[1] The majority of studies suggest that HCM has a prevalence of approximately 1 in 500 adults and disease is recognized in Caucasians, Africans and Asians.[2] Inheritance is usually autosomal dominant with variable clinical penetrance. In adults the majority of cases are familial, caused by a mutation in one of the cardiac sarcomeric protein genes.[3,4] Recent studies indicate that HCM in toddlers and children is also caused by a mutation in the same sarcomeric genes.[3] Approximately 50-70% of adults and 50% of children have a mutation in one of eight genes that encode different components of the cardiac sarcomere: β-myosin heavy chain, cardiac myosin-binding protein C, cardiac troponin T, cardiac troponin I, α-tropomyosin, the essential and regulatory myosin light chains, and cardiac actin.[4,5] Mutations in three other sarcomeric protein genes (titin, troponin C, and α-cardiac myosin heavy chain) have also been reported.[4,6,7]

Other non-sarcomeric gene mutations may cause a HCM (like phenotype): human muscle LIM protein,[8] LAMP-2 (Danon disease)[9] and phospholamban promoter.[10] There are also non-sarcomeric diseases which can cause LVH, such as Anderson-Fabry disease,[11] mitochondrial disease,[12] glycogen storage diseases[13] and a phenotype that includes LVH, Wolff-Parkinson-White syndrome and premature conduction disease, associated with mutations in the gene encoding the Á-subunit of AMP-kinase.[14] In sarcomeric HCM the hypertrophy most commonly affects the interventricular septum, but may involve any myocardial segment, while the histology typically shows myocyte and myofibrillar disarray with increased loose connective tissue. LVH which is truly concentric is more likely to be a phenocopy caused by a storage or mitochondrial disorder with histological features of the specific storage disorder and fibrosis without myocyte disarray.

The clinical course and outcome in HCM varies greatly: some patients may have profound exercise limitation and/or recurrent arrhythmias, whereas the majority has little or no discernible cardiovascular symptoms. The overall risk of disease-related complications such as sudden cardiac death (SCD), advanced heart failure and fatal stroke is approximately 1-2% per year, but the absolute risk in individuals varies as a function of age, underlying genetic abnormality, myocardial histopathology and other pathophysiological abnormalities, such as impaired peripheral vascular responses.[1]

One of the major clinical challenges in HCM is the identification of the small number of patients who are prone to rapid disease progression, serious complications and sudden cardiac death.

1   Characteristics of sudden cardiac death in HCM

Although HCM is the most common cause of sudden death in the young and in young athletes, most contemporary survival studies of HCM cohorts report low annual mortality rates. It also appears that some patient cohorts have very similar overall survival to that of age-matched controls.[15] A recent meta-analysis reveals that survival rates of patients with HCM have improved over the last fifty years, with a reduction in annual sudden cardiac death mortality from ~3% to <1%.[16] Possible explanations for this downward trend include earlier diagnosis, patient selection with a less severe clinical profile, as well as the impact of modern management strategies. Despite these reassuring data, prevention of sudden death in HCM remains a major focus of clinical management. Sudden death can occur throughout life, but there is a peak in incidence during late adolescence and young adulthood, while middle-aged and elderly patients are at increased risk of death from heart failure and stroke.[15,16]

2   Pathophysiology of sudden cardiac death in HCM

Hypertrophic cardiomyopathy can be considered a prototype substrate for ventricular arrhythmia. LVH causes dispersion of repolarization and refractoriness, leading to increased vulnerability of the myocardium to triggered arrhythmias, while myocyte disarray, expansion of the interstitial compartment and replacement fibrosis may create areas of conduction block and predispose to reentry arrhythmia.[17] Furthermore, abnormalities in ion fluxes during cardiomyocyte repolarization may cause after-depolarizations and triggered activity.[18] In adults, myocardial ischemia, maladaptive autonomic responses, diastolic dysfunction and left ventricular outflow tract obstruction contribute to modulate the complex arrhythmogenic substrate in HCM.[19,20]

In patients known to have HCM, sudden cardiac death usually happens during mild exertion or sedentary activities, but it occurs also during or immediately after strenuous exertion.[21] In the past, it was assumed that brief runs of ventricular tachycardia or the sudden onset of atrial fibrillation were the precipitating cause for ventricular fibrillation in the majority of episodes of cardiac arrest, but data obtained from implantable cardioverter-defibrillators (ICD) have shown that ventricular fibrillation in HCM patients often arises directly from sinus rhythm.[22,23] These data illustrate the vulnerability of the myocardium in hypertrophic cardiomyopathy and the powerful influence of other physiological modulators.[24]

3   Risk assessment in HCM

Many clinical features have been associated with an increased risk of sudden cardiac death, but most have only modest positive predictive value[7,25] (see figure 1). The present approach to risk stratification for SCD in HCM (see table 1) relies on non-invasive assessment of a number of clinical features which reflect the severity of the underlying myocardial disease. In the current guidelines,[7] prior cardiac arrest, spontaneous sustained ventricular tachycardia, family history of SCD, abnormal blood pressure response to exercise, maximal wall thickness ≥30 mm, non-sustained ventricular tachycardia on 24-hour ECG, and unexplained syncope are considered "major" risk factors, while myocardial ischemia, specific mutations (for example troponin T), competitive exercise, extensive late gadolinium enhancement in cardiac magnetic resonance imaging, LV outflow tract obstruction and atrial fibrillation are ranked as "possible".

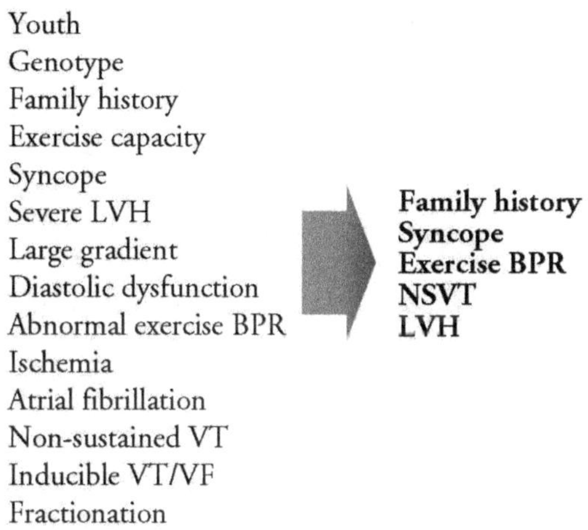

Figure 1. Risk factors in hypertrophic cardiomyopathy.

Risk factors for SCD	
Established	*Possible in individual patients*
• Prior cardiac arrest	• Severe LV outflow tract obstruction
• Spontaneous sustained VT	• Myocardial ischemia
• Unexplained syncope	• Extensive late enhancement on MRI
• Family history of premature SCD	• Specific mutations (troponin T and I)
• LV wall thickness ≥30 mm	• Intense physical exertion
• Abnormal BP response to exercise	• Atrial fibrillation
• Non-sustained ventricular tachycardia	

Table 1. Risk factors for sudden cardiac death.
Adapted from ACC/AHA/ESC guidelines J Am Coll Cardiol 2003; 42: 1687-713.

Nevertheless, with the exception of an aborted cardiac arrest, there is little evidence to suggest that any one single risk factor is more predictive than another.[24] The presence of more than one risk factor, however, does appear to confer greater risk. A cohort in whom risk assessment was performed prospectively had annual sudden death rates of 3-6% with two or more risk factors versus 0.2-1.2% with one or no risk factors[23] (see table 2). Importantly, patients with no risk factors for sudden death had a good prognosis and do not require aggressive primary prevention.[7,25] An ICD registry in which risk assessment was collected retrospectively did not identify this difference perhaps because the most sensitive risk markers in the young (exercise blood pressure response) and adults (24-hour ECG) were not systematically evaluated.[26] Exercise blood pressure response data were excluded from the analysis because data were available in only a minority of patients, while 24-hour ECG data were missing in ~20% of patients.

The management of patients with a single risk factor, however, is more complex: 25% of HCM patients have a single major risk factor, however, only a minority of patients with a single major risk factor will die suddenly (6-year survival rate of 93%).[7,24,25] The clinical challenge is to identify which patients with a single risk factor are at greatest risk for sudden death.

Sudden death and risk markers	
Risk factors	*Sudden death/year*
≥3 (5%)	6% (4-16)
2 (20%)	3% (0.7-5.5)
1 (25%)	1.2% (0.2-2.2)
0 (50%)	0.8% (0.2-1.5)
Cox model – 368 patients	

Table 2. Sudden death and risk markers.
Adapted from Elliott PM et al. JACC 2000; 36: 2212-8.

4 Limitations of current approach to risk stratification

One of the problems in risk evaluation of HCM patients is accurate assessment of the two major aspects of the patient history: a family history of premature and sudden cardiac death and a history of syncope. The interpretation of sudden death in a family has limitations: the cause of death is frequently unknown and may be impossible to determine retrospectively if a postmortem examination was not performed. In some cases, the presence of co-morbidities may add uncertainty. Furthermore, the presence of a single (perhaps unclear) episode of sudden death in a family is unlikely to be comparable in risk to a "malignant family history", with multiple sudden cardiac deaths at a young age.

The assessment of "unexplained" syncope can also be a major challenge. Many potential mechanisms for loss of consciousness need to be considered: peripheral vasodilatation caused by abnormal vascular reflexes, left ventricular outflow tract obstruction and arrhythmia, including supraventricular and ventricular tachycardia as well as bradyarrhythmia caused by conduction disease. The circumstances may provide clues to the potential mechanism (e.g., unheralded syncope during mild exertion or at rest might suggest an arrhythmia as the cause, while repeated episodes during exercise might be caused by provocable left ventricular outflow tract obstruction, ischemia or exertion related mitral regurgitation). It is often difficult to identify retrospectively the mechanism responsible for syncope, even when an extensive clinical assessment is performed. Unpublished data suggest that occult arrhythmia detected by prolonged ECG monitoring (that is paroxysmal atrial fibrillation, conduction disease) are important causes when routine investigations do not reveal abnormalities.

Standard investigations (echocardiography, ambulatory electrocardiographic monitoring and upright exercise testing) provide the other markers of increased sudden death risk. The application of severe LVH ≥30 mm has limitations with respect to accuracy of the wall thickness measurements, as well as the current use of binary ROC generated cutoffs to define risk. LVH may be overestimated by inclusion of a tendon or right ventricular structures in the measurement or by measuring from even mildly off-axis views. The prognostic power of this risk marker is greatest in the young, low in adults and markedly increased by the presence of other risk factors.[27,28] The same problem of accuracy of measurements and the use of ROC generated cutoffs to define risk is present in determining the presence and severity of dynamic left ventricular outflow tract obstruction and the blood pressure response during upright exercise testing. Failure of systolic blood pressure to rise by more than 25 mmHg from baseline is associated with an increased risk of sudden death.[25,29,30] However, many mechanisms may account for this abnormal response: early interruption of the test because of inadequate effort or other co-morbidities, as well as the effect of medications, should be considered when interpreting blood pressure responses to exercise. Furthermore, as to the severity of hypertrophy, the clinical significance of an abnormal blood pressure response during exercise can vary with age, being higher in younger (age 40 years or less) than in older patients.[25] Anecdotal data suggest an increased risk in individuals with an abnormal exercise blood pressure response who carry a troponin T mutation.

Finally, it is well established that the presence of one or more runs of non-sustained ventricular tachycardia (NSVT) at a rate 120 beats/minute during ambulatory electrocardiography is associated with a relative risk for sudden cardiac death of around 2–3.[31,32] Again, age is an important modifier, with a fourfold relative risk in patients younger than 30 years of age.[33] Occasionally, the differentiation between NSVT and aberrancy in patients with paroxysmal atrial fibrillation may also be a problem.

5   ICD in hypertrophic cardiomyopathy

Observational non-randomized series represent the major sources of evidence for most treatments in patients with HCM, partly because of the relative infrequency of the disease in clinical practice. The absence of prospective trials in hypertrophic cardiomyopathy has become particularly relevant since the development of the implantable cardioverter-defibrillator. While in patients with heart failure due to coronary artery disease and dilated cardiomyopathy large randomized trials have shown that the ICD improves survival (compared to antiarrhythmic drugs, such as amiodarone), in patients with HCM similar comparative data are not available.

Amiodarone has been shown useful in prevention of sudden death in some non-randomized studies,[21,34] while other studies have suggested symptomatic improvement but have not shown reduced mortality.[35,36]

Data from multicenter studies report a ~10% per year ICD appropriate intervention rate for ventricular fibrillation or rapid ventricular tachycardia in patients with a history of aborted sudden death, and approximately 4% per year in high risk patients without previous cardiac arrest[22,26] (see figure 2). Current guidelines recommend ICD implantation in patients with HCM and a sustained ventricular arrhythmia or prior cardiac arrest (secondary prophylaxis). For primary prophylaxis, ICD is recommended in those patients with multiple risk factors and in selected patients with a single risk factor judged to be at high risk.[37] There is general agreement that the presence of multiple risk factors warrants serious consideration of primary prophylaxis with an ICD, while the absence of risk markers permits reassurance. Management of patients with a single risk factor, however, requires more detailed evaluation of the overall risk profile taking into account the strength of the risk marker, age of the patient and level of risk which is acceptable to the patient/family. The presence of a single risk factor is associated with approximately 1% annual sudden death rate. This may be acceptable in the later decades, but not in the young. In addition, the confidence limits range from 0.2-2.2%, which indicates that risk varies widely and hence the need to refine the risk algorithm in the setting[7,25] (see figure 3). In referral centers, approximately 25% of patients with hypertrophic cardiomyopathy will have one risk factor and therefore the notion that ICD may be justified in patients with a single marker of increased risk raises some important clinical questions. ICDs are often associated with significant lifelong morbidity and limitations in quality of life, particularly in young patients. It is therefore very important to identify those patients with a single risk factor who may be at high risk of sudden death and therefore candidates for an ICD.

How do we identify which patient with a single risk factor is at sufficient risk to warrant an ICD? In this clinical setting, it is particularly important to individualize the management, taking into account the entire clinical spectrum of disease. The presence of other clinical features such as myocardial ischemia, left ventricular outflow tract obstruction, or extensive myocardial scar detected by cardiovascular magnetic resonance imaging (MRI) may favor more aggressive management.

Figure 4 summarizes a potential management approach in patients with a single risk factor. As shown in figure 4A, when assessing a HCM patient who has NSVT on 24-hour ECG, it is

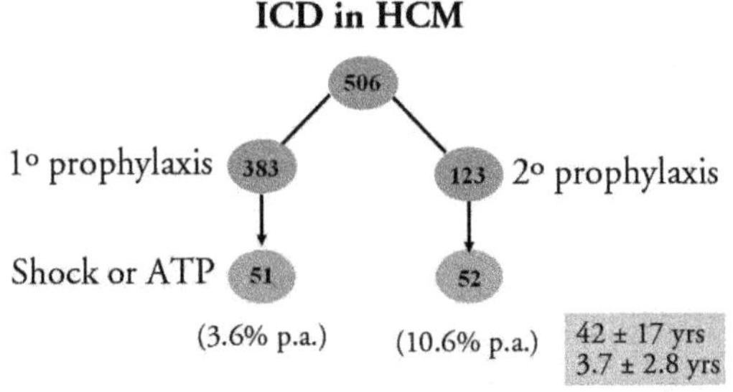

Figure 2. ICD in hypertrophic cardiomyopathy.
Adapted from Maron B et al. JAMA 2007; 298: 405-12.

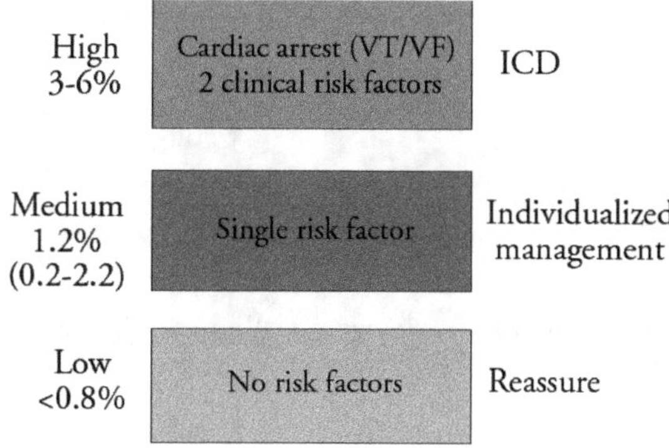

Figure 3. Risk and treatment in hypertrophic cardiomyopathy.

relevant to determine the characteristics (rate, number of beats and association with symptoms)[38] of the NSVT, but age is perhaps more important as it has been shown that the major discriminator is the age of the patient ≤30 years.[33] The recommendation in this context is to have a low threshold for ICD in adolescents and the young, while in older adults it is important to exclude other causes of NSVT (e.g., CAD) and treat them.

With regard to LVH ≥3 cm as a single risk factor (see figure 4B), the suggestion is, in the first instance, to ensure the accuracy of measurements, consider if the severe hypertrophy is localised or diffuse and to repeat assessment of established (24-hour ECG, exercise blood pressure response) and potential risk factors such as LV obstruction, ischemia and late enhancement on MRI. Young age, extensive distribution of LVH and additional (conventional or not) risk factors are in favor of ICD implantation, while older age and localized distribution allow reassurance; LVH ≥3 cm in isolation is rarely sufficient to warrant an ICD.

For flat or hypotensive exercise blood pressure response, again age is an important discriminator as the risk is highest in patients ≤40 years[25] (see figure 4C). It is fundamental to define the cause of abnormal exercise blood pressure response and exclude inadequate exercise, obstruction, ischemia or mitral regurgitation as possible treatable causes. Abnormal vascular responses, together with troponin T mutation, warrant a careful consideration for ICD in the young.

A family history of SCD as a single risk factor generally raises high anxiety. In this context, it is important to obtain an accurate family tree and to consider that the presence of multiple episodes of SCD occurred at young age ("malignant" families) have a higher positive predictive value compared to a single event or an unclear episode of SCD. The recommendation in both later cases is to periodically repeat the assessment of established and potential risk factors and to maintain a low threshold for ICD in presence of additional risk factors, even if borderline (see figure 4D).

Unexplained syncope as a single risk factor warrants intensive efforts to identify the mechanism of the syncope. Prolonged ECG monitoring (e.g., seven days ECG tape or reveal device) may be required to exclude paroxysmal atrial fibrillation or occult conduction disease, and exercise echocardiogram is useful to exclude exercise-induced ischemia, obstruction or mitral regurgitation, which may be the underlying causes of syncope and may require specific treatment (see figure 4E).

A

Single risk factor: NSVT on 24-h ECG

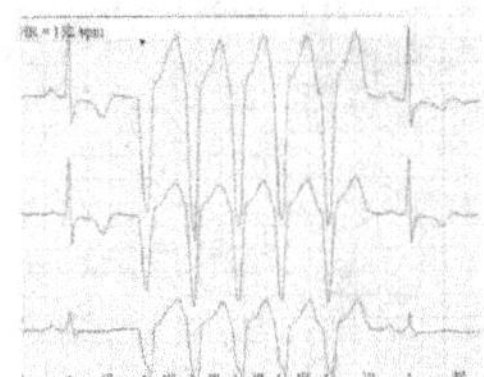

Fast?
Prolonged?
Associated with
symptoms?

Spirito et al., Circulation 1994 Dec; 90(6): 2743-7.

- Major discriminator: age
- Relative risk of SCD highest
  in patients ≤30 years
    Age 15 – relative risk 6
    Age 50 – relative risk 2

<u>Recomendations:</u>
– In adolescent/young → ICD
– In adult/elderly:
  Exclude other causes of NSVT
  (e.g., CAD)
  No treatment, or beta-blockers

Montserrat et al., JACC 2003; 42: 873-9.

B

Single risk factor: severe LVH ≥3 cm

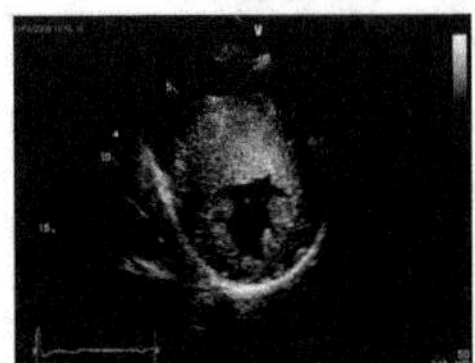

- Ensure accuracy of measurements
- Check distribution of LVH
  (diffuse versus localized)
- Repeat assessment of established and
  potential risk factors (e.g., LVOTO, late
  enhancement on MRI, ischemia)

ICS

Pros
- Extensive distribution
- Young age
- Additional risk factors

Cons
- Localized distribution
- Adult/older age
- LVH ≥3 cm alone is insufficient
  to warrant an ICD

Spirito P et al., N Engl J Med 2000; 342: 1778-85
Elliott PM et al., Lancet 2001; 357: 420-4

C

Single risk factor: abnormal exercise BP response

Flat of hypotensive BPR, risk highest in patients ≤40 years:
    Age 15 – relative risk 2-3
    Age 50 – relative risk < 2

Define cause of abnormal BPR

– Inadequate exercise
– Obstruction
– Ischemia
– MR

– Abnormal vascular responses
  +
– Troponim T mutation

Treat the specific problem   **Consider ICD**

Data from Elliott PM, J Am Coll Cardiol 2000; 36: 2212-8.

*Figure 4. Approaches to the patient with single risk factor: individualization
of risk assessment (continues on next page).*

D

Single risk factor: family history of sudden cardiac death

- High anxiety
- Risk heterogeneous even within "malignant" families

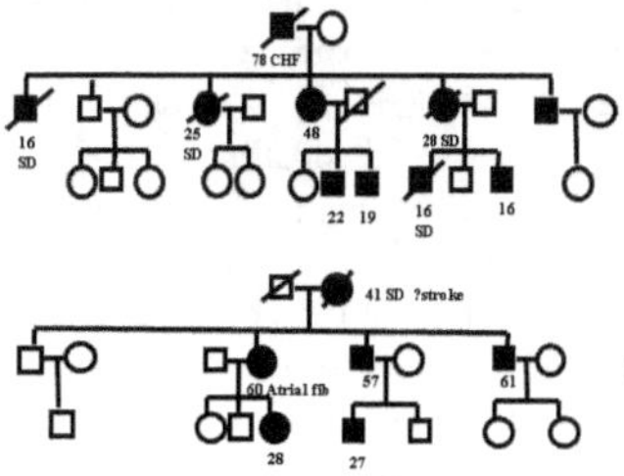

Multiple SD in young age
positive predictive value
\>15%

Single SD (?)
positive predictive value
<10%

<u>**Recommendations:**</u>

- Repeat risk assessment
- Low threshold for ICD if borderline/additional risk factors

E

Single risk factor: unexplained syncope

Key: careful evaluation of circumstances of syncope

Try to identify mechanism of syncope

<u>Prolonged ECG monitoring</u>
to exclude:

<u>Exercise echocardiogram</u>
to exclude:

Paroxysmal atrial fibrillation

Exercise-induced obstruction

Occult conduction disease

Exercise-induced ischemia

Exercise-induced MR

<u>Treat the specific mechanism(s)</u>

Figure 4. Approaches to the patient with single risk factor: individualization of risk assessment.

Conclusion

In the evaluation of the hypertrophic cardiomyopathy patient for sudden death risk, the absence of conventional risk factors accurately identifies the low risk cohort, while the presence of multiple risk factors identifies the high risk cohort.

The presence of a single risk factor identifies individuals at increased risk who warrant careful consideration for ICD.

Though adequate prospective data is lacking, mutation analysis and extensive myocardial scarring detected by cardiovascular magnetic resonance imaging may contribute to the risk profile.

References

1. Elliott P, McKenna WJ. Hypertrophic cardiomyopathy. Lancet 2004; 363: 1881-91.

2. Elliott P, Andersson B, Arbustini E *et al*. Classification of the cardiomyopathies: a position statement from the European Society of Cardiology Working Group on Myocardial and Pericardial Diseases. Eur Heart J 2008; 29: 270-76.

3. Morita H, Rehm HL, Menesses A *et al*. Shared genetic causes of cardiac hypertrophy in children and adults. N Engl J Med 2008; 358: 1899-908.

4. Seidman JG, Seidman C. The genetic basis for cardiomyopathy: from mutation identification to mechanistic paradigms. Cell 2001; 104: 557-67.

5. Richard P, Charron P, Carrier L *et al*. Hypertrophic cardiomyopathy: distribution of disease genes, spectrum of mutations, and implications for a molecular diagnosis strategy. Circulation 2003; 107: 2227-232.

6. Sanbe A, Nelson D, Gulick J *et al*. In vivo analysis of an essential myosin light chain mutation linked to familial hypertrophic cardiomyopathy. Circ Res 2000; 87: 296-302.

7. Maron BJ, McKenna WJ, Danielson GK *et al*. American College of Cardiology/European Society of Cardiology Clinical Expert Consensus Document on Hypertrophic Cardiomyopathy. A report of the American College of Cardiology Foundation Task Force on Clinical Expert Consensus Documents and the European Society of Cardiology Committee for Practice Guidelines. Eur Heart J 2003; 24: 1965-991.

8. Geier C, Perrot A, Ozcelik C *et al*. Mutations in the human muscle LIM protein gene in families with hypertrophic cardiomyopathy. Circulation 2003; 107: 1390-5.

9. Charron P, Villard E, Sebillon P *et al*. Danon's disease as a cause of hypertrophic cardiomyopathy: a systematic survey. Heart 2004; 90: 842-6.

10. Minamisawa S, Sato Y, Tatsuguchi Y *et al*. Mutation of the phospholamban promoter associated with hypertrophic cardiomyopathy. Biochem Biophys Res Commun 2003; 304: 1-4.

11. Sachdev B, Takenaka T, Teraguchi H *et al*. Prevalence of Anderson-Fabry disease in male patients with late onset hypertrophic cardiomyopathy. Circulation 2002; 105: 1407-11.

12. DiMauro S, Schon EA. Mitochondrial respiratory-chain diseases. N Engl J Med 2003; 348: 2656-68.

13. Arad M, Maron BJ, Gorham JM *et al*. Glycogen storage diseases presenting as hypertrophic cardiomyopathy. N Engl J Med 2005; 352: 362-72.

14. Blair E, Redwood C, Ashrafian H *et al*. Mutations in the gamma (2) subunit of AMP-activated protein kinase cause familial hypertrophic cardiomyopathy: evidence for the central role of energy compromise in disease pathogenesis. Hum Mol Genet 2001; 10: 1215-20.

15. Maron BJ, Casey SA, Poliac LC *et al*. Clinical course of hypertrophic cardiomyopathy in a regional United States cohort. JAMA 1999; 281: 650-55.

16. Elliott PM, Gimeno JR, Thaman R *et al*. Historical trends in reported survival rates in patients with hypertrophic cardiomyopathy. Heart 2006; 92: 785-91.

17. Hughes SE. The pathology of hypertrophic cardiomyopathy. Histopathology 2004; 44: 412-27.

18. Tsoutsman T, Lam L, Semsarian C. Genes, calcium and modifying factors in hypertrophic cardiomyopathy. Clin Exp Pharmacol Physiol 2006; 33: 139-45.

19. Counihan PJ, Fei L, Bashir Y *et al*. Assessment of heart rate variability in hypertrophic cardiomyopathy. Association with clinical and prognostic features. Circulation 1993; 88: 1682-90.

20. Cecchi F, Olivotto I, Gistri R *et al*. Coronary microvascular dysfunction and prognosis in hypertrophic cardiomyopathy. N Engl J Med 2003; 349: 1027-35.

21. Maron BJ, Roberts WC, Epstein SE. Sudden death in hypertrophic cardiomyopathy: a profile of 78 patients. Circulation 1982; 65: 1388-94.

22. Maron BJ, Shen WK, Link MS *et al*. Efficacy of implantable cardioverter-defibrillators for the prevention of sudden death in patients with hypertrophic cardiomyopathy. N Engl J Med 2000; 342: 365-73.

23. Woo A, Monakier D, Harris L, *et al*. Determinants of implantable defibrillator discharges in high-risk patients with hypertrophic cardiomyopathy. Heart 2007; 93: 1044-5.

24. Elliott P, Spirito P. Prevention of hypertrophic cardiomyopathy-related deaths: theory and practice. Heart 2008; 94: 1269-75.

25. Elliott PM, Poloniecki J, Dickie S *et al*. Sudden death in hypertrophic cardiomyopathy: identification of high risk patients. J Am Coll Cardiol 2000; 36: 2212-8.

26. Maron BJ, Spirito P, Shen WK *et al*. Implantable cardioverter-defibrillators and prevention of sudden cardiac death in hypertrophic cardiomyopathy. JAMA 2007; 298: 405-12.

27. Spirito P, Bellone P, Harris KM *et al*. Magnitude of left ventricular hypertrophy and risk of sudden death in hypertrophic cardiomyopathy. N Engl J Med 2000; 342: 1778-85.

28. Elliott PM, Gimeno B, Jr., Mahon NG *et al*. Relation between severity of left-ventricular hypertrophy and prognosis in patients with hypertrophic cardiomyopathy. Lancet 2001; 357: 420-4.

29. Sadoul N, Prasad K, Elliott PM *et al*. Prospective prognostic assessment of blood pressure response during exercise in patients with hypertrophic cardiomyopathy. Circulation 1997; 96: 2987-91.

30. Olivotto I, Maron BJ, Montereggi A *et al*. Prognostic value of systemic blood pressure response during exercise in a community-based patient population with hypertrophic cardiomyopathy. J Am Coll Cardiol 1999; 33: 2044-51.

31. McKenna WJ, Oakley CM, Krikler DM *et al*. Improved survival with amiodarone in patients with hypertrophic cardiomyopathy and ventricular tachycardia. Br Heart J 1985; 53: 412-16.

32. Adabag AS, Casey SA, Kuskowski MA *et al*. Spectrum and prognostic significance of arrhythmias on ambulatory

Holter electrocardiogram in hypertrophic cardiomyopathy. J Am Coll Cardiol 2005; 45: 697-704.

33. Monserrat L, Elliott PM, Gimeno JR *et al.* Non-sustained ventricular tachycardia in hypertrophic cardiomyopathy: an independent marker of sudden death risk in young patients. J Am Coll Cardiol 2003; 42: 873-79.

34. McKenna WJ, Harris L, Rowland E *et al.* Amiodarone for long-term management of patients with hypertrophic cardiomyopathy. Am J Cardiol 1984; 54: 802-10.

35. Gilligan DM, Missouris CG, Boyd MJ *et al.* Sudden death due to ventricular tachycardia during amiodarone therapy in familial hypertrophic cardiomyopathy. Am J Cardiol 1991; 68: 971-3.

36. Fananapazir L, Leon MB, Bonow RO *et al.* Sudden death during empiric amiodarone therapy in symptomatic hypertrophic cardiomyopathy. Am J Cardiol 1991; 67: 169-74.

37. Zipes DP, Camm AJ, Borggrefe M *et al.* ACC/AHA/ESC 2006 guidelines for management of patients with ventricular arrhythmias and the prevention of sudden cardiac death—executive summary: A report of the American College of Cardiology/American Heart Association Task Force and the European Society of Cardiology Committee for Practice Guidelines (Writing Committee to Develop Guidelines for Management of Patients with Ventricular Arrhythmias and the Prevention of Sudden Cardiac Death) Developed in collaboration with the European Heart Rhythm Association and the Heart Rhythm Society. Eur Heart J 2006; 27: 2099-140.

38. Spirito P, Rapezzi C, Autore C, *et al.*, Prognosis of asymptomatic patients with hypertrophic cardiomyopathy and nonsustained ventricular tachycardia. Circulation 1994; 90(6): 2743-7.

Chapter 17. Diagnosis and therapy in Brugada syndrome: how to transform complex questions into simple answers

O. Campuzano,[1] B. Benito,[2] A. Iglesias,[1] P. Brugada,[3] J. Brugada,[4] R. Brugada[1]

[1]Cardiovascular Genetics Center
Universitat de Girona
Girona, Spain

[2]Montreal Heart Institute
Montreal, Canada

[3]Thorax Institute
Hospital Clínic of Barcelona
Barcelona, Spain

[4]Heart Rhythm Management Centre
UZ Brussels, VUB
Brussels, Belgium

Address for correspondence:
University of Girona
Cardiovascular Genetics Center UdG-IDIBGI
Dr. Ramon Brugada
ramon@brugada.org

Introduction

The Brugada syndrome (BrS) was published in 1992 as a new disorder characterized by a typical electrocardiogram pattern (right bundle branch block and persistent ST-segment elevation in right precordial leads) causing unexpected sudden cardiac death (SCD).[1] The original publication was followed up by several publications which focused on the clinical characteristics,[2-8] genetics, molecular basis and cellular etiology of the disease.[9-13] Major advances in clinical and mechanistic knowledge have provided very valuable information about the disease, but remaining questions still generate important research activity on the subject.

1 Clinical criteria

The BrS is an inherited rare genetic disease with an autosomal dominant pattern of transmission. To date, 4-12% of total sudden death (SD) cases and 20% of SD in patients with structurally normal hearts can be attributed to BrS. Arrhythmias in Brugada syndrome are mainly due to polymorphic ventricular tachycardia (PVT) or ventricular fibrillation (VF).[5,8]

1.1 The electrocardiogram

The BrS is diagnosed by the presence of ST-segment elevation in the right precordial leads (V1-V3) of the electrocardiogram (ECG). The diagnosis of BrS is based on this electrocardiographic criteria, but it may be difficult to detect because of incomplete penetrance. In spite of the disease being originally described as "persistent ST elevation with right bundle branch block (RBBB)", persistency is no longer necessary for its diagnosis, and further patient recruitment has shown that it may present without RBBB.[1,5]

In the meeting to define the ECG criteria for the BrS diagnosis, three repolarization patterns were described:[14] *a)* type-1 ECG pattern, in which a coved ST-segment elevation ≥2 mm is followed by a negative T-wave, with little or no isoelectric separation, this feature being present in >1 right precordial leads (from V1 to V3); *b)* type-2 ECG pattern, also characterized by an ST-segment elevation but followed by a positive or biphasic T-wave that results in a saddle back configuration; *c)* type-3 ECG pattern, a right precordial ST-segment elevation ≤1mm, either with a coved-type or a saddle-back morphology.

Although all the three ECG patterns have been described in BrS, only type 1 is accepted as a diagnostic ECG (BrS type 1) (see figure 1). Therefore, at present, the BrS can be only definitely diagnosed when a type-1 ECG pattern is observed in >1 right precordial lead (V1 to V3), in conjunction with one of the following: documented VF, PVT, a family history of SD at <45 years old, the presence of coved-type ECG in family members, inducibility of ventricular arrhythmias with programmed electrical stimulation, syncope, or nocturnal agonal respiration.[15] This pattern may be spontaneously evident or it may be induced by a provocative pharmaco-

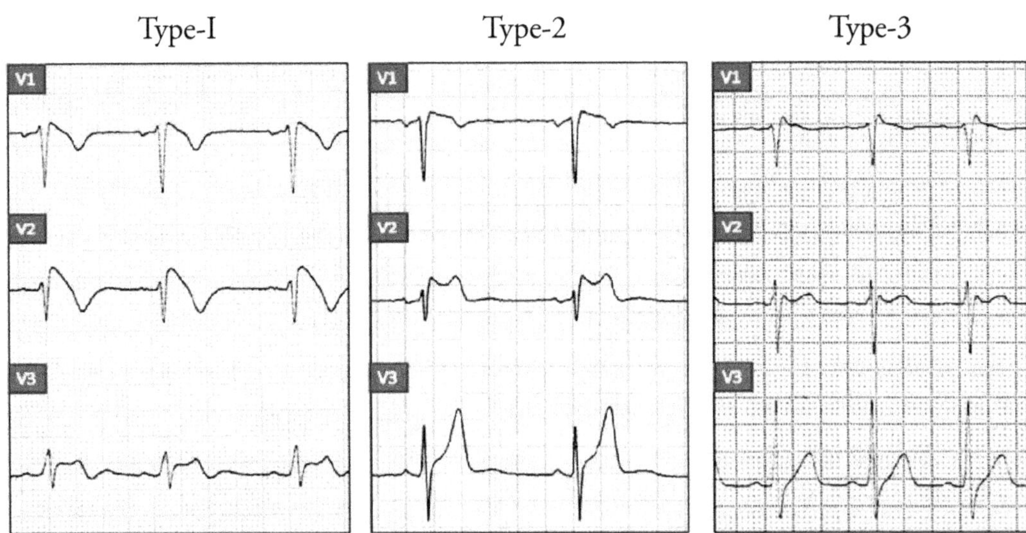

Figure 1. Three different ECG patterns in right precordial leads frequently observed in patients with BrS. Type-1 or otherwise called coved-type ECG pattern, in which a descendant ST-segment elevation is followed by negative T-waves. Type-2 or saddle-back pattern, an ST-segment elevation followed by positive or biphasic T-waves. Type-3, either a coved-type or saddle-back morphology with ST-segment elevation < 1 mm. A type-1 ECG pattern is required to establish the definite diagnosis of BrS.

logical test with intravenous application of sodium channel blockers (ajmaline or flecainide).[16] Note that patients displaying the characteristic type-1 ECG without further clinical criteria should be referred as having an idiopathic Brugada ECG pattern and not a BrS.[14]

1.2 Prevalence

The prevalence of BrS is difficult to estimate because the pattern is not always recognized or because it may transiently normalize. Nevertheless, it is believed to be in the range of 1 to 5 in every 10,000,[15] although this rate should be taken cautiously, first, because many patients present concealed forms of the disease, thus making it likely that the real prevalence is higher, and second, because important ethnic and geographic differences have been described. For example, whereas in a Japanese study, a type-1 ECG pattern was observed in 12 of 10,000 inhabitants,[17] the few available data on North American and European populations point to a much lower prevalence.[18,19] Its prevalence is higher in Southeast Asia where it has long been recognized as the so-called sudden unexplained death syndrome (SUDS), also known as Bangungut (in Philippines), Pokkuri (in Japan) or Lai Tai (in Thailand), which today are known to be phenotypically, genetically and functionally the same disorder as the BrS.[20] SUDS is considered to be endemic in these countries and one of the leading causes of death in males <50 years.[21]

The disease is more common in males than in females (8:1), especially in Southeast Asia. The average age of diagnosis is usually around age 40, however, there have been descriptions of affected individuals who range in age from 1 to 84. BrS has even been described as responsible for sudden infant death syndrome (SIDS).[22] Cardiac events typically occur at rest, during sleep. Some episodes of syncope or SCD may be triggered by hyperpyrexia, large meals (even leading to the suggestion of a "full stomach test" as a diagnostic test in the BrS), cocaine, excessive alcohol consumption and sodium blockers.[23-25] In some of these induced cases a genetic predisposition has been identified.[26]

2 Genetics

Inheritance in the BrS occurs via an autosomal dominant pattern of transmission and variable penetrance.[20] In up to 60% of patients the disease can be sporadic, that is, absent in parents and other relatives.[27] The BrS was classified as genetically determined with the identification in 1998 of the first mutations in *SCN5A*, which encodes the alpha subunit of the cardiac voltage-gated sodium channel Nav1.5, depolarizing current responsible for inward sodium, I_{Na}.[9] On average 15-30% of cases of BrS can be attributed to mutations in *SCN5A*.[15,28] Since then, many BrS-associated mutations have been described in *SCN5A*. Functional studies performed with expression systems have demonstrated, for most of the mutations, a loss of function of the sodium-channel current (I_{Na}), which is achieved either through a quantitative decrease in the sodium channels due to a failure in their expression or through a qualitative dysfunction of the sodium channels due to impaired kinetics (a shift in the voltage- and time-dependent activation, inactivation or reactivation; an entry into an intermediate state of inactivation; or an accelerated inactivation).[9,12,13,20,27,29-31]

Four distinct loss-of-function mechanisms were suggested in BrS mutant *SCN5A* channels: *1)* the mutation results in non-functional channels and thus in haploinsufficiency. A reduced Na^+ current can either result from a single point mutation or from two heterozygous mutations causing an additive effect on the peak current amplitude.[29] All nonsense and frame-shift mutations usually produce truncated and thus non-functional channel proteins. Missense mutations may result in no or strongly reduced Na^+ currents by causing trafficking defects, inability for the channel to reach the cellular membrane; *2)* loss-of-function due to either a negative shift of steady-state inactivation leading to decreased channel availability at the resting membrane potential or due to a positive shift of steady-state activation leading to an increased threshold for action potential generation and depending on the extent of this shift also to a reduced I_{Na};[32] *3)* an accelerated inactivation consistent with a reduced net Na^+ influx during the early plateau phase. A faster current decay is indeed found in many BrS mutant channels; *4)* an enhanced intermediate/slow inactivation.[33] These mutant channels undergo excessive intermediate/slow inactivation during a sustained depolarizing pulse. This causes an accumulation of inactivated channels and thus a reduction in Na^+ inward current especially at higher stimulation frequencies.

Since the identification of *SCN5A*, a few other genes have also been found to be responsible for the disease. Most mutations occur in genes related to Na^+ current, although other channels may also be implicated (see table 1).

In 2002, mutations in a second gene named *GPD1-L,* located in chromosome 3 (3p22-p24), was identified in a large family with BrS.[34] This gene encodes the protein glycerol 3-phosphate dehydrogenase 1-like (G3PD1L), and it affects the trafficking to the cell surface of the cardiac Na^+ channel. In 2007, the mutation (A280V)[35] and the novel SIDS-associated mutation (E83K)[36] were both shown to decrease cardiac I_{Na} amplitude. A280V reduces inward sodium currents by 50% and *SCN5A* cell surface by 31% approximately.[35] This decrease could account for their arrhythmogenesis.

Additionally to *SCN5A* alterations, mutations in the genes *SCN1B* (sodium channel beta-1 subunit)[37] and *SCN3B* (beta-3 subunit of the cardiac sodium channel)[38] have been recently described (see table 1). The sodium current-related genes *SCN1B* and *SCN3B* encode small ,-subunits ,1 and ,1b, and ,3, respectively, of the Nav complexes.[39] The ,-subunits have several functions, including interaction with ankyrin-B and -G. The gene *SCN1B* encodes the ,1-sub-

BrS	Gene	Locus	Protein	Ionic Channel	Function
BrS 1	*SCN5A*	3p21–p23	Nav1.5	Subunit-I_{Na}	
BrS 2	*GPD-1L*	3p24	G3PD1L	Interaction Subunit-I_{Na}	Loss
BrS 3	*CACNA1C*	12p13.3	Cav1.2	Subunit-I_{Ca}	Loss
BrS 4	*CACNB2*	10p12.33	Cav?2	Subunit-I_{Ca}	Loss
BrS 5	*SCN1B*	19q13.1	Nav?1/?1b	Subunit-I_{Na}	Loss
BrS 6	*KCNE3*	11q13–q14	MiRP2	Subunit-I_{Ks}/I_{To}	Gain
BrS 7	*SCN3B*	11q24.1	Nav?3	Subunit-I_{Na}	Loss

Table 1. Brugada syndrome (BrS) types.

unit of the cardiac sodium channel conducting the I_{Na} current. In the heart, the biophysical function of the ,1- and ,1b-subunits is to modify the function of Nav1.5, by increasing the I_{Na}.[37] The *SCN3B* gene encodes the ,3-subunit of the cardiac sodium channel conducting the I_{Na} current. The recently described mutation in *SCN3B* (L10P) was expressed in TSA201 cells together with *SCN5A* and *SCN1B*, and the mutation induced a defective trafficking of Nav1.5 and reduced I_{Na}.[38]

It is not only mutations leading to a loss of function in the sodium channel that can cause BrS: 11-12% of cases are attributable to loss-of-function mutations in the cardiac calcium channel *CACNA1c* (Cav1.2) and its ??subunit, *CACNB2b* (Cav2b),[40] can also be responsible for a syndrome overlapping shorter than normal QT intervals and the Brugada ECG pattern.[41] These genes encode proteins that participate directly or indirectly in the formation of the cardiac action potential (see table 1). *CACNA1C* gene encodes the pore-forming 1-subunit of the long-lasting (L-type) voltage gated Ca^{2+} channel (Cav1.2).[42] Cav1.2 is activated upon depolarization of the cardiomyocyte, and is responsible for the depolarizing influx of Ca^{2+}, the L-type Ca^{2+} current ($I_{L,Ca}$), that inactivates so slowly that it is of major significance for maintaining the plateau phase of the AP. Furthermore, it represents a coupling between excitation and contraction by inducing release of Ca^{2+} from the sarcoplasmic reticulum. The Cav1.2 channel is the most important source of intracellular calcium and inhibition of the channel function. Gain-of-function mutations in *CACNA1C* have previously been associated with Timothy syndrome (TS),[43] a dominantly inherited genetic condition characterized by prolonged QT-interval, multiple malformations, and a very poor prognosis due to lethal cardiac arrhythmias. These mutations result in complete loss of voltage-dependent inactivation of Cav1.2, resulting in Ca^{2+} overload and delayed repolarization due to prolonged Ca^{2+} inward current during the plateau phase of the AP.[43] The other calcium BrS-related gene, *CACNB2*, encodes for 2-subunit (Cav2) of Cav1.2,[44] which modifies gate and increase the I_{Ca} current.[45] *CACNB2* is composed of 14 exons and is located at chromosome 10p12.[46] Cav2 functions as a chaperone for the -subunit of Cav1.2, ensuring its transport to the plasma membrane.[47]. It is the dominantly expressed Cav1.2 -subunit in the heart. In *CACNB2*, a missense mutation (S481L) was identified.[41] The mutation is located in the C-terminal part of Cav2 close to the Cav1.2 binding domain. As the mutation is located in close proximity to the DI–DII linker of Cav1.2, interference with the stimulatory role of Cav2 on I_{Ca} is a likely pathogenic mechanism for this mutation. The mechanism of BrS4 involves a reduction of the depolarizing I_{Ca}.

To date, the seventh BrS-related gene is *KCNE3* (see table 1). This gene encodes MiRP2, one of five homologous auxiliary -subunits (KCNE peptides) of voltage-gated potassium ion channels.[48-50] The KCNE peptides modulate several potassium currents in the heart,[51,52] including I_{Ks},[53] I_{Kr},[54] and possibly I_{to}.[55] *KCNE3* codify for a regulatory beta subunit of the transient outward potassium channel, I_{to}.[37,38,55]

Given our limited knowledge on the genetic determinants of this syndrome, the management and risk stratification of BrS patients should be performed on a clinical basis. Nonetheless, genetic testing, when successful, allows confirmation of the diagnosis in borderline cases and identification of silent carriers.

3 Genetic modulators

Polymorphisms have recently acquired more importance in the explanation of certain phenotypes of genetic diseases. In the *SCN5A* locus, the common H558R polymorphism has been shown to partially restore the sodium current impaired by other simultaneous mutations causing either cardiac conduction disturbances (T512I)[56] or BrS (R282H).[57] Thus, this polymorphism seems to give rise to less severe phenotypes by reducing the effects of nearby mutations and its lack is associated with longer QRS complex duration in lead II, higher J-point elevation in lead V2, higher "aVR sign" and a trend towards more symptoms than AG or GG carriers. Thus, this common variant H558R seems to be a genetic modulator of BrS among carriers of an *SCN5A* mutation, in whom the presence of the less common allele makes BrS less severe.[58]

Genetic variants in the *SCN5A* promoter region may also have a pathophysiological role in BrS. A haplotype of six polymorphisms in the *SCN5A* promoter has been identified and functionally linked to a reduced expression of the sodium current. This variant was found among patients of Asian origin and it could play a role in modulating the expression of BrS in Far Eastern countries.[59,60] In another study,[61,62] a combination of two BrS mutations (R1232W and T1620), each of which can produce functional but biophysically defective sodium channels, blocked protein trafficking of the channel. This finding offers an explanation for the severity of the disease.

A recently published study has proposed the genetic data as a tool for risk stratification in BrS. In this study a genotype-phenotype correlation was performed according to the type of *SCN5A* mutation (missense, truncated). Patients and relatives with a truncated protein had a more severe phenotype and more severe conduction disorders.[63]

The identification of several triggering factors of arrhythmias in patients with a genetic predisposition to Brugada syndrome has raised the question as to what role the environment plays in this disease. Precipitating factors for the Brugada ECG pattern and syndrome of SCD include fever, cocaine, electrolyte disturbances, class I antiarrhythmic medications, as well as a number of other non-cardiac medications.[64] Most importantly, in some of these cases, usually young individuals, the presence of the induced ECG pattern has been associated with sudden cardiac death. While the pathophysiological mechanisms behind this association remain largely unknown, acute measures are critical in patients with the ECG pattern under these inducers.

4   Brugada syndrome associated with other genetic diseases

In certain situations, BrS and atrial fibrillation (AF) coexist in the same patient. Approximately 10–20% of patients of BrS develop supraventricular arrhythmias, especially AF.[65,66] Therefore, ICD devices need to be carefully programmed in BrS patients in order to avoid inappropriate shocks. Additionally, mutations in L-type Ca^{2+} channel (*CACNA1C*) or its 2b-subunit (*CACNB2b*) have been reported in BrS patients with shorter QT intervals[41,67] (see table 2).

5   Clinical manifestations of the Brugada syndrome

Patients with BrS usually remain asymptomatic. However, syncope or cardiac arrest has been described in up to 17-42% of diagnosed individuals.[68-71] This rate probably overestimates the real prevalence of symptoms among BrS patients, given that most asymptomatic patients remain underdiagnosed. The age of symptom occurrence is consistently around the fourth decade of life in all the series (especially cardiac arrest),[68-71] with no definite explanation for this observation thus far. Previous syncope may be present in up to 23% of patients who present with cardiac arrest.[69]

Channel	Disease	Inheritance	Locus	Gene
Sodium	BrS	Autosomic dominant	3p21-p24	*SCN5A*
	BrS	Autosomic dominant	3p22.3	*GPD1-L*
	BrS	Autosomic dominant	19q13.1	*SCN1b*
	BrS	Autosomic dominant	11q24.1	*SCN3b*
Potassium	AF and BrS	Autosomic dominant	11q13-q14	*KCNE3*
Calcium	BrS and Shorter QT	Autosomic dominant	2p13.3	*CACNA1c*
	BrS and Shorter QT	Autosomic dominant	10p12.33	*CACNB2b*

Table 2. Ion channels diseases associated with Brugada syndrome (BrS).
AF = atrial fibrillation.

Up to 20% of patients with BrS may present supraventricular arrhythmias,[72] and thus complain of palpitations and/or dizziness. An increased atrial vulnerability to both spontaneous and induced AF has been reported in patients with BrS.[65] The electrophysiological basis could be an abnormal atrial conduction.[65] Whether atrial vulnerability is correlated to an increased susceptibility for ventricular arrhythmias is thus far unknown. Other symptoms, such as neurally mediated syncope have been also recently associated to BrS, but their implications for prognosis have not yet been established.[73]

As in the case of other Na^+ channel-related disorders as type-3 long-QT syndrome (LQTS), ventricular arrhythmias in the BrS typically occur at rest, especially during sleep, suggesting that vagal activity may play an important role in the arrhythmogenesis of BrS.[74] Indeed, recent data on cardiac autonomic nervous system assessed by positron emission tomography confirm that BrS patients display a certain degree of sympathetic autonomic dysfunction, with increased presynaptic norepinephrine recycling and thus a decrease in the concentration of norepinephrine at the synaptic cleft, this imbalance facilitating arrhythmogenicity by decreasing intracellular levels of 3-5-cyclic adenosine monophosphate.[75,76]

5.1 Children

Although 3 of the 8 patients reported in the first description of the disease were within pediatric ages, little information has been thus far available on the behavior of the BrS during childhood. Probst *et al.* recently provided data from a multicenter study including 30 Brugada patients aged less than 16 years (mean age 8±5).[22] More than half (n=17) had been diagnosed during family screening, but symptoms were present in 11 patients (1 aborted SD and 10 syncope). Interestingly, 10 of the 11 symptomatic patients displayed spontaneous type-1 ECG, and in five of them, symptoms were precipitated by fever illnesses. Five patients received an ICD and four were treated with hydroquinidine.[22] During a mean follow-up period of 37±23 months, three patients (10% of the population) experienced SD (n=1) or appropriate shock by ICD (n=2). Importantly, all the three patients had presented with syncope at the time of diagnosis and displayed spontaneous type-1 ECG. The four patients on quinidine remained asymptomatic during the 28±24 months of follow-up.[22] In accordance with these results, a study of 58 pediatric patients with BrS was published in 2008 which provided further data on prognosis markers during childhood.[77] Cardiac events occurred more frequently among patients with spontaneous type-1 ECG and among those with inducible VF at the EPS, but, in our series, a symptom at diagnosis was the strongest variable to predict events during follow-up.

Though small, these studies suggest that: *1)* Brugada syndrome can manifest during childhood; *2)* symptoms may appear particularly during febrile episodes; *3)* symptomatic patients, especially if they present spontaneous type-1 ECG, may be at a high risk of cardiac events in a relatively short period of follow-up; *4)* patients at risk can be protected with an ICD, although quinidine could be an option in certain patients, particularly the youngest.

6 Prognosis and risk stratification

Prognosis and risk stratification are probably the most controversial issues in BrS. The main clinical studies arising from the largest databases differ on the risk of SD or VF in the population with BrS, and particularly on defining the specific risk markers with regard to prognosis.

In order to update population with BrS coming from the international registry, a recent study described that the percentage of patients who experienced SD or VF throughout their lifetime was 25%, and mean age at cardiac events was 42±15 years.[78] Of course, such a high rate might have been influenced by a baseline high risk population referred to the international registry and included in this analysis. These results are lower from the first patients included in the registry [5] to the most recent published series,[68,70,79] the change probably reflecting the inherent bias during the first years after the description of a novel disease, in which particularly severe forms of the disease are most likely to be diagnosed. It is important to note that in the global series, the lifetime probability of having a cardiac event a varied widely (from 3-45%) depending on the baseline characteristics of the individuals. Thus, a careful risk stratification of every individual seems mandatory.

Several clinical variables have been demonstrated to predict a worse outcome in patients with BrS. In all the analysis of our series over time, the presence of symptoms before diagnosis, a spontaneous type-1 ECG at baseline, the inducibility of ventricular arrhythmias at the EPS and male sex have consistently been shown to be related to the occurrence of cardiac events in follow-up.[5,68,70,79]

Little controversy exists on the value of a previous cardiac arrest as a risk marker for future events. Our data state that up to 62% of patients recovered from an aborted SD are at risk for a new arrhythmic event within the following 54 months.[68] Thus, these patients should be protected with an ICD irrespective of the presence of other risk factors (indication class I).[15] Because there is not such a general agreement on the best approach toward patients who have never developed VF, we conducted a prospective study including 547 individuals with BrS and no previous cardiac arrest.[70,79] Of those (mean age, 41±45 years; 408 males), 124 (22.7%) had presented with syncope, and 423 (77.3%) were asymptomatic and had been diagnosed during routine ECG or family screening. The baseline ECG showed a type-1 ECG pattern spontaneously in 391 patients (71.5%) and after a Na^+ channel blocker challenge in 156 (28.5%). During a mean follow-up of 24±32 months, 45 individuals (8.2%) developed a first cardiac event (documented VF or SD).[70] By univariate analysis, a previous history of syncope (HR,

2.79; 95% CI, 1.5-5.1; P=0.002), a spontaneous type-1 ECG (HR 7.69; 95% CI, 1.9-33.3; P=0.0001), male sex (HR 5.26; 95% CI, 1.6-16.6; P=0.001), and inducibility of ventricular arrhythmias at the EPS (HR 8.33; 95% CI, 2.8-25; P=0.0001) were significantly related to VF or SD in follow-up. Multivariate analysis identified previous syncope and inducibility of VF as the only independent risk factors for the occurrence of events in follow- up.[70] Logistic regression analysis allowed the definition of eight categories of risk, of which asymptomatic patients with normal ECG at baseline and no inducible VF at the EPS would represent the lowest-risk population, and patients with syncope, spontaneous type-1 ECG, and inducibility at EPS would have the worst outcome. Further analysis indicated that EPS was particularly useful in predicting cardiac events among asymptomatic patients with no family history of SD (so-called fortuitous cases, n = 167).[79] Indeed, 11 (6%) of 167 patients presented with VF during follow-up, and the only independent predictor was inducibility at EPS, whereas the lack of an EPS was shown to be predictive of effective SD (P=0.002).[79] Other groups agree that previous symptoms and a spontaneous type-1 ECG are risk factors, although they have found a much lower incidence of arrhythmic events for the whole population (6.5% in 34±44 months of follow-up in the work of Priori *et al.* [69] and 4.2% in 40±50 months of follow-up in that of Eckardt *et al.*[71]). The worse outcome in our series may probably reflect a more severely ill baseline population.[71] The other large registries also agree that EPS inducibility is greatest among patients with previous SD or syncope,[69,71] but failed to demonstrate a value of the EPS in predicting outcome. Several reasons could explain this discrepancy:[79] *1)* the use of multiple testing centers with no standardized stimulation protocols; *2)* the inclusion of patients with type-2 and type-3 ST-segment elevation (and not type-1) in some series, suggesting that they may contain individuals who do not have the syndrome; *3)* the lack of events during follow-up in the other registries. The latter might change when longer follow-ups are available because events can only increase in follow-up and so does the positive predictive value.[79] Because this issue is a source of ongoing controversy, we are currently performing a prospective study to determine the role of EPS in the risk stratification of BrS. Male sex has consistently shown a trend to present more arrhythmic events in all the studies, and even has been defined as an independent predictor for a worse outcome in a published meta-analysis.[80] A very recent study by our group indicates that males with BrS display a higher risk profile than females, and thus present a worse prognosis during follow-up.[77] Multiple ECG parameters have been assessed in the search for new risk markers, of which a prolonged QTc in right precordial leads, the aVR sign, the presence of T-wave alternans, and probably a wide QRS complex seem to be the most important (see ECG and Modulating Factors). Interestingly, a positive family history of SD or the presence of an *SCN5A* mutation have not been proven to be risk markers in any of the large studies conducted thus far.[68-71,80]

7   Treatment

7.1   Implantable cardioverter defibrillator

The ICD is the only proven effective treatment of the BrS thus far. On the basis of available clinical and basic science data, the consensus conference focused on risk stratification schemes and approaches to therapy.[15] Briefly, symptomatic patients should always receive an ICD. The EPS in these patients could be performed to better assess the sensitivity and specificity of the test to predict outcome, and also for the study of supraventricular arrhythmias. Asymptomatic patients may benefit from EPS for risk stratification: ICD should be implanted in those with inducible VF having a spontaneous type-1 ECG at baseline or a Na⁺ channel blocker-induced ECG with a positive family history of SD. Finally, asymptomatic patients who have no family history of SD and who develop a type-1 ECG only after sodium channel blockade should be closely followed up, without enough evidence existing for the usefulness of EPS or a direct indication for ICD.[15]

From the two main retrospective studies conducted on patients with BrS who have received primary prophylactic ICD, it can be concluded that ICD is an effective therapy for patients at risk[81,82] which can have an annual rate of appropriate shocks of up to 3.7%.[82] It is important to note that this rate is not only comparable to ICD trials[83,84] dealing with other cardiac diseases, but also is affecting young and otherwise healthy people, whose life expectancy could be more than 30 years. Therefore, should this rate remain constant in time, it seems that most patients would be likely to experience an appropriate shock in a lifetime. However, perhaps just due to the young age, a noteworthy rate of inappropriate shocks by the device has also been reported. In a published study, 45 (20%) out of 220 patients had inappropriate shocks in a follow-up.[81] In our series, the rate was even higher (36%).[82] The reasons for inappropriate therapies were mainly sinus tachycardia, supraventricular arrhythmias, T-wave over sensing, and lead failure in both studies.[81,82] On the basis of these results and because ICD is not affordable worldwide, there is growing effort to find pharmacological approaches to help treat the disease.

7.2 Pharmacological options

With the aim of rebalancing the ion channel currents active during phase 1 of the action potential, so as to reduce the magnitude of the notch, two main pharmacological approaches have been assessed: *1)* drugs that decrease outward positive currents, such as I_{to} inhibitors; *2)* drugs that increase inward positive currents (I_{Ca}, I_{Na}).

Quinidine, a drug with I_{to}- and I_{Kr}-blocking properties, has been the most assayed drug in clinical studies. In a work by Belhassen *et al.*,[85] 25 patients with inducible VF were treated with quinidine (1483±240 mg orally). After treatment, 22 (88%) of 25 patients were no longer inducible at the EPS, and none of the 19 patients with ongoing medical therapy with oral quinidine developed arrhythmias during follow-up (56±67 months).[85] However, 36% of the patients had transient side effects that led to drug discontinuation.[85] Preliminary data have also proven quinidine to be a good adjunctive therapy in patients with ICD and multiple shocks[86] and as an effective treatment of electrical storms associated with BrS.[87] More recently, quinidine has been proposed as a good alternative to ICD implantation in children with the syndrome and at high risk for malignant arrhythmias.[22] However, large randomized controlled clinical trials assessing the effectiveness of quinidine (which should be addressed in patients who have already received an ICD) are still lacking. ,-adrenergic agents, through an increase in I_{Ca} currents, decrease transmural dispersion of repolarization and epicardial dispersion of repolarization in experimental models.[11] Clinically, they have proven effectiveness in the treatment of electrical storms associated to BrS.[88] Recently, phosphodiesterase III inhibitors have appeared as a new appealing option because they would increase I_{Ca} and decrease I_{to}. Indeed, cilostazol was effective in preventing ICD shocks in a patient with recurrent episodes of VF.[89] However, a recent publication reports the failure of such a drug in another patient with multiple ICD discharges despite sustained therapy.[90] Dimethyl lithospermate B, an extract of Danshen, a traditional Chinese herbal remedy that slows inactivation of I_{Na}, has recently been assayed in experimental models, demonstrating a reduction of both transmural and epicardial dispersion of repolarization and abolishing phase 2 reentry-induced extrasystoles and VT/ VF in 9 of 9 preparations. Clinical data with this agent are, however, not yet available, but the results of experimental studies suggest that this agent could be a new candidate for the pharmacological treatment of BrS.[21]

Conclusion

Nowadays, more than 15 years after its original description, several major aspects of BrS remain unanswered. At present, there is strong agreement on the fact that the ICD is recommended in secondary prevention of cardiac arrest and in primary prevention of cardiac arrest in patients presenting a spontaneous type I ECG and history of symptoms. However, a critical issue is the approach to the asymptomatic patient, which remains a matter of controversy. Likewise in the basic science field, an important percentage of the cases of BrS have yet to be genotyped. Several genes have been identified in recent years, however, most account for a small portion of the total cases. The etiology of the BrS is likely multifactorial, both genetic and environmental. In the years to come, an increased effort will be placed on the discovery of these environmental factors and of genetic defects, genetic modulators and genotype-phenotype correlations to attempt to better define the role that genetic background plays in risk stratification.

References

1. Brugada P, Brugada J. Right bundle branch block, persistent ST segment elevation and sudden cardiac death: a distinct clinical and electrocardiographic syndrome. A multicenter report. J Am Coll Cardiol 1992; 20(6): 1391-6.
2. Ferracci A, Fromer M, Schlapfer J, *et al.* Primary ventricular fibrillation and early recurrence: apropos of a case of association of right bundle branch block and persistent ST segment elevation. Arch Mal Coeur Vaiss 1994; 87(10): 1359-62 (in french).
3. Proclemer A, Facchin D, Feruglio GA, *et al.* Recurrent ventricular fibrillation, right bundle-branch block and persistent ST segment elevation in V1-V3: a new arrhythmia syndrome? A clinical case report. G Ital Cardiol 1993; 23(12): 1211-8 (in italian).
4. Brugada J, Brugada P. Further characterization of the syndrome of right bundle branch block, ST segment elevation, and sudden cardiac death. J Cardiovasc Electrophysiol 1997; 8(3): 325-31.
5. Brugada J, Brugada R, Brugada P. Right bundle-branch block and ST-segment elevation in leads V1 through V3: a marker for sudden death in patients without demonstrable structural heart disease. Circulation 1998; 97(5): 457-60.
6. Alings M, Wilde A. "Brugada" syndrome: clinical data and suggested pathophysiological mechanism. Circulation 1999; 99(5): 666-73.
7. Priori SG, Napolitano C, Gasparini M, *et al.* Clinical and genetic heterogeneity of right bundle branch block and ST-

segment elevation syndrome: A prospective evaluation of 52 families. Circulation 2000; 102(20): 2509-15.
8. Brugada P, Brugada R, Brugada J. Sudden death in patients and relatives with the syndrome of right bundle branch block, ST segment elevation in the precordial leads V(1)to V(3)and sudden death. Eur Heart J 2000; 21(4): 321-6.
9. Chen Q, Kirsch GE, Zhang D, *et al.* Genetic basis and molecular mechanism for idiopathic ventricular fibrillation. Nature 1998; 392(6673): 293-6.
10. Dumaine R, Towbin JA, Brugada P, *et al.* Ionic mechanisms responsible for the electrocardiographic phenotype of the Brugada syndrome are temperature dependent. Circ Res 1999; 85(9): 803-9.
11. Yan GX, Antzelevitch C. Cellular basis for the Brugada syndrome and other mechanisms of arrhythmogenesis associated with ST-segment elevation. Circulation 1999; 100(15): 1660-6.
12. Rook MB, Bezzina Alshinawi C, Groenewegen WA, *et al.* Human SCN5A gene mutations alter cardiac sodium channel kinetics and are associated with the Brugada syndrome. Cardiovasc Res 1999; 44(3): 507-17.
13. Deschenes I, Baroudi G, Berthet M, *et al.* Electrophysiological characterization of SCN5A mutations causing long QT (E1784K) and Brugada (R1512W and R1432G) syndromes. Cardiovasc Res 2000; 46(1): 55-65.
14. Wilde AA, Antzelevitch C, Borggrefe M, *et al.* Proposed diagnostic criteria for the Brugada syndrome: consensus report. Circulation 2002; 106(19): 2514-9.

15. Antzelevitch C, Brugada P, Borggrefe M, *et al.* Brugada syndrome: report of the second consensus conference: endorsed by the Heart Rhythm Society and the European Heart Rhythm Association. Circulation 2005; 111(5): 659-70.

16. Brugada R, Brugada J, Antzelevitch C, *et al.* Sodium channel blockers identify risk for sudden death in patients with ST-segment elevation and right bundle branch block but structurally normal hearts. Circulation 2000; 101(5): 510-5.

17. Miyasaka Y, Tsuji H, Yamada K, *et al.* Prevalence and mortality of the Brugada-type electrocardiogram in one city in Japan. J Am Coll Cardiol 2001; 38(3): 771-4.

18. Donohue D, Tehrani F, Jamehdor R, *et al.* The prevalence of Brugada ECG in adult patients in a large university hospital in the western United States. Am Heart Hosp J 2008; 6(1): 48-50.

19. Hermida JS, Lemoine JL, Aoun FB, *et al.* Prevalence of the brugada syndrome in an apparently healthy population. Am J Cardiol 2000; 86(1): 91-4.

20. Vatta M, Dumaine R, Varghese G, *et al.* Genetic and biophysical basis of sudden unexplained nocturnal death syndrome (SUNDS), a disease allelic to Brugada syndrome. Hum Mol Genet 2002; 11(3): 337-45.

21. Antzelevitch C. Brugada syndrome. Pacing Clin Electrophysiol 2006; 29(10): 1130-59.

22. Probst V, Denjoy I, Meregalli PG, *et al.* Clinical aspects and prognosis of Brugada syndrome in children. Circulation 2007; 115(15): 2042-48.

23. Ikeda T, Abe A, Yusu S, *et al.* The full stomach test as a novel diagnostic technique for identifying patients at risk of Brugada syndrome. J Cardiovasc Electrophysiol 2006; 17(6): 602-7.

24. Ortega-Carnicer J, Bertos-Polo J, Gutierrez-Tirado C. Aborted sudden death, transient Brugada pattern, and wide QRS dysrrhythmias after massive cocaine ingestion. J Electrocardiol 2001; 34(4): 345-9.

25. Littmann L, Monroe MH, Svenson RH. Brugada-type electrocardiographic pattern induced by cocaine. Mayo Clin Proc 2000; 75(8): 845-9.

26. Vernooy K, Sicouri S, Dumaine R, *et al.* Genetic and biophysical basis for bupivacaine-induced ST segment elevation and VT/VF. Anesthesia unmasked Brugada syndrome. Heart Rhythm 2006; 3(9): 1074-8.

27. Schulze-Bahr E, Eckardt L, Breithardt G, *et al.* Sodium channel gene (SCN5A) mutations in 44 index patients with Brugada syndrome: different incidences in familial and sporadic disease. Hum Mutat 2003; 21(6): 651-2.

28. Schott JJ, Alshinawi C, Kyndt F, *et al.* Cardiac conduction defects associate with mutations in SCN5A. Nat Genet 1999; 23(1): 20-1.

29. Cordeiro JM, Barajas-Martinez H, Hong K, *et al.* Compound heterozygous mutations P336L and I1660V in the human cardiac sodium channel associated with the Brugada syndrome. Circulation 2006; 114(19): 2026-33.

30. Pfahnl AE, Viswanathan PC, Weiss R, *et al.* A sodium channel pore mutation causing Brugada syndrome. Heart Rhythm 2007; 4(1): 46-53.

31. Casini S, Tan HL, Bhuiyan ZA, *et al.* Characterization of a novel SCN5A mutation associated with Brugada syndrome reveals involvement of DIIIS4-S5 linker in slow inactivation. Cardiovasc Res 2007; 76(3): 418-29.

32. Mok NS, Priori SG, Napolitano C, *et al.* A newly characterized SCN5A mutation underlying Brugada syndrome unmasked by hyperthermia. J Cardiovasc Electrophysiol 2003; 14(4): 407-11.

33. Veldkamp MW, Viswanathan PC, Bezzina C, *et al.* Two distinct congenital arrhythmias evoked by a multidysfunctional Na(+) channel. Circ Res 2000; 86(9): E91-7.

34. Weiss R, Barmada MM, Nguyen T, *et al.* Clinical and molecular heterogeneity in the Brugada syndrome: a novel gene locus on chromosome 3. Circulation 2002; 105(6): 707-13.

35. London B, Michalec M, Mehdi H, *et al.* Mutation in glycerol-3-phosphate dehydrogenase 1 like gene (GPD1-L) decreases cardiac Na+ current and causes inherited arrhythmias. Circulation 2007; 116(20): 2260-8.

36. Van Norstrand DW, Valdivia CR, Tester DJ, *et al.* Molecular and functional characterization of novel glycerol-3-phosphate dehydrogenase 1 like gene (GPD1-L) mutations in sudden infant death syndrome. Circulation 2007; 116(20): 2253-9.

37. Watanabe H, Koopmann TT, Le Scouarnec S, *et al.* Sodium channel beta1 subunit mutations associated with Brugada syndrome and cardiac conduction disease in humans. J Clin Invest 2008; 118(6): 2260-8.

38. Hu D, Barajas-Martinez H, Burashnikov E, *et al.* A mutation in the beta 3 subunit of the cardiac sodium channel associated with Brugada ECG phenotype. Circ Cardiovasc Genet 2009; 2(3): 270-8.

39. Meadows LS, Isom LL. Sodium channels as macromolecular complexes: implications for inherited arrhythmia syndromes. Cardiovasc Res 2005; 67(3): 448-458.

40. Cordeiro JM, Marieb M, Pfeiffer R, *et al.* Accelerated inactivation of the L-type calcium current due to a mutation in CACNB2b underlies Brugada syndrome. J Mol Cell Cardiol 2009; 46(5): 695-703.

41. Antzelevitch C, Pollevick GD, Cordeiro JM, *et al.* Loss-of-function mutations in the cardiac calcium channel underlie a new clinical entity characterized by ST-segment elevation, short QT intervals, and sudden cardiac death. Circulation 2007; 115(4): 442-9.

42. Takimoto K, Li D, Nerbonne JM, *et al.* Distribution, splicing and glucocorticoid-induced expression of cardiac alpha 1C and alpha 1D voltage-gated Ca2+ channel mRNAs. J Mol Cell Cardiol 1997; 29(11): 3035-42.

43. Splawski I, Timothy KW, Decher N, *et al.* Severe arrhythmia disorder caused by cardiac L-type calcium channel mutations. Proc Natl Acad Sci USA 2005; 102(23): 8089-96; discussion 8086-8.

44. Van Petegem F, Clark KA, Chatelain FC, *et al.* Structure of a complex between a voltage-gated calcium channel beta-subunit and an alpha-subunit domain. Nature 2004; 429(6992): 671-5.

45. Catterall WA, Perez-Reyes E, Snutch TP, *et al.* International Union of Pharmacology. XLVIII. Nomenclature and structure-function relationships of voltage-gated calcium channels. Pharmacol Rev 2005; 57(4): 411-25.

46. Allen TJ, Mikala G. Effects of temperature on human L-type cardiac Ca2+ channels expressed in Xenopus oocytes. Pflugers Arch 1998; 436(2): 238-47.

47. Cornet V, Bichet D, Sandoz G, *et al.* Multiple determinants in voltage-dependent P/Q calcium channels control their retention in the endoplasmic reticulum. Eur J Neurosci 2002; 16(5): 883-95.

48. Abbott GW, Butler MH, Bendahhou S, *et al.* MiRP2 forms potassium channels in skeletal muscle with Kv3.4 and is associated with periodic paralysis. Cell 2001; 104(2): 217-31.

49. Abbott GW, Goldstein SA, Sesti F. Do all voltage-gated potassium channels use MiRPs? Circ Re 2001; 88(10): 981-3.

50. McCrossan ZA, Lewis A, Panaghie G, *et al.* MinK-related peptide 2 modulates Kv2.1 and Kv3.1 potassium channels in mammalian brain. J Neurosci 2003; 23(22): 8077-91.

51. Lewis A, McCrossan ZA, Abbott GW. MinK, MiRP1, and MiRP2 diversify Kv3.1 and Kv3.2 potassium channel gating. J Biol Chem 2004; 279(9): 7884-92.

52. Grunnet M, Rasmussen HB, Hay-Schmidt A, *et al.* KCNE4 is an inhibitory subunit to Kv1.1 and Kv1.3 potassium channels. Biophys J 2003; 85(3): 1525-37.

53. Bendahhou S, Marionneau C, Haurogne K, *et al.* In vitro molecular interactions and distribution of KCNE family with KCNQ1 in the human heart. Cardiovasc Res 2005; 67(3): 529-38.

54. Abbott GW, Goldstein SA. Disease-associated mutations in KCNE potassium channel subunits (MiRPs) reveal promiscuous disruption of multiple currents and conservation of mechanism. Faseb J 2002; 16(3): 390-400.

55. Delpon E, Cordeiro JM, Nunez L, *et al.* Functional effects of KCNE3 mutation and its role in the development of Brugada syndrome. Circ Arrhythm Electrophysiol 2008; 1(3): 209-18.

56. Viswanathan PC, Benson DW, Balser JR. A common SCN5A polymorphism modulates the biophysical effects of an SCN5A mutation. J Clin Invest 2003; 111(3): 341-6.

57. Poelzing S, Forleo C, Samodell M, *et al.* SCN5A polymorphism restores trafficking of a Brugada syndrome mutation on a separate gene. Circulation 2006; 114(5): 368-76.

58. Lizotte E, Junttila MJ, Dube MP, *et al.* Genetic modulation of brugada syndrome by a common polymorphism. J Cardiovasc Electrophysiol 2009; 20(10): 1137-41.

59. Bezzina CR, Shimizu W, Yang P, *et al.* Common sodium channel promoter haplotype in asian subjects underlies variability in cardiac conduction. Circulation 2006; 113(3): 338-44.

60. Ito H, Yano K, Chen R, *et al.* The prevalence and prognosis of a Brugada-type electrocardiogram in a population of middle-aged Japanese-American men with follow-up of three decades. Am J Med Sci 2006; 331(1): 25-9.

61. Baroudi G, Acharfi S, Larouche C, *et al.* Expression and intracellular localization of an SCN5A double mutant R1232W/T1620M implicated in Brugada syndrome. Circ Res 2002; 90(1): E11-6.

62. Makita N, Mochizuki N, Tsutsui H. Absence of a trafficking defect in R1232W/T1620M, a double SCN5A mutant responsible for Brugada syndrome. Circ J 2008; 72(6): 1018-9.

63. Meregalli PG, Tan HL, Probst V, *et al.* Type of SCN5A mutation determines clinical severity and degree of conduction slowing in loss-of-function sodium channelopathies. Heart Rhythm 2009; 6(3): 341-8.

64. Francis J, Antzelevitch C. Brugada syndrome. Int J Cardiol 2005; 101(2): 173-8.

65. Morita H, Kusano-Fukushima K, Nagase S, *et al.* Atrial fibrillation and atrial vulnerability in patients with Brugada syndrome. J Am Coll Cardiol 2002; 40(8): 1437-44.

66. Bordachar P, Reuter S, Garrigue S, et al. Incidence, clinical implications and prognosis of atrial arrhythmias in Brugada syndrome. Eur Heart J 2004; 25(10): 879-84.

67. Antzelevitch C. Genetic basis of Brugada syndrome. Heart Rhythm 2007; 4(6): 756-7.

68. Brugada J, Brugada R, Antzelevitch C, *et al.* Long-term follow-up of individuals with the electrocardiographic pattern of right bundle-branch block and ST-segment elevation in precordial leads V1 to V3. Circulation 2002; 105(1): 73-8.

69. Priori SG, Napolitano C, Gasparini M, *et al.* Natural history of Brugada syndrome: insights for risk stratification and management. Circulation 2002; 105(11): 1342-7.

70. Brugada J, Brugada R, Brugada P. Determinants of sudden cardiac death in individuals with the electrocardiographic pattern of Brugada syndrome and no previous cardiac arrest. Circulation 2003; 108(25): 3092-6.

71. Eckardt L, Probst V, Smits JP, *et al.* Long-term prognosis of individuals with right precordial ST-segment-elevation Brugada syndrome. Circulation 2005; 111(3): 257-63.

72. Eckardt L, Kirchhof P, Loh P, *et al.* Brugada syndrome and supraventricular tachyarrhythmias: a novel association? J Cardiovasc Electrophysiol 2001; 12(6): 680-5.

73. Makita N, Sumitomo N, Watanabe I, *et al.* Novel SCN5A mutation (Q55X) associated with age-dependent expression of Brugada syndrome presenting as neurally mediated syncope. Heart Rhythm 2007; 4(4): 516-9.

74. Matsuo K, Kurita T, Inagaki M, *et al.* The circadian pattern of the development of ventricular fibrillation in patients with Brugada syndrome. Eur Heart J 1999; 20(6): 465-70.

75. Wichter T, Matheja P, Eckardt L, *et al.* Cardiac autonomic dysfunction in Brugada syndrome. Circulation 2002; 105(6): 702-6.

76. Kies P, Wichter T, Schafers M, *et al.* Abnormal myocardial presynaptic norepinephrine recycling in patients with Brugada syndrome. Circulation 2004; 110(19): 3017-22.

77. Benito B, Sarkozy A, Mont L, *et al.* Gender differences in clinical manifestations of Brugada syndrome. J Am Coll Cardiol 2008; 52(19): 1567-73.

78. Benito B, Brugada R, Brugada J, *et al.* Brugada syndrome. Prog Cardiovasc Dis 2008; 51(1): 1-22.

79. Brugada P, Brugada R, Brugada J. Should patients with an asymptomatic Brugada electrocardiogram undergo pharmacological and electrophysiological testing? Circulation 2005; 112(2): 279-92; discussion 279-92.

80. Gehi AK, Duong TD, Metz LD, *et al.* Risk stratification of individuals with the Brugada electrocardiogram: a meta-analysis. J Cardiovasc Electrophysiol 2006; 17(6): 577-83.

81. Sacher F, Probst V, Iesaka Y, *et al.* Outcome after implantation of a cardioverter-defibrillator in patients with Brugada syndrome: a multicenter study. Circulation 2006; 114(22): 2317-24.

82. Sarkozy A, Boussy T, Kourgiannides G, *et al.* Long-term follow-up of primary prophylactic implantable cardioverter-defibrillator therapy in Brugada syndrome. Eur Heart J 2007; 28(3): 334-44.

83. Maron BJ, Shen WK, Link MS, *et al.* Efficacy of implantable cardioverter-defibrillators for the prevention of sudden death in patients with hypertrophic cardiomyopathy. N Engl J Med 2000; 342(6): 365-73.

84. Bardy GH, Lee KL, Mark DB, *et al.* Amiodarone or an implantable cardioverter-defibrillator for congestive heart failure. N Engl J Med 2005; 352(3): 225-37.

85. Belhassen B, Glick A, Viskin S. Efficacy of quinidine in high-risk patients with Brugada syndrome. Circulation 2004; 110(13): 1731-7.

86. Hermida JS, Denjoy I, Clerc J, *et al.* Hydroquinidine therapy in Brugada syndrome. J Am Coll Cardiol 2004; 43(10): 1853-60.

87. Mok NS, Chan NY, Chiu AC. Successful use of quinidine in treatment of electrical storm in Brugada syndrome. Pacing Clin Electrophysiol 2004; 27(6 Pt 1): 821-3.

88. Ohgo T, Okamura H, Noda T, *et al.* Acute and chronic management in patients with Brugada syndrome associated with electrical storm of ventricular fibrillation. Heart Rhythm 2007; 4(6): 695-700.

89. Tsuchiya T, Ashikaga K, Honda T, *et al.* Prevention of ventricular fibrillation by cilostazol, an oral phosphodiesterase inhibitor, in a patient with Brugada syndrome. J Cardiovasc Electrophysiol 2002; 13(7): 698-701.

90. Abud A, Bagattin D, Goyeneche R, *et al.* Failure of cilostazol in the prevention of ventricular fibrillation in a patient with Brugada syndrome. J Cardiovasc Electrophysiol 2006; 17(2): 210-2.

Chapter 18. Arrhythmogenic right ventricular cardiomyopathy/dysplasia: diagnosis and management

D. Corrado, M. Perazzolo, I. Rigato,
C. Basso, G. Thiene

**Division of Cardiology
Department of Cardiac,
Thoracic and Vascular Sciences
Cardiovascular Pathology Department
of Medical-Diagnostic Sciences
University of Padua
Padua, Italy**

Address for correspondence:
Department of Cardiac, Thoracic
and Vascular Sciences
University of Padua Medical School
Dr. Domenico Corrado
domenico.corrado@unipd.it

Introduction

Arrhythmogenic right ventricular cardiomyopathy/dysplasia (ARVC/D) is an inheritable heart muscle disease that is characterized by fibrofatty replacement of the right ventricular (RV) myocardium. The most common clinical manifestations of ARVC/D consist of ventricular arrhythmias of RV origin, which may lead to sudden death mostly in young people and athletes, right precordial ECG depolarization/repolarization changes, and morphofunctional alterations of the RV.

Later in the disease evolution, progression and extension of RV muscle disease and left ventricular involvement may result in right or biventricular heart failure. The diagnosis of ARVC/D may be difficult due to several problems with specificity of ECG abnormalities, different potential etiologies of ventricular arrhythmias with a left bundle branch morphology, assessment of RV structure and function, and interpretation of endomyocardial biopsy findings. Standardized diagnostic criteria have been proposed by an International Task Force. According to current guidelines, the diagnosis of ARVC/D is based on the presence of major and minor criteria encompassing ECG, arrhythmic, morphofunctional, histopathological, and genetic factors. The assessment of sudden death risk is still not well established and there are no definitive recommendations for patient management. Therapeutic options include beta-blockers, antiarrhythmic drugs, catheter ablation and implantable cardioverter defibrillator (ICD). The ICD has proven to be the most effective safeguard against arrhythmic sudden death. In patients in whom ARVC has progressed to severe RV or biventricular systolic dysfunction, treatment consists of traditional therapy for heart failure including heart transplantation.

Arrhythmogenic right ventricular cardiomyopathy/dysplasia (ARVC/D) is an inheritable heart muscle disease that predominantly affects the right ventricle (RV).[1-5] It is characterized pathologically by myocardial atrophy and fibro-fatty replacement of the right ventricular myocardium.[2,3,5] Clinical manifestations develop most often between the second and third decade of life and are related to ventricular tachycardia (VT) or ventricular fibrillation (VF) which may lead to sudden death, mostly in young people. Ventricular arrhythmias are worse during or immediately after exercise, and participation in competitive athletics has been associated with an increased risk for sudden death.[6] Later in the natural history, the RV may become more diffusely involved and the left ventricle (LV) progressively affected with subsequent biventricular heart failure.[4] Clinical diagnosis of ARVC/D is often difficult due to the non-specific nature of disease features and the broad spectrum of phenotypic manifestation, ranging from severe to concealed forms. Early detection and preventive therapy of young individuals at highest risk of experiencing sudden cardiac death may modify the natural history of the disease.

The extraordinary advances of molecular genetics provided significant insights in our understanding of the etiopathogenesis of ARVC/D. According to current perspectives, the disease is the result of a genetically determined and progressive atrophy of the RV myocardium, which becomes symptomatic in adolescents and young adults.[7] On the basis of its nature of genetic heart muscle disease, ARVC/D has been appropriately included among the cardiomyopathies.[8]

1   Diagnosis

The estimated prevalence of ARVC/D in the general population ranges from 1 in 2,000 to 1 in 5,000. A familial background has been demonstrated in >50% of cases. The disease affects men more frequently than females (ratio of 3:1), and becomes clinically overt most often in adolescents or young adults[5] (see figure 1). The clinical picture varies considerably ranging from asymptomatic family members with concealed RV structural abnormalities and no arrhythmias to patients experiencing arrhythmic cardiac arrest or undergoing cardiac transplantation due to right or biventricular heart failure.[1-4,9-14]

In 1994 the ARVC/D study group of the Working Group of Myocardial and Pericardial Disease of the European Society of Cardiology and the Scientific Council on Cardiomyopathies of the International Society and Federation of Cardiology proposed standardized diagnostic criteria.[15,16] The purpose of the Task Force was to provide diagnostic guidelines helping to overcome several problems with specificity of the ECG abnormalities, different potential etiologies of ventricular arrhythmias with a left bundle branch morphology, assessment of the RV structure and function, and interpretation of endomyocardial biopsy findings. The strategy consists of achieving clinical diagnosis by combining multiple sources of diagnostic information, such as genetic, electrocardiographic, arrhythmic, morphofunctional and histopathological findings (see table 1). Diagnosis of ARVC/D would be fulfilled in the presence of two major criteria or one major plus two minor or four minor criteria from different groups.

Since their publication in 1992, the Task Force criteria have been extremely useful in providing a standardized approach to clinical diagnosis of ARVC/D. Criteria were initially designed to guarantee an adequate specificity for ARVC/D among index cases with overt clinical manifestations. Task Force guidelines have actually helped cardiologists to avoid misdiagnosis of ARVC/D in patients with dilated cardiomyopathy or idiopathic RV outflow tract tachycar-

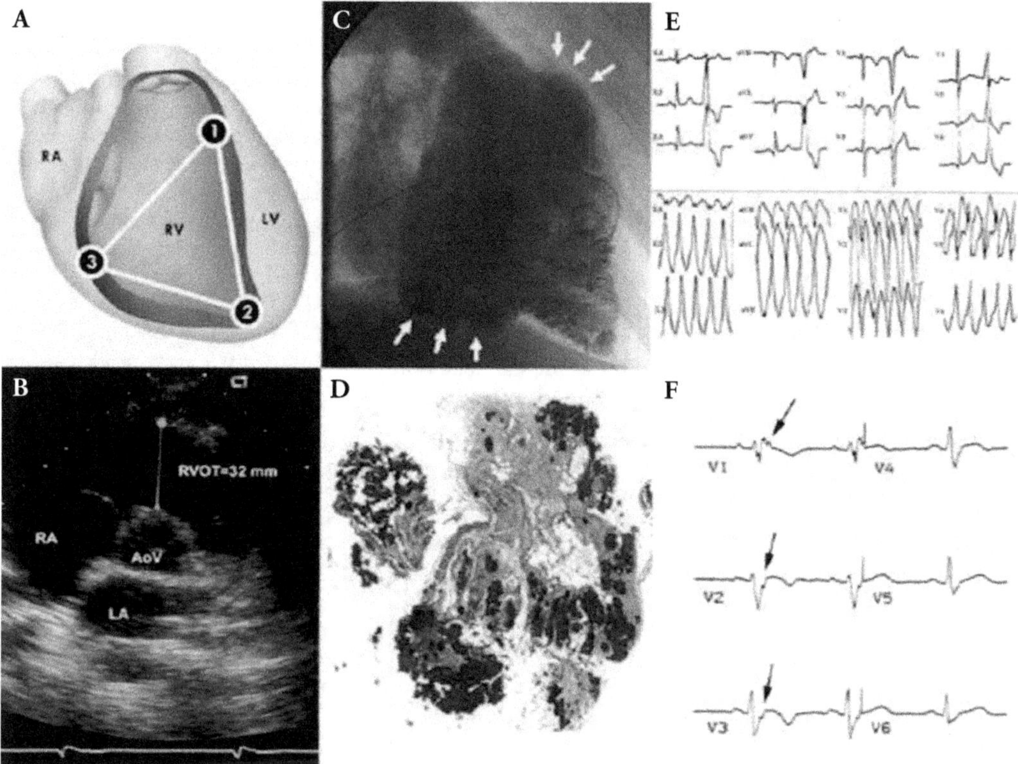

Figure 1. Morphofunctional, electrocardiographic and tissue characterization diagnostic features of ARVC/D.
A. Diagram of the "triangle of dysplasia" which illustrates the characteristic areas for structural and functional abnormalities of the RV.
RA = right atrium; RV = right ventricle; LV = left ventricle.
B. 2D echocardiography showing RV outflow tract enlargement from the parasternal short axis view.
AoV = aortic valve; RA = right atrium; LA = left atrium; RVOT = right ventricle outflow tract.
C. Right ventricular contrast angiography (30° right anterior oblique view) demonstrating a localized RV outflow tract aneurysm (arrows) as well as inferobasal akinesia (arrows) with mild tricuspid regurgitation.
D. Endomyocardial biopsy sample with extensive myocardial atrophy and fibrofatty replacement (trichrome; original x6) (from Corrado D *et al.*, reference number 60, modified).
E. 12-lead ECG with inverted T-waves (V1, V2, V3) with LBBB morphology premature ventricular beats and VT.
F. ECG tracing showing post-excitation epsilon wave in precordial leads V1, V2, V3 (arrows).
Modified from reference number 1.

dia. However, diagnostic criteria have shown to lack sensitivity for identification of early/minor phenotypes, particularly in the setting of familial ARVC/D. Hence, a revision of such diagnostic guidelines has been proposed with the aim to make a proper diagnosis in first degree relatives with incomplete phenotypic expression.[17,18] According to modified criteria, the presence of any one of right precordial T-wave inversion, late potentials on SAECG, a left bandle branch block pattern VT, premature ventricular beats ≥200 over 24 hours or mild morphofunctional

Group	Major	Minor
1. Global and/or regional dysfunction and structural alterations	– Severe dilatation and reduction of right ventricular ejection fraction with no (or only mild) left ventricular involvement – Localized right ventricular aneurysms (akinetic or dyskinetic areas with diastolic bulgings) – Severe segmental dilatation of the right ventricle	Mild global right ventricular dilatation and or ejection fraction reduction with normal left ventricle Mild segmental dilatation of the right ventricle Regional right ventricular hypokinesia
2. Tissue characteristics of walls	Fibrofatty replacement of myocardium on endomyocardial biopsy	
3. ECG depolarization/ conduction abnormalities	Epsilon waves or localized prolongation (≥110 ms) of the QRS complex in the right precordial leads (V1-V3)	Late potentials seen on signal averaged electrocardiography
4. ECG repolarization abnormalities		Inverted T-waves in right precordial leads (V2 and V3) in people >12 years and in the absence of right bundle branch block
5. Arrhythmias		– Sustained or nonsustained left bundle branch block type ventricular tachycardia documented on the electrocardiography, Holter monitoring or during exercise testing – Frequent ventricular extrasystoles (>1,000/24 hours on Holter monitoring)
6. Family history	Familial disease confirmed at necropsy or surgery	Family history of premature sudden death (<35 years) due to suspected ARVC/D Family history (clinical diagnosis based on present criteria)

*Table 1. Task Force criteria for diagnosis of ARVC.**

* Diagnosis of ARVC in probands is made when two major criteria or one major plus two minor or four minor criteria from different groups are met. According to the proposed revision, the diagnosis of probable ARVC in a first degree family member would be fulfilled by the presence of a single minor criteria from group 1, 3, 4 and 5.

Modified from reference 5.

RV abnormalities is considered to be itself diagnostic, in the setting of family screening of probands with clinically or pathologically proven ARVC/D. Indeed, the chance that such isolated ECG, arrhythmic, or echocardiographic features represent a clinical manifestation of ARVC/D is definitively higher in family members who have a 50% probability of defective gene trasmission. A further limitation of current Task Force criteria is the lack of quantitative cut-off values for proper grading of RV dilatation/dysfunction and fibrofatty myocardial replacement.[15] Besides a visual evaluation of RV wall motion and structural abnormalities, a quantitative assessment including measurements of end-diastolic cavity dimensions (inlet, outlet, and mean RV ventricular body), wall thickness, volume and function, either global or regional, is mandatory to enhance the diagnostic accuracy. Revised guidelines for ARVC/D diagnosis will provide quantitative imaging and histopathological measurement cut points for defining a normal RV and categorize the various degree of morphofunctional RV abnormalities.[19]

1.1   Genetics

Recent availability of genetic testing for screening ARVC/D-causing mutations offers the potential to identify genetically affected individuals by DNA characterization.[7,19-21] The inherited nature of the disease has been recognized since 1982 when Marcus *et al.* described 24 affected cases, two in the same family.[1,5] In 1988 a report on eight Italian families suggested the autosomal dominant pattern of inheritance with incomplete penetrance and variable expression.[22] The first chromosomal locus (14q23-q24) was published in 1994 after clinical evaluation of a large Venetian family.[21] Subsequently, linkage analysis provided evidence for genetic heterogeneity with sequential discovery of several ARVC/D loci on chromosome 1 (1q42-q43), chromosome 2 (2q32.1-q32.2), chromosome 3 (3p23), chromosome 6 (6p24), chromosome 10 (10p12-p14 and 10q22) and chromosome 14 (14q12-q22).[7] Other families analyzed with markers linked to these loci failed to show linkage, indicating further genetic heterogeneity. An autosomal recessive variant of ARVC/D (so-called Naxos disease) in which there is a cosegregation of cardiac (ARVC/D), skin (palmoplantar keratosis) and hair (woolly hair) abnormalities has been mapped on chromosome 17 (locus 17q21). The first disease-causing gene, the JUP gene, was identified by McKoy *et al.* in patients with Naxos disease.[23] The gene encodes desmosomal protein plakoglobin, which is the major constituent of cell adhesion junction. Its discovery suggested that ARVC/D is a cell-to-cell junction disease and stimulated the research for other related genes (see figure 2). Subsequently, mutations in desmosomal protein genes have been shown also to cause the more common (non-syndromic) autosomal dominant form of the disease (see table 2). Desmoplakin was the first defective gene to be associated with autosomal dominant ARVC/D by Rampazzo *et al.*[24] Thus, Gerull *et al.* identified 25 different mutations in the gene encoding plakophilin-2 (PKP2) in 32 out of 120 ARVC/D probands (27%).[25] More recently, mutations of the gene encoding for desmoglein-2 and desmocollin-2 have been involved in the disease pathogenesis.[26,27]

How the mutations of desmosomal protein genes cause disease remains to be elucidated. It has been hypothesized that the lack of the protein or the incorporation of mutant protein into cardiac desmosomes may provoke detachment of myocytes at the intercalated discs, particularly under condition of mechanical stress (like that occurring during competitive sports activity). As a consequence, there is a progressive myocyte degeneration and death with subsequent repair by fibrofatty replacement.[20,23] Life-threatening ventricular arrhythmias may occur either during the "hot phase" of myocyte death as abrupt VF or later in the form of scar-related macro-reentrant VT.[28]

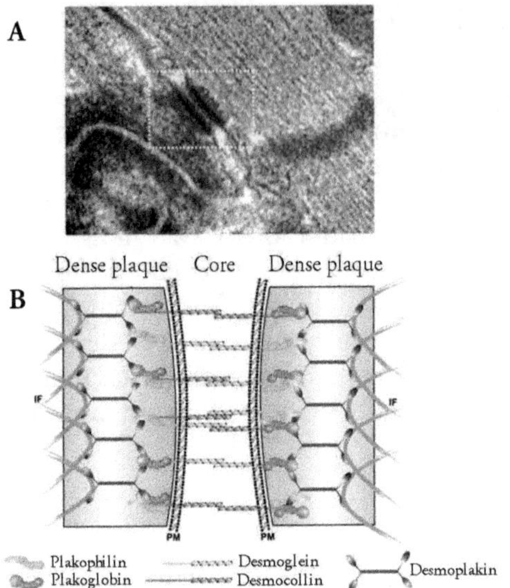

Figure 2. Intercellular mechanical junction (desmosome) of the cardiomyocyte.
A. Transmission electron microscopy of cardiomyocyte desmosome (boxed area, original x80,000).
B. Schematic representation of the desmosome components. It consists of a core region, which
mediates cell-cell adhesion, and a dense plaque, which provides attachment to the intermediate filaments.
There are three major groups of desmosomal proteins: *1)* transmembrane proteins (i.e., desmosomal
cadherins) including desmocollins and desmogleins; *2)* desmoplakin, a plakin family protein
that binds directly to intermediate filaments (desmin in the heart); *3)* linker proteins (i.e., armadillo
family proteins) including plakoglobin and plakophilins which mediate interactions between the
desmosomal cadherin tails and desmoplakin.
IF = intermediate filaments; PM =plasma membrane.
Reproduced from reference 1, with permission of the publisher.

Extradesmosomal genes implicated in ARVC/D include the cardiac ryanodyne-2 receptor, the transforming growth factor β3, and the TMEM43 genes.[29-31]

1.2 Depolarization/repolarization abnormalities

ECG abnormalites are detected in up to 90% of ARVC/D patients.[5,29] T-wave inversion in the precordial leads exploring the right ventricle (V1-V3) is the most common finding. These repolarizations are not pathognomonic of ARVC/D since may be a normal variant in females and in children younger than 14 years, or may be secondary to a right bundle branch block, either isolated or in the setting of a congenital heart disease accounting for a RV overload.[15,16] The ECG abnormalities resulting from delayed RV activation include complete or incomplete right bundle branch block, prolongation of right precordial QRS duration (≥110 ms), and post-excitation epsilon waves, namely small amplitude potentials occurring after the QRS complex at the beginning of the ST segment[1,4,5] (see figure 1). Prolongation of right precordial QRS duration is often the result of a delayed S-wave upstroke (>55 msec).[30] Although epsilon waves

Designation (pattern of inheritance)	Chromosomal locus	Gene mutations
ARVD1 (AD)	14q23-q24	Transforming growth factor-β3 (TGF,3)
ARVD2 (AD)	1q42-q43	Cardiac ryanodine receptor (RyR2)
ARVD3 (AD)	14q12-q22	?
ARVD4 (AD)	2q32.1-q32.3	?
ARVD5 (AD)	3p23	Transmembrane 43 (TMEM43)
ARVD6 (AD)	10p12-p14	?
ARVD7 (AD)	10q22	?
Naxos disease (AR)	17q21	Plakoglobin (JUP)
ARVD8 (AD)	6p24	Desmoplakin (DSP)
ARVD 9 (AD)	12p11	Plakophilin-2 (PKP2)
ARVD 10 (AD)	18q12.1	Desmoglein-2 (DSG2)
ARVD 11 (AD)	18q12.1	Desmocollin-2 (DSC2)
ARVD 12 (AD)	17q21	Plakoglobin (JUP)

Table 2. Chromosomal loci and disease-causing genes in ARVC/D.
AD = autosomal dominant; AR = autosomal recessive.
Modified from reference number 5.

are uncommon on standard 12-lead ECG, they can be frequently detected in the form of late potentials in the terminal portion of the QRS complex by signal averaging techniques. Both epsilon waves and late potentials reflect areas of slow intraventricular conduction which may predispose to reentrant ventricular arrhythmias. The underlying substrate consists of islands of surviving myocardium interspersed with fatty and fibrous tissue, accounting for fragmentation of the electrical activation of the ventricular myocardium.[2-4,29,31,32] In ARVC/D, late potentials are correlated with the extension of RV involvement and with the disease progression.

1.2.1　Ventricular arrhythmias

The spectrum of ventricular arrhythmias in ARVC/D ranges from isolated premature ventricular beats to sustained VT or VF leading to sudden cardiac arrest.[1-5] The arrhythmia severity varies both from patients to patients and during the course of the disease. The distinctive QRS morphology of ventricular arrhythmias is left bundle branch block which indicates an origin from the right ventricle; moreover, the mean QRS axis suggests the site of origin: inferior axis the RV outflow tract, superior axis the RV inferior wall or the apex. Patients with advanced and widespread ARVC/D may show several morphologies of VT, indicating multiple RV arrhythmogenic foci. VTs with LBBB pattern are not specific for ARVC/D: differential diagnosis include RV tachycardias complicating congenital heart disease, such as repaired tetralogy of Fallot, Ebstein anomaly, atrial septal defect, and partial anomalous venous return; acquired disease such as tricuspid valve disease, pulmonary hypertension and RV infarction; bundle branch reentry often associated with a dilated cardiomyopathy; Mahaim-preexcitated AV reentry tachycardia; and idiopathic RV outflow tract tachycardia.[33] It is often difficult to differentiate ARVC/D from the latter condition, which is usually benign and non-familial. It is still debated whether a subset of RV outflow tract tachycardia represents a forme fruste of ARVC/D, as suggested by the underlying RV structural abnormalities detected by either cardiac MR or endocardial voltage mapping.[34]

VF is relatively rare in patients with known ARVC undergoing medical treatment of symptomatic ventricular tachycardia, although some cases of rapid, hemodinamically unstable or prolonged ventricular tachycardia may degenerate into VF.[5] On the other hand, abrupt VF is the most likely mechanism of instantaneous sudden death in previously asymptomatic young people and athletes with ARVC/D.[6,35] Whether VF in this subset of patients is related to an acute phase of disease progression, either due to myocyte necrosis-apoptosis, or inflammation remains to be established.[5]

1.2.2   *Imaging of morphofunctional ventricular abnormalities*

Echocardiography and contrast ventriculography are the standard imaging techniques for diagnosing ARVC/D.[1,5,9,33,36] Relevant structural abnormalities include global RV dilatation with or without ejection fraction reduction and LV involvement; segmental RV dilatation with or without dyskinesia (aneurysms and bulgings); and wall motion abnormalities such as hypoakinesia or dyskinesia.[15] RV angiography is usually regarded as the gold standard for the diagnosis. Angiographic evidence of akinetic or dyskinetic bulgings localized in infundibular, apical and subtricuspidal regions has a high diagnostic specificity (over 90%).[11] Large areas of dilatation-akinesia with an irregular and "mamillated" aspect, most often involving the inferior RV wall, are also significantly associated with the diagnosis of ARVC/D. Compared with contrast angiography, echocardiography is a non-invasive and widely spread technique, and represents the first-line imaging approach in evaluating patients with suspected ARVC/D or in screening family members.[5,9,18] Echocardiography also allows serial examinations aimed to assess the disease progression during the follow-up of affected patients. Other than a visual assessment of wall motion and structural abnormalities, a quantitative echocardiographic evaluation of the RV including measurements of endiastolic cavity dimensions (inlet, outlet, and mean ventricular body), wall thickness, volume and function is mandatory in order to enhance the diagnostic accuracy.[18,36]

Although echocardiographic demonstration of typical RV morphofunctional abnormalities is diagnostic, borderline or apparently normal findings in patients with suspected ARVC require further examination by cardiac MR.[37-40] Cardiac MR allows an accurate RV morphofunctional analysis and has the unique ability to detect intramyocardial fatty deposition by spin-echo technique.[37] However, it has been implicated in overdiagnosis of ARVC/D based on the low specificity of qualitative findings such as increased myocardial fat and wall thinning. Moreover, significant interobserver variability in the interpretation of segmental contraction analysis of the RV free wall has been reported. A cardiac MR study demonstrated a 93.1%

prevalence of RV wall motion abnormalities in normal subjects, including areas of apparent dyskinesia (75.9%) and bulging (27.6%).[41] There is an emerging role of contrast-enhanced cardiac MR for detection of myocardial fibrofatty scar in both the RV and left ventricle (LV). Tandri *et al.*[39] first reported that RV delayed enhancement is found in 67% of patients with ARVC/D and correlate with both inducibility of VT at programmed ventricular stimulation and fibrofatty myocardial replacement at endomyocardial biopsy. Sen-Chowdhry *et al.*[40] confirmed that LV late enhancement is a common finding in patients with ARVC/D and provides higher diagnostic sensitivity and specificity than RV late-enhancement. In ARVC/D patients, LV late-enhancement predominantly involves the inferolateral and inferoseptal regions, and, unlike subendocardial distribution of ischemic scar, is characteristically localized in the subepicardial or midwall layers, similarly to the histological pattern of fibrofatty myocardial replacement found at post-mortem examination (see figure 3). Prominent LV late-enhancement with ventricular dilatation/dysfunction and no or mild RV involvement may be observed in "left-dominant" form of ARVC, which are characteristically related to desmoplakin-gene defects.[42] Other clinical markers of this disease variant include ECG abnormalities suggesting an LV involvement, such as T-wave inversion in the leads exploring the LV (V5, V6, L1 and aVL), and ventricular arrhythmias of LV origin (with a right bundle branch block morphology). The frequent and early finding of LV involvement in ARVC/D and the identification of a predominantly left-sided variant of the disease, led to the evolving concept that ARVC is a genetically determined heart muscle disease extending across the entire heart.

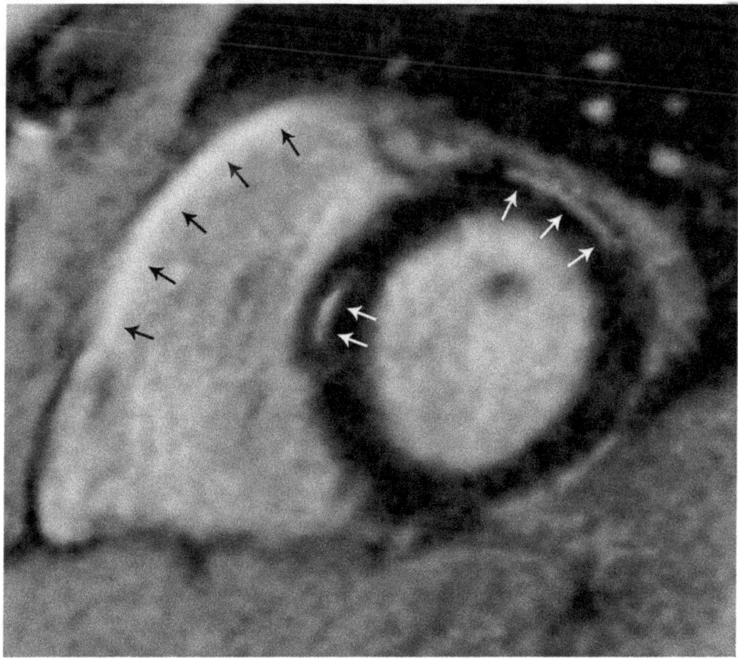

Figure 3. Short axis image after gadolinium injection in an ARVC patient with biventricular involvement.
The image shows delayed hyperenhancement on the anteroinfundibular wall of the right ventricle (black arrows),
as well as on the interventricular septum and the free wall of the left ventricle (white arrows).
Reproduced from reference 5, with permission of the publisher.

Computed tomography and radionuclide angiography are also accurate noninvasive imaging techniques with good diagnostic concordance with RV angiography in delineating RV anatomy and function.[1,5,42] Three-dimensional electroanatomical voltage mapping by CARTO system can reveal low voltage areas that correspond to fibrofatty myocardial replacement and may assist in the differential diagnosis with diseases that can mimic ARVC/D, such as inflammatory cardiomyopathy and idiopathic RV outflow tract tachycardia[32,34] (see figure 4).

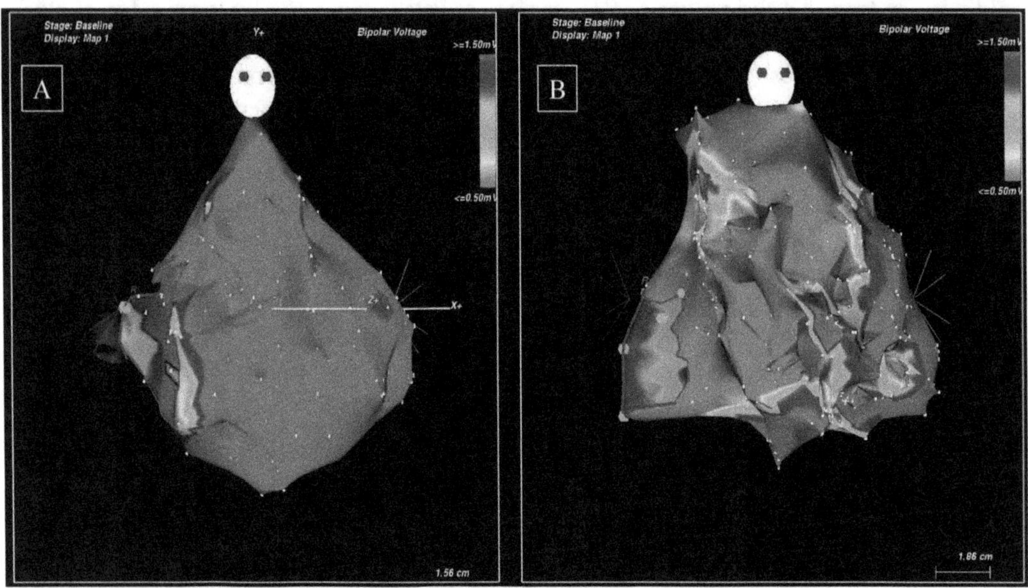

Figure 4. Representative normal and abnormal 3D electroanatomic voltage maps. Voltages are color coded according to corresponding color bars. Color range is identical for all subsequent figures: purple represents signal amplitudes >1.5 mV ("electroanatomic normal myocardium"); red <0.5 mV ("electroanatomic scar tissue"); and range between purple and red 0.5 to 1.5 mV ("electroanatomic border zone").
A. Anteroposterior view of the RV bipolar voltage map from one control subject entirely represented by normal bipolar voltages; B. Anteroposterior view of the RV bipolar voltage map from a patient with ARVC/D showing diffuse low-amplitude electrical activity involving anterior, lateral, inferobasal, anteroapical and infundibular regions.
Reproduced from reference 5, with permission of the publisher.

1.2.3   *Endomyocardial biopsy*

In selected patients transvenous endomyocardial biopsy can validate the diagnosis of ARVC/D by demonstrating fibrofatty replacement (see figure 1) and allowing exclusion of phenocopies, such as myocarditis and sarcoidosis.[43-46] Since the ventricular septum is usually spared, to increase the sensitivity samples should be obtained from the RV free wall, preferably under echo/MR guidance. Myocardial atrophy, with a residual amount of myocardium <60% due to fibrofatty replacement, has been shown to be a very accurate diagnostic marker.[47]

2   Management

2.1   Risk stratification

The clinical outcome of patients with ARVC/D is related to the ventricular electrical instability which can precipitate life-theratening ventricular arrhythmias at any time during the disease course and to progressive myocardial loss that may induce ventricular dysfunction and heart failure.[1-5] The available data suggest that young age, prior cardiac arrest, fast and poorly tolerated VT with different morphologies, syncope, severe right ventricular dysfunction, heart failure with left ventricular involvement, and familial occurrence of juvenile sudden death are the major determinants in predicting sudden death and worse outcome.[1,5,21,48] Whether genotyping is able to predict phenotype and/or prognosis on the basis of characterization of malignant versus benign mutations remains to be established by studies on genotype-phenotype correlations.[7] The role of electrophysiological study with programmed ventricular stimulation in identifying patients at risk of lethal ventricular arrhythmias is debated. Three recent, separate studies reported different results. The largest study by Corrado *et al.*[28] reported that the incidence of appropriate ICD discharge did not differ between patients who were and were not inducible at programmed ventricular stimulation for either primary and secondary prevention of arrhythmic sudden death, regardless of indication for ICD implant. In this study, the type of ventricular tachyarrhythmia inducible at the time of electrophysiological study did not appear to predict the occurrence of ventricular fibrillation during follow-up. The results of this study indicate that the electrophysiological study is of limited value in identifying patients at risk of lethal ventricular arrhythmias because of a low predictive accuracy (approximately 50% of both false-positive and false-negative results). This finding is in agreement with the limitation of electrophysiological study for arrhythmic risk stratification of other non-ischemic heart disease such as hypertrophic and dilated cardiomyopathy. In the study by Wichter *et al.,*[49] in which patients with a history of cardiac arrest or sustained VT were enrolled, inducibility of VT or VF at preimplant electrophysiological study demonstrated a trend toward statistical significance for subsequent appropriate device interventions. Roguin *et al.*[50] reported that VT induction was the most significant independent predictor of appropriate ICD firing in their cohort of ARVC patients. Further studies on a large patient population are needed to establish whether electrophysiological study with programmed ventricular stimulation may identify those ARVC/D patients with no prior spontaneous ventricular tachycardia or ventricular fibrillation, in whom the probability of sudden arrhythmic death is sufficienty high to warrant an ICD for primary prevention.

2.2   Therapy

The first objective of management therapy in patients with ARVC/D is to prevent sudden death. Therapeutic options include beta-blockers, antiarrhythmic drugs, catheter ablation, and ICD. The current data indicate that asymptomatic ARVC/D patients do not require any prophylactic treatment. They should be followed up on a regular basis by non-invasive cardiac evaluations for early identification of warning symptoms and demonstration of disease progression or ventricular arrhythmias. Importantly, asymptomatic and healthy gene carriers should be prudently advised to refrain from participating in physical exercise and sport activity, which is associated with an increased risk of ventricular arrhythmias and disease worsening. Whether prophylactic beta-blockers therapy may reduce the rate of ARVC/D progression and arrhythmic complications in asymptomatic patients and gene carriers remains to be proven. Antiarrhythmic drug therapy is the first choice treatment of patients with well tolerated and not life-threatening ventricular arrhythmias.[51,52] The evidence available suggests that either sotalol or amiodarone (alone or in combination with beta-blockers) are the most effective drugs with a relatively low proarrhythmic risk, although their ability to prevent sudden death has not been proven.

Catheter ablation of the VT reentry circuit has acute success rates of 60%-90%.[52-54] However, VT relapses are frequent (up to 85% of the cases) and have been attributed to development of new arrhythmogenic zones because of the progressive nature of the underlying disease. Therefore, catheter ablation should be reserved for particular clinical conditions such as drug refractory incessant VT or frequent recurrences of VT after ICD implantation, in whom it is the only option available.[5]

ICD is the most logical therapeutic strategy for patients with ARVC/D, whose natural history is primarily characterised by the risk of sudden arrhythmic death and, only secondarily, by contractile dysfunction leading with progressive heart failure. The results of published trials strongly suggest an improvement in long-term prognosis by ICD therapy in high-risk patients with ARVC/D.[28,49,50] Although ICD confers optimal protection against sudden death,

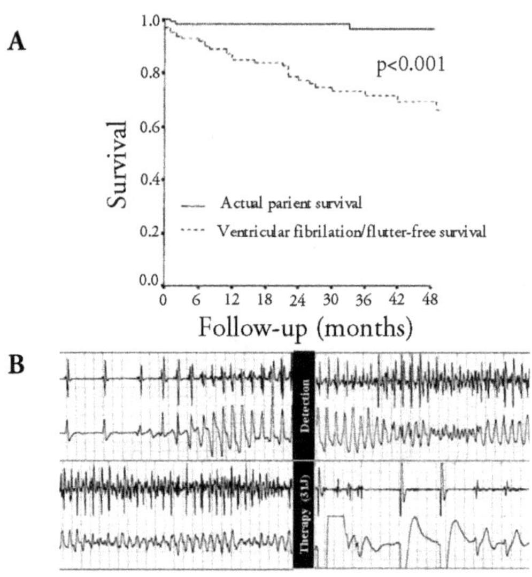

Figure 5. ICD therapy in ARVC.
A. Projected survival of 132 ARVC patients with ICD. The Kaplan-Meier analysis compares actual patient survival (continuous line) with survival free from either VF or ventricular flutter (dotted line) that would have been fatal in the absence of an appropriate ICD intervention. The divergence between curves reflects the estimated survival benefit conferred by ICD therapy. At 36 months, actual total patient survival was 96%, compared with 72% VF and ventricular flutter survival.
B. Stored intracardiac electrogram in an ARVC/D patient. This shows one episode of VF, followed by appropriate detection and successful ICD discharge followed by sinus rhythm.
Modified from reference 28, with permission of the publisher.

the significant rate of inappropriate interventions and complications as well as the psychological repercussions mostly in the younger age group argue strongly against indiscriminate device implantation.

The best candidates for ICD therapy are patients with prior cardiac arrest, VT with hemodynamic compromise, and extensive right/left ventricular involvement. Unexplained syncope is also considered a predictor of sudden death and appears to be an indication for ICD implantation. In this high risk group of patients the ICD intervention rate is approximately 10% per year and the estimated mortality reduction at 36 months of follow-up ranges from 24-35%[28,49] (see figure 5). In contrast, patients with well-tolerated VT and localized RV myocardial disease appear to have a good long-term prognosis. In this subgroup of patients, antiarrhythmic drug therapy (including beta-blockers) and/or catheter ablation seem to be a reasonable first-line therapy.

In asymptomatic patients and gene carriers there is no general indication for prophylactic ICD implantation because of their overall favorable prognosis and the high rate of device and electrode-related complications observed during the follow-up.[1,5] ICD therapy in patients with multiple risk factors, familial sudden death, or VT/VF inducibility at programmed ventricular stimulation is controversial and the decision to implant should be made on a case-by-case basis.

In patients with RV or biventricular heart failure, treatment consists of diuretics, angiotensin-converting-enzyme inhibitors and digitalis, as well as anticoagulants.[55] Heart transplantation is the final therapeutic option in case of refractory congestive heart failure and/or untreatable ventricular arrhythmias.[56]

References

1. Basso C, Corrado D, Marcus FI, *et al.* Arrhythmogenic right ventricular cardiomyopathy. Lancet 2009; 373: 1289-300.

2. Thiene G, Nava A, Corrado D, *et al.* Right ventricular cardiomyopathy and sudden death in young people. N Engl J Med 1988; 318: 129-133.

3. Basso C, Thiene G, Corrado D, *et al.* Arrhythmogenic right ventricular cardiomyopathy. Dysplasia, dystrophy, or myocarditis? Circulation 1996; 94: 983-991.

4. Corrado D, Basso C, Thiene G, *et al.* Spectrum of clinicopathologic manifestations of arrhythmogenic right ventricular cardiomyopathy/dysplasia: a multicenter study. J Am Coll Cardiol 1997; 30: 1512-20.

5. Corrado D, Basso C, Thiene G. Arrhythmogenic right ventricular cardiomyopathy: an update. Heart 2009; 95: 766–773.

6. Corrado D, Thiene G, Nava A, *et al.* Sudden death in young competitive athletes: clinicopathologic correlation in 22 cases. Am J Med 1990; 89: 588-596.

7. Corrado D, Thiene G. Arrhythmogenic right ventricular cardiomyopathy/dysplasia: clinical impact of molecular genetic studies. Circulation 2006; 113: 1634-7.

8. Maron BJ, Towbin JA, Thiene G, *et al.*; American Heart Association; Council on Clinical Cardiology, Heart Failure and Transplantation Committee; Quality of Care and Outcomes Research and Functional Genomics and Trans-

lational Biology Interdisciplinary Working Groups; Council on Epidemiology and Prevention. Contemporary definitions and classification of the cardiomyopathies: an American Heart Association Scientific Statement from the Council on Clinical Cardiology, Heart Failure and Transplantation Committee; Quality of Care and Outcomes Research and Functional Genomics and Translational Biology Interdisciplinary Working Groups; and Council on Epidemiology and Prevention. Circulation 2006; 113: 1807-16.

9. Blomstrom-Lundqvist C, Beckman-Suurkula M, Wallentin I, *et al.* Ventricular dimensions and wall motion assessed by echocardiography in patients with arrhythmogenic right ventricular dysplasia. Eur Heart J 1988; 9:1291-302

10. Menghetti L, Basso C, Nava A, *et al.* Spin-echo nuclear magnetic resonance for tissue characterization in arrhythmogenic right ventricular cardiomyopathy. Heart 1996; 76: 467-470.

11. Daliento L, Rizzoli G, Thiene G, *et al.* Diagnostic accuracy of right ventriculography in arrhythmogenic right ventricular cardiomyopathy. Am J Cardiol 1990; 66: 741-5.

12. Angelini A, Basso C, Nava A, *et al.* Endomyocardial biopsy in arrhythmogenic right ventricular cardiomyopathy. Am Heart J 1996; 132: 203-206.

13. Tandri H, Saranathan M, Rodriguez ER, *et al.* Noninvasive detection of myocardial fibrosis in arrhythmogenic right ventricular cardiomyopathy using delayed-en-

hancement magnetic resonance imaging. J Am Coll Cardiol 2005; 45: 98-103.

14. Corrado D, Basso C, Leoni L, *et al.* Three-dimensional electroanatomical voltage mapping and histologic evaluation of myocardial substrate in right ventricular outflow tract tachycardia. J Am Coll Cardiol 2008; 51: 731-9.

15. McKenna WJ, Thiene G, Nava A, *et al.* Diagnosis of arrhythmogenic right ventricular dysplasia/cardiomyopathy. Br Heart J 1994; 71: 215-218.

16. Corrado D, Fontaine G, Marcus FI, *et al.* Arrythmogenic right ventricular dysplasia / cardiomyopathy. Need for an international registry. Circulation 2000; 101: e101-e106.

17. Hamid MS, Norman M, Quraishi A, *et al.* Prospective evaluation of relatives for familial arrhythmogenic right ventricular cardiomyopathy/dysplasia reveals a need to broaden diagnostic criteria. J Am Coll Cardiol. 2002; 40(8): 1445-50.

18. Nava A, Bauce B, Basso C, *et al.* Clinical profile and long-term follow-up of 37 families with arrhythmogenic right ventricular cardiomyopathy. J Am Coll Cardiol 2000; 36: 2226-33.

19. Marcus FI, McKenna WJ, Sherill D, *et al.* Diagnosis of arrhythmogenic right ventricular cardiomyopathy/dysplasie (ARVC/D); Proposed Modifications of the Task Force Criteria. Circulation 2010; (in press).

20. Sen-Chowdhry S, Syrris P, Mckenna WJ. Genetics of right ventricular cardiomyopathy. J Cardiovasc Electrophysiol 2005; 16: 927-935.

21. Sen-Chowdhry S, Syrris P, McKenna WJ. Role of genetic analysisin the management of patients with arrhythmogenic right ventricular dysplasia/cardiomyopathy. J Am Coll Cardiol 2007; 50: 1813–21.

22. Rampazzo A, Nava A, Danieli GA, *et al.* The gene for arrhythmogenic right ventricular cardiomyopathy maps to chromosome 14q23-q24. Hum Mol Genet 1994; 3: 959-62.

23. McKoy G, Protonotarios N, Crosby A, *et al:* Identification of a deletion in plakoglobin in arrhythmogenic right ventricular cardiomyopathy with palmoplantar keratoderma and woolly hair (Naxos disease). Lancet 2000; 355: 2119-2124.

24. Rampazzo A, Nava A, Malacrida S, *et al.* Mutation in human desmoplakin domain binding to plakoglobin causes a dominant form of arrhythmogenic right ventricular cardiomyopathy. Am J Hum Genet 2002; 71: 1200-1206.

25. Gerull B, Heuser A, Wichter T, *et al.* Mutations in the desmosomal protein plakophilin-2 are common in arrhythmogenic right ventricular cardiomyopathy. Nat Genet 2004; 36: 1162-1164.

26. Pilichou K, Nava A, Basso C, *et al.* Mutations in Desmoglein-2 gene are associated to arrhythmogenic right ventricular cardiomyopathy. Circulation 2006; 113(9): 1171-9.

27. Syrris P, Ward D, Evans A, *et al.* Arrhythmogenic right ventricular dysplasia/cardiomyopathy associated with mutations in the desmosomal gene desmocollin-2. Am J Hum Genet 2006; 79: 978-84.

28. Corrado D, Leoni L, Link MS, *et al.* Implantable cardioverter-defibrillator therapy for prevention of sudden death in patients with arrhythmogenic right ventricular cardiomyopathy/dysplasia. Circulation 2003; 108: 3084-91.

29. Marcus FI, Fontaine G, Guiraudon G, *et al.* Right ventricular dysplasia. A report of 24 adult cases. Circulation 1982; 65: 384-398.

30. Nasir K, Bomma C, Tandri H, et al. Electrocardiographic features of arrhythmogenic right ventricular dysplasia/cardiomyopathy according to disease severity: a need to broaden diagnostic criteria. Circulation 2004; 110: 1527–34.

31. Turrini P, Corrado D, Basso C, *et al.* Dispersion of ventricular depolarization-repolarization: a noninvasive marker for risk stratification in arrhythmogenic right ventricular cardiomyopathy. Circulation 2001; 103: 3075-80.

32. Corrado D, Basso C, Leoni L, *et al.* Three-dimensional electroanatomic voltage mapping increases accuracy of diagnosing arrhythmogenic right ventricular cardiomyopathy/displasia. Circulation 2005; 111: 3042-3050.

33. Corrado D, Basso C, Thiene G. Arrhythmogenic right ventricular cardiomyopathy: diagnosis, prognosis, and treatment. Heart 2000; 83: 588-595.

34. Corrado D, Basso C, Leoni L, *et al.* Three-dimensional electroanatomic voltage mapping increases accuracy of diagnosing arrhythmogenic right ventricular cardiomyopathy/dysplasia. Circulation 2005; 111: 3042-3050.

35. Corrado D, Basso C, Pavei A, *et al.* Trends in sudden cardiovascular death in young competitive athletes after implementation of a preparticipation screening program. JAMA 2006; 296: 1593-1601.

36. Yoerger DM, Marcus F, Sherrill D, *et al.* Multidisciplinary Study of Right Ventricular Dysplasia Investigators. Echocardiographic findings in patients meeting task force criteria for arrhythmogenic right ventricular dysplasia: new insights from the multidisciplinary study of right ventricular dysplasia. J Am Coll Cardiol 2005; 45: 860-5.

37. Bluemke DA, Krupinski EA, Ovitt T, *et al.* MR imaging of arrhythmogenic right ventricular cardiomyopathy: morphologic findings and interobserver reliability. Cardiology 2003; 99: 153-62.

38. Tandri H, Macedo R, Calkins H, *et al.* Role of magnetic resonance imaging in arrhythmogenic right ventricular dysplasia: insights from the North American arrhythmogenic right ventricular dysplasia (ARVD/C) study. Am Heart J 2008; 155: 147-53.

39. Tandri H, Saranathan M, Rodriguez ER, *et al.* Noninvasive detection of myocardial fibrosis in arrhythmogenic right ventricular cardiomyopathy using delayed-enhancement magnetic resonance imaging. J Am Coll Cardiol 2005; 45: 98-103.

40. Sen-Chowdhry S, Prasad SK, Syrris P, *et al.* Cardiovascular magnetic resonance in arrhythmogenic right ventricular cardiomyopathy revisited: comparison with task force criteria and genotype. J Am Coll Cardiol 2006; 48: 2132-40.

41. Sievers B, Addo M, Franken U, *et al.* Right ventricular wall motion abnormalities found in healthy subjects by cardiovascular magnetic resonance imaging and characterized with a new segmental model. J Cardiovasc Magn Reson 2004; 6: 601-608.

42. Sen-Chowdhry S, Syrris P, Ward D, *et al.* Clinical and genetic characterization of families with arrhythmogenic

right ventricular dysplasia/cardiomyopathy provides novel insights into patterns of disease expression. Circulation 2007; 115: 1710-20.

43. Angelini A, Basso C, Nava A, *et al.* Endomyocardial biopsy in arrhythmogenic right ventricular cardiomyopathy. Am Heart J 1996; 132: 203-6.

44. Ott P, Marcus FI, Sobonya RE. Cardiac sarcoidosis masquerading as right ventricular dysplasia. Pacing Clin Electrophysiology 2003; 26: 1498–503.

45. Chimenti C, Pieroni M, Maseri A, *et al.* Histologic findings in patients with clinical and instrumental diagnosis of sporadic arrhythmogenic right ventricular dysplasia. J Am Coll Cardiol 2004; 43: 2305–13.

46. Corrado D, Thiene G. Cardiac sarcoidosis mimicking arrhythmogenic right ventricular cardiomyopathy/dysplasia: the renaissance of endomyocardial biopsy? J Cardiovasc Electrophysiol 2009; 20: 477-9.

47. Basso C, Ronco F, Marcus F, *et al.* Quantitative assessment of endomyocardial biopsy in arrhythmogenic right ventricular cardiomyopathy/dysplasia: an in vitro validation of diagnostic criteria. Eur Heart J 2008; 29: 2760-71.

48. Buja G, Estes NA 3rd, Wichter T, *et al.* Arrhythmogenic right ventricular cardiomyopathy/dysplasia: risk stratification and therapy. Prog Cardiovasc Dis 2008; 50: 282-93.

49. Wichter T, Paul M, Wollmann C, *et al.* Implantable cardioverter/defibrillator therapy in arrhythmogenic right ventricular cardiomyopathy: single-center experience of long-term follow-up and complications in 60 patients. Circulation 2004; 109: 1503-8.

50. Roguin A, Bomma CS, Nasir K, *et al.* Implantable cardioverter-defibrillators in patients with arrhythmogenic right ventricular dysplasia/cardiomyopathy. J Am Coll Cardiol 2004; 43: 1843–52.

51. Wichter T, Borggrefe M, Hoverkamp W, *et al.* Efficacy of antiarrhythmic drugs in patients with arrhythmogenic right ventricular disaese. Results in patients with inducible and noninducible ventricular tachycardia. Circulation 1992; 86: 29-37.

52. Wichter T, Hindricks G, Kottkamp H, *et al.* Catheter ablation of ventricular tachycardia. In: A Nava, L Rossi, G Thiene, eds. Arrhythmogenic right ventricular cardiomyopathy- dysplasia. Elsevier, Amsterdam 1997; 376-91.

53. Verma A, Kilicaslan F, Schweikert RA, *et al.* Short- and long-term success of substrate-based mapping and ablation of ventricular tachycardia in arrhythmogenic right ventricular dysplasia. Circulation 2005; 111: 3209-16.

54. Dalal D, Jain R, Tandri H, *et al.* Long-term efficacy of catheter ablation of ventricular tachicardia in patients with arrhythmogenic right ventricular dysplasia/cardiomyopathy. J Am Coll Cardiol 2007; 50: 432-40.

55. Wlodarska EK, Wozniak O, Konka M, *et al.* Thromboembolic complications in patients with arrhythmogenic right ventricular dysplasia/cardiomyopathy. Europace 2006; 8: 596–600.

56. Thiene G, Angelini A, Basso C, *et al.* Novel heart diseases requiring transplantation. Adv Clin Path 1998, 2: 65–73.